Complex Cases with LASIK

with

LASIK

Advanced Techniques
and Complication Management

Complex Cases with LASIK

with

Advanced Techniques
and Complication Management

Louis E. Probst

Medical Director, TLC Laser Eye Center
Windsor, Ontario
Chicago, Illinois and Madison, Wisconsin

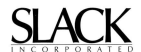

6900 Grove Road • Thorofare, NJ • 08086

Publisher: John H. Bond
Editorial Director: Amy E. Drummond
Assistant Editor: Lauren Biddle Plummer

The procedures and practices described in this book should be implemented in a manner consistent with the professional standards set for the circumstances that apply in each specific situation. Every effort has been made to confirm the accuracy of the information presented and to correctly relate generally accepted practices. The author, editor, and publisher cannot accept responsibility for errors or exclusions or for the outcome of the application of the material presented herein. There is no expressed or implied warranty of this book or information imparted by it.

Care has been taken to ensure that drug selection and dosages are in accordance with currently accepted/recommended practice. Due to continuing research, changes in government policy and regulations, and various effects of drug reactions and interactions, it is recommended that the reader review all materials and literature provided for each drug, especially those that are new or not frequently used.

Any review or mention of specific companies or products is not intended as an endorsement by the author or the publisher.

Probst, Louis E.
    Complex cases with LASIK: Advanced Techniques and Complication Management/Louis E. Probst.
        p. cm.
    ISBN 1-55642-404-3 (alk. paper)
     1. Cornea--Laser surgery--Complications--Case studies I. Title.
    [DNLM: 1. Myopia--Surgery. 2. Cornea--surgery. 3. Astigmatism surgery. 4. Laser surgery--adverse effects. 5. Corneal Transplantation. 6. Case Report. WW 320 P962c 1999]
    RE336 .P76 1999
    617.7'19059 21--dc21

                                   99-040823

Published by: SLACK Incorporated
                 6900 Grove Road
                 Thorofare, NJ 08086-9447 USA
                 Telephone: 856-848-1000
                 Fax: 856-853-5991
                 World Wide Web: http://www.slackinc.com

Contact SLACK Incorporated for more information about other books in this field or about the availability of our books from distributors outside the United States.

Last digit is print number: 10 9 8 7 6 5 4 3 2 1

DEDICATION

To my wife Kate,
for her ongoing love and support.

CONTENTS

ACKNOWLEDGMENTS

The most profound influence on my development as a refractive surgeon has been Jeffery J. Machat, MD who taught me that LASIK is both psychological and technical. Jeff's unique focus on LASIK, along with his superhuman work ethic and tremendous ability, has demonstrated that nothing is impossible with the appropriate dedication and commitment. He has set the example I will always aspire to emulate.

I must also acknowledge the support and assistance of the entire SLACK team both with *The Art of LASIK* textbook and CD as well as this current effort. John Bond, Amy Drummond, Jennifer Cahill, Jennifer Stewart, Viktoria Kristiansson, and Lauren Plummer have all worked with tremendous efficiency to assemble this textbook in record time while maintaining the highest level of quality. Without their concerted efforts, this book could not have come to fruition.

ABOUT THE AUTHOR

In 1995, Louis Probst began performing LASIK in Canada with the Chiron 116 excimer laser. Since that time, he has performed over 18,000 excimer laser procedures and 16,000 LASIK procedures using the Bausch and Lomb Technolas 217, Nidek EC 5000, LaserSight LSX, and the VISX Star and S2 Smoothscan excimer lasers. As Medical Director for TLC Chicago and TLC Madison in the United States, and Medical Director of TLC Windsor and Assistant Professor of Ophthalmology at the University of Western Ontario in Canada, he is one of the most experienced LASIK surgeons in North America. Dr. Probst currently performs between 100 to 200 LASIK procedures per week.

Dr. Probst has also coauthored the LASIK reference textbook titled *The Art of LASIK*, used by refractive surgeons and eye care professionals worldwide. He has also completed a companion CD with instructional surgical videos to be used along with *The Art of LASIK* for refractive surgeons. He has published over 40 articles in peer-reviewed journals, written 35 book chapters on refractive surgery, and given over 100 lectures and courses on LASIK. As a leader in LASIK, Dr. Probst has developed several instruments specifically designed for LASIK with the Hansatome and pioneered the design of disposable LASIK instruments.

Contributing Authors

Amar Agarwal, MS, FRCS, FRCOphth(Lon)
Chennai and Bangalore, India

Athiya Agarwal, MD, FRSH(Lon), DO
Chennai and Bangalore, India

Sunita Agarwal, MS, FSVH(Germ), DO
Chennai and Bangalore, India

Sergio Belloni, MD
Milan, Italy

Lucio Buratto, MD
Milan, Italy

Charlotte Burns, OD, MS
Madison, Wisconsin

Y. Ralph Chu, MD
Maplewood, Minnesota

John F. Doane, MD
Independence, Missouri

Richard Duffey, MD
Mobile, Alabama

James D. Ferguson, OD
Westchester, Illinois

Jose Güell, MD
Barcelona, Spain

David R. Hardten, MD
Minneapolis, Minnesota

Douglas Katz, MD
Minneapolis, Minnesota

Michael C. Knorz, MD
Mannheim, Germany

Michiel S. Kritzinger, MD
Cresta, South Africa

Stephen S. Lane, MD
Stillwater, Minnesota

Michael Lawless, MBBS, FRACO, FRACS, FRCOphth
Chatswood, Australia

Richard L. Lindstrom, MD
Minneapolis, Minnesota

Eric J. Linebarger, MD
Minneapolis, Minnesota

Jeffery J. Machat, MD
Windsor, Ontario

Susana Oscherow, MD
Mendosa, Argentina

Ioannis G. Pallikaris, MD
Crete, Greece

Theokliti Papadaki, MD
Crete, Greece

Nelson Preschel, MD
Minneapolis, Minnesota

Louis E. Probst, MD
Windsor, Ontario

Giselle Ricur, MD
Mendosa, Argentina

Dimitrios S. Siganos, MD
Crete, Greece

Stephen G. Slade, MD
Houston, Texas

Ted Smith, OD
Windsor, Ontario

Gerard Sutton, FRACO, FRACS
Sydney, Australia

Remato Valeri, MD
Milan, Italy

Sue Webber, BSc(Hons), FRCOphth
Chatswood, Australia

Jonathan Woolfson, MD
Greenville, South Carolina

Roberto Zaldivar, MD
Mendosa, Argentina

FOREWORD

Refractive surgery has finally entered its adolescence.

It has been an awkward child, but is now being embraced not only by refractive surgeons, but ophthalmologists generally and by patients worldwide.

Refractive surgery, given current technology, is difficult to perform well, but highly worthwhile. It is like playing a musical instrument. It can be complex, but when performed by an expert can be made to look easy. The more you know about the subject the more you appreciate the nuances and complexities, and learn to have respect for what an expert musician and instrument can do. Refractive surgery is an art, a craft and a science, and all aspects need to be mastered.

We know a lot, but there is much to discover. What is the relevance of posterior corneal curvature? What is the minimal bed thickness? What are the optical limits of positive asphericity? How will corneal imaging evolve in the next few years and what is the real potential of customized ablations?

One of the first rules is to work out which cases are complex so as to avoid problems, deal with complications and enhance results. Louis Probst, MD, has been able to convince the leading refractive surgeons in the world to contribute to this textbook. Getting these busy people together is an achievement in itself, but getting them to talk about problem cases, difficulties they have encountered, and how they have wrestled with clinical problems in LASIK, is a major achievement. Ophthalmologists need this information and this book will be closely scrutinized by ophthalmologists and others in the field of refractive surgery. It is ophthalmology's attempt to deal with a maturing refractive surgical specialty, and is the first attempt that I know of in a textbook to present not just new data, techniques or technology, but to deal with the complexities and complications that arise perioperatively in refractive surgery.

We all have an interest in making refractive surgery better. It will become so common that it will have major public health ramifications apart from its significance in private medicine. Avoiding complications, understanding difficult clinical situations, recognizing problems when they do arise and dealing with them expertly is what this textbook is all about. It is the first of a kind and will be the gold standard for any book that follows.

Louis Probst, MD, and his coauthors are to be congratulated on an extraordinary achievement in bringing this textbook to fruition. It could not have occurred without the drive of Louis Probst, MD, as well as his intelligence and dedication to refractive surgery. I am grateful to have been allowed to play a small part.

Michael A. Lawless, MBBS, FRACO, FRACS, FRCOphth
Medical Director
The Eye Institute, Sydney, Australia

INTRODUCTION

Complex Cases with LASIK presents a comprehensive review of LASIK complications and their management as well as the most advanced LASIK techniques as presented by the world experts in refractive surgery with experience with over 100,000 cases of LASIK. This book includes 88 complex cases with over 400 illustrations.

Each case begins with the single page complex case form, which describes the preoperative characteristics of the eye, the procedures performed, and the postoperative outcome. The complex case form has been standardized for each case so that the reader will become accustomed to the format after the first few cases. This concise synopsis of the case history allows the reader to assimilate the important factual details and the areas of interest in less than a minute.

Following the complex case form, each author has provided a detailed narrative account of the complex case. This includes his or her own personal and insightful comments that allow the reader to appreciate the "atmosphere" of the case. In this portion, the complexities of the case are discussed along with descriptions of the patients themselves. This portion is presented as a doctor would describe the case to another doctor.

Multiple illustrations are provided with pre- and postoperative topographies as well as clinical and intraoperative photographs. These illustrations provide the clinical background to support the complex case form and the narrative account. The presentation of this material puts the reader "in the room" with the patient and his or her eye care professional.

Finally, every case in the textbook is completed with the Editor's comments by Louis Probst, MD, who has performed over 16,000 LASIK procedures, including hundreds of "complex cases". These comments may be an evaluation of the technique used, a summary of the current concepts involving the case, or a description of the "pearls and pitfalls" of that particular situation. The Editor's comments provide a consistent train of thought that ties this multi-authored textbook together into a complete and comprehensive package.

Louis E. Probst, MD

PREFACE

Why do we need a book on complex cases with LASIK? Because the exponential growth of the popularity of LASIK guarantees that every refractive surgeon will need to deal with complex LASIK cases for either consultations or their own complications. The degree of confidence and knowledge that the eye care professional conveys about these complex LASIK situations will, in many ways, define the success of that LASIK practice.

Complex Cases with LASIK has been designed to provide all the information that would be typically available when evaluating a patient for LASIK. The refractive data, photographs, and topographies are included. The complex case form is provided for each case to allow an easy grasp of the key data. The narrative account provides the more personal description of the case both from the view of the doctor and the patient. Finally, the editor's comments outline some pearls and pitfalls of each case. The preoperative and the postoperative results are all illustrated, described, and discussed allowing the reader to evaluate the results.

The goal of this textbook is to create the "complex cases environment" so that readers feel like they have indirectly experienced the case themselves. When the reader then encounters one of these complex cases in his or her own practice, he or she will be able the avoid much of the indecision and anxiety that can be associated with the atypical patient with an imperfect outcome. I hope that many of the potential problems in LASIK will be avoided because of the concepts illustrated in this textbook.

Louis E. Probst, MD

COMPLEX PREOPERATIVE LASIK CONSIDERATIONS

1

SUMMARY NOTES

COMPLEX PREOPERATIVE LASIK CONSIDERATIONS - SUMMARY NOTES

ANTERIOR BASEMENT MEMBRANE DYSTROPHY

Clinical

Anterior basement membrane dystrophy (ABMD) will often lead to epithelial defects with laser in situ keratomileusis (LASIK). Epithelial defects are generally evident as soon as the keratectomy is performed. They most commonly form along the superior aspect of the keratectomy edge with both the Bausch and Lomb Automated Corneal Shaper (ACS) and Hansatome. Epithelial defects will cause postoperative pain, as well as a foreign body sensation. Once an epithelial defect occurs, the risk of epithelial ingrowth increases as epithelial healing and growth has been stimulated.

Etiology of Epithelial Defects

- ABMD
- history of recurrent corneal erosions
- epithelial toxicity from topical anesthesia
- operative trauma/manipulation
- advanced age

Complications Associated with Epithelial Defects

- significant pain
- prolonged visual recovery
- epithelial ingrowth
- flap melt
- infection
- LASIK interface inflammation (sands of the Sahara)

Management

Patients should be given copious lubrication, a topical prophylactic antibiotic drop to guard against infection, and followed daily until the defect heals. Small epithelial defects (less than 3 mm) will generally heal quickly so a postoperative nonsteroidal drop and a good sleep will restore the eye comfort. Larger epithelial defects are best treated with a contact lens that will reduce the postoperative pain, lacrimation, and eyelid squeezing. The contact lens can generally be removed in 1 to 2 days. Patients with epithelial defects should be followed weekly for 1 month to monitor for epithelial ingrowth.

Prevention

LASIK should be avoided with ABMD as they will commonly develop epithelial defects. Patients with loose epithelium, such as those with ABMD or a history of recurrent corneal erosions, are best treated with photorefractive keratectomy (PRK). All the preparatory and procedural aspects of LASIK should be performed with the goal of preserving the integrity of the corneal epithelium. Topical anesthesia should be used sparingly to avoid any epithelial toxicity. In cases with questionable epithelium, extra lubrication with a drop of Celluvisc (Allergan Pharmaceuticals, Irvine, Calif) on the cornea prior to the keratectomy can help to minimize epithelial defects.

PREOPERATIVE IRREGULAR ASTIGMATISM AND FORME FRUSTE KERATOCONUS

Clinical

While all patients will have some degree of irregular astigmatism on the preoperative topography, any significant degree of irregularity should be considered a contraindication for LASIK. The excimer laser performs a standard ablation based on the programmed correction so any unique irregularities of the cornea will persist after LASIK. This irregular surface will cause irregular astigmatism with a reduction in the uncorrected visual acuity (UCVA) and the best corrected visual acuity (BCVA). Contact lenses must be removed prior to LASIK to allow the cornea to resume it's nature shape. Any change in refraction or irregularity of topography should be followed for stability prior to performing LASIK. A forme fruste keratoconus pattern identified on topography should be followed for resolution with the contact lenses out prior to LASIK.

Causes of Preoperative Irregular Astigmatism
- hard contact lens use
- soft contact lens use
- forme fruste keratoconus
- pellucid marginal degeneration
- previous corneal surgery
- corneal scars
- dry eyes (artifact)

Guidelines for Cessation of Contact Lenses Prior to LASIK
- soft contact lenses   4 to 7 days
- soft toric lenses   2 weeks
- hard contact lenses   6 weeks for each 10 years of hard contact lens use

Management

Topographic irregular astigmatism that persists despite prolonged contact removal is a contraindication for LASIK with the standard ablation patterns. The preoperative BCVA may already be reduced so the risk for a postoperative reduction is much greater. If the astigmatism measured on topography does not correspond to the refractive astigmatism, the results should be carefully reviewed prior to LASIK. Forme fruste keratoconus is a form of progressive corneal instability, which could be exacerbated by thinning procedure such as LASIK. Topography-assisted LASIK offers the best hope for the treatment of irregular astigmatism in the future

CASE A, ANTERIOR BASEMENT MEMBRANE DYSTROPHY

Ted Smith, OD, and Jeffery J. Machat, MD

Main Concern: ABMD with LASIK flap epithelial defects
Patient Age: 52

INITIAL PREOPERATIVE INFORMATION

	OD	OS	COMMENTS
Preoperative Refraction	+2.00 – 1.75 X 60	+2.25 – 1.50 X 110	ABMD
UCVA	20/60	20/60	
BCVA	20/20	20/20	
Topography Details	44.12/43.00 X 57	43.12/42.12 X 154	
Sim Keratometry (K) Values	1.23	1.08	
Pachymetry	610 μm	627 μm	

PROCEDURES PERFORMED

	OD	OS	COMMENTS
1. Date/type	12/11/98 H-LASIK	12/11/98 H-LASIK	epithelial defects OU
Laser/keratome/plate	Technolas 217/	Technolas 217/	
	Hansatome/180	Hansatome/180	

CURRENT POSTOPERATIVE INFORMATION

	OD	OS	COMMENTS
Time Postoperative	2 months	3 months	
Postoperative Refraction	plano (pl) – 0.50 X 125	pl – 0.25 X 085	
UCVA	20/25+	20/20	
BCVA	20/20	20/20	
Topography Details	n/a	n/a	
SimK Values	n/a	n/a	
Pachymetry	n/a	n/a	
Visual Complaints	none	none	
Medications	none	none	
Refractive Correction	none	none	

This 52-year-old white female had bilateral LASIK performed on December 11, 1998. Preoperative topography was normal (Figure 1A-1). An attempt to fully correct OD +2.00 – 1.75 X 060 and OS +2.25 – 1.50 X 110 using the Hansatome (Chiron Vision Corporation, Claremont, Calif) with a 180 μm flap and the Chiron Technolas 217 (Chiron Vision Corporation, Claremont, Calif) was made. Prior to surgery, there was a mild, ABMD OU in the region of the superior cornea from 11 to 1 o'clock. During LASIK flap manipulation, an epithelial defect occurred in the left superior cornea (Figure 1A-2). The flap was replaced gently. A bandage contact lens was not indicated. The right cornea also sustained a small epithelial defect much smaller than the left eye. The right eye stabilized well with a UCVA of 20/25+ with Rx pl – 0.50 X 125 giving 20/20 at 2 months postoperatively.

At 1 month postoperatively, the comanaging doctor found 1.5 mm progression of ingrowth beneath the area of the flap where the epithelial defect occurred in the left eye. Over the next month, the ingrowth stabilized with no further progression. At 3 months postoperatively, there was a minimal residual Rx OS of pl – 0.25 X 085 and an unaided acuity of 20/20. The epithelium of the corneal flap was healthy and smooth. The patient had occasional symptoms of irritation and dryness OU, which was managed with Genteal prn (Ciba Vision Ophthalmics, Atlanta, Ga).

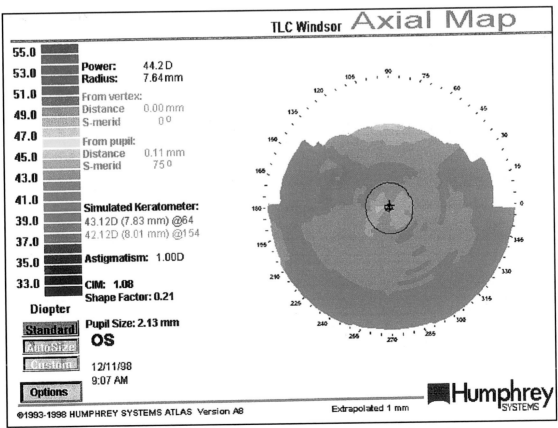

Figure 1A-1. Preoperative topography OS demonstrates a regular pattern.

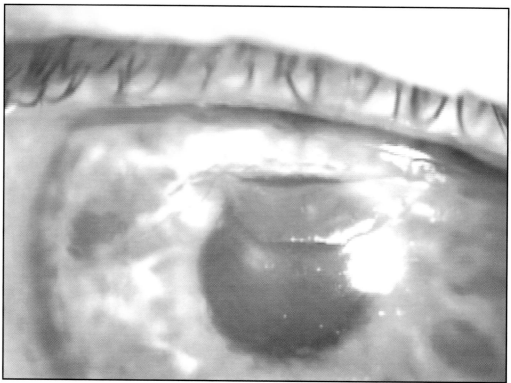

Figure 1A-2. Superior epithelial defect immediately after a LASIK on a patient with ABMD.

Editor's Notes

ABMD significantly increases the risk of epithelial defects during the LASIK procedure. Epithelial defects following LASIK increase the incidence of epithelial ingrowth, as well as increase the postoperative discomfort that can add to the risk of flap striae from eye squeezing or rubbing.

ABMD should be considered a relative contraindication for LASIK. In cases of questionable or mild ABMD, several measures can be taken to reduce the risk of epithelial defects. Minimal topical anaesthetic should be used, such as 1 drop of proparacaine 1 minute before LASIK. Celluvisc can be applied to the cornea prior to performing the keratectomy in order to provide the smoothest cut possible. Finally, the microkeratome can be advanced for the keratectomy but not reversed. The suction is released and the microkeratome, as well as the suction cup, are slid away from the eye so there is no movement of the blade as the microkeratome is retracted across the flap.

This case demonstrates that not all cases of epithelial ingrowth need to be treated. This patient had a 1.5 mm ingrowth which did not progress, and therefore did not require further management. Epithelial ingrowth that is progressive, causing a flap melt (greater than 2 mm from the flap edge), should be treated.

CASE B, PREVIOUS TREATMENT OF FORME FRUSTE KERATOCONUS

Michiel S. Kritzinger, MD

Main Concern: Fluctuating Refraction Postoperatively

INITIAL PREOPERATIVE INFORMATION

	OD	OS	COMMENTS
Preoperative Refraction	+2.25/-3.25 X 80	+3.25/-6.50 X 80	referring center
BCVA	20/20	20/20	forme fruste
			keratoconus

PROCEDURES PERFORMED

	OD	OS	COMMENTS
1. Date/type	LASIK	LASIK	mixed pattern
Laser/keratome/plate			
2. Date/type	H-LASIK	H-LASIK	
	enhancement	enhancement	
3. Date/type		LASIK	
		enhancement	

CURRENT POSTOPERATIVE INFORMATION

	OD	OS	COMMENTS
Time Postoperative	10 months	10 months	after retreatment
Postoperative Refraction	+1.00 – 1.25 X 095	+2.00 – 1.50 X 084	
UCVA	20/25	20/30	
BCVA	20/20	20/20	

This patient was referred to me after having a LASIK procedure done at another eye center. Original condition of both eyes before any eye surgery was:

	OD	OS
Refraction	+2.25 / -3.25 X 80	+3.25 / -6.50 X 80
BCVA	20/20	20/20
Treatment:		
Sphere	+2.00	+3.00
Cylinder	-4.00	-6.00
Cylinder Axis	85	83
Zone	3.8 mm	3.8 mm

Two months after the first refractive surgical attempt, the patient came to seek advice. He was very depressed and visually frustrated, because of the severe hyperopia iatrogenically induced, as well as the residual astigmatism. The previous surgeon did not take the following into account:

• 20% of the negative cylinder value that has an effect on the sphere treated.

• No refractive transposition was attempted to reduce the tissue removal and treatment time during ablation.

• Too small of an optical zone was selected for treatment. The "expected" overcorrection post-treatment was the reason why he consulted me 2 months after initial treatment. Examination revealed the following:

	OD	OS
Refraction	+4.75/-2.75 X 85	+5.75/-3.50 X 87
BCVA	20/25	20/20
Topography	Figure 1B-1 (bow-tie forme fruste keratoconus)	Figure 1B-2 (bow-tie forme fruste keratoconus)
SimK value	42.6 X 11/39.0 X 101	42.7 X 17/37.0 X 84
Pachymetry	535 μm	527 μm

An enhancement procedure was done by myself on this patient using a positive cylinder transposition treatment method. The Chiron Technolas 217 was programmed as follows:

	OD		OS	
	Preoperative	Treatment	Preoperative	Treatment
Sphere	+4.50	+2.47	+6.00	+3.30
Cylinder	-2.25	+2.47	-3.25	+3.57
Cylinder Axis	8	175	87	177
Zone diameter (Sphere/Cyl)		5 mm		5 mm

Postoperative visual results were satisfactory with a happier patient. Refractive result was:

	OD	OS
UCVA	20/25	20/40
BCVA	20/20	20/20
Refraction	+0.25/-0.25 X 138	+3.00/-2.75 X 54
Topography	Figure 1B-3	Figure 1B-4

Another LASIK procedure was performed on the left eye 5 months later. Once again a positive cylinder transposition method was used:

	OS	
	Preoperative	Treatment
Sphere	+3.25	plano
Cylinder	-3.50	+3.90
Cylinder Axis	61	151
Zone diameter		5mm

The last assessment was done 10 months after I started treatment. Results were:

	OD	OS
Refraction	+1.00/-1.25 X 95	+2.00/-1.50 X 84
BCVA	20/20	20/20
UCVA	20/25	20/30
Topography	Figure 1B-5	Figure 1B-6

No corrective eyewear was prescribed for distance vision. Only a reading prescription was given.

Conclusion

The patient is now much happier than the first day I assessed him. Enhancement surgery is planned for the future, once the refraction has stabilized (if it ever will, because of the forme fruste keratoconus).

This patient will be an ideal candidate for TopoLink customized ablation in the future, if he insists on further treatment.

The lesson in this story is to *not* LASIK/PRK a forme fruste keratoconus, but rather to try other refractive options. By thinning the cornea you create constantly fluctuating vision and can induce real keratoconus.

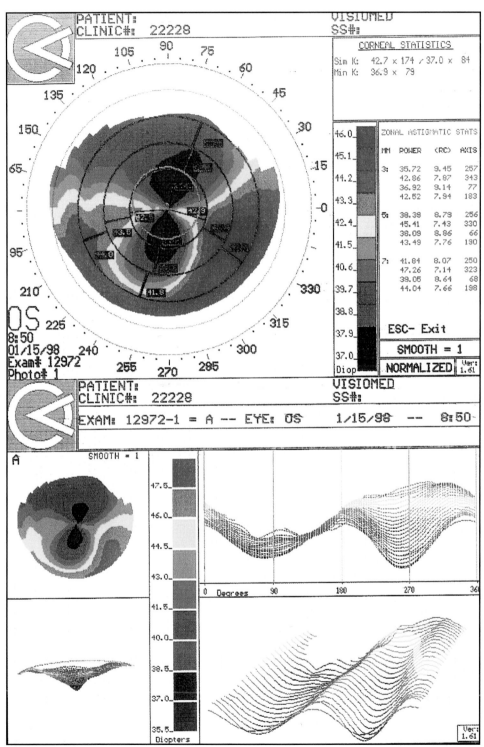

Figure 1B-1. Bow-tie pattern of astigmatism OD associated with inferior corneal steepening.

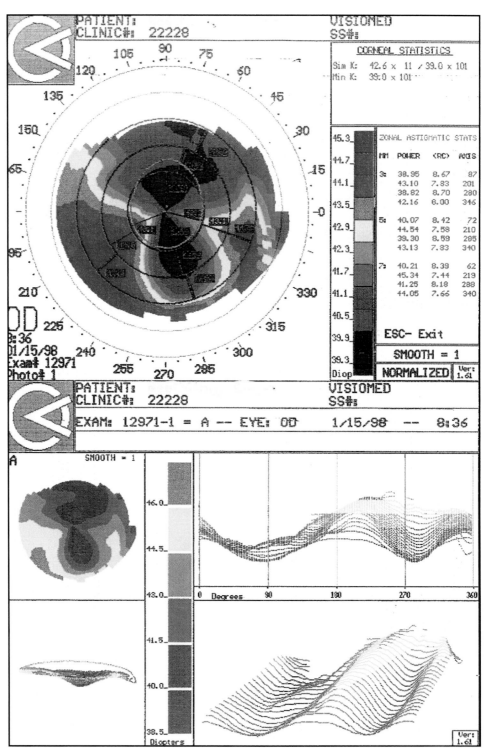

Figure 1B-2. Bow-tie pattern of astigmatism OS associated with inferior corneal steepening.

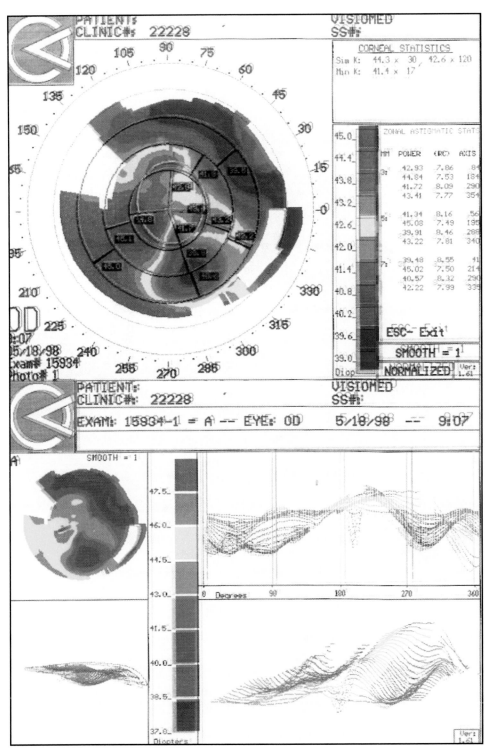

Figure 1B-3. Irregular pattern OD with persistent inferior steepening extending into visual axis.

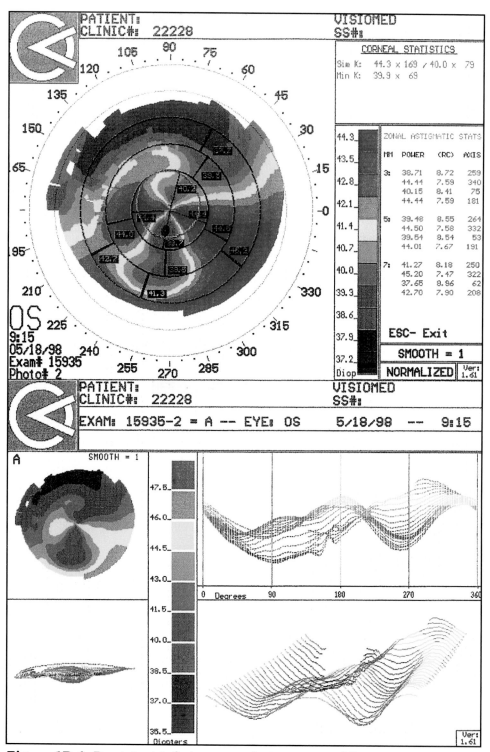

Figure 1B-4. Persistent inferior corneal steepening, OS.

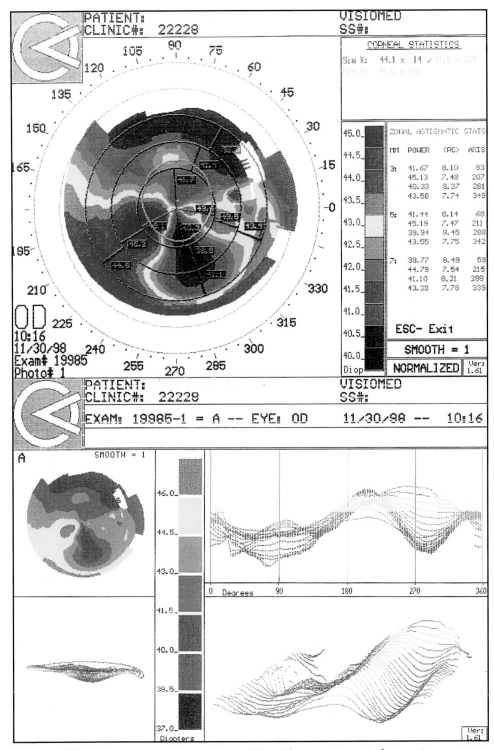

Figure 1B-5. A more regular pattern OD with persistent inferior steepening.

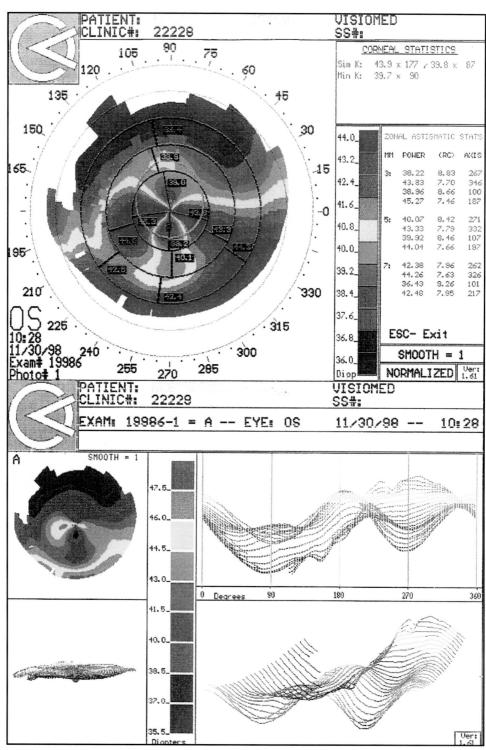

Figure 1B-6. Persistent inferior steepening OS after second enhancement procedure.

Editor's Notes

The high degree of astigmatism in this case should immediately draw suspicion to the diagnosis of keratoconus. The inferior steepening on the preoperative topography associated with this degree of preoperative astigmatism contraindicates LASIK. Corneal pachymetry performed both superiorly and inferiorly in the cornea may also yield useful information. When the corneal thickness is less inferiorly this may also support a diagnosis of form fruste keratoconus. Patients with forme fruste keratoconus have an unpredictable refractive result, and therefore should be considered poor candidates for LASIK. Patients that have normal corneal thickness, a stable refraction with little astigmatism, and a mild forme fruste keratoconus picture on topography may be reasonable candidates for LASIK in selected cases.

This patient is fortunate that two enhancement procedures could be performed in the left eye because of adequate corneal thickness. Often when treating high levels of astigmatism using a scanning laser, large amounts of tissue are ablated and repeat enhancement procedures are not possible. In this case the positive cylinder transposition treatment was used, which preserved some of the central cornea.

Although the final result was quite impressive, with a UCVA of 20/25 OD and 20/30 OS, the postoperative topographies are perhaps more informative. The topography of the right eye indicates an irregular pattern with inferior steepening. The topography in the left eye is more remarkable, with significant irregularity and inferior steepening. While this patient's refractive results appear to be relatively stable at present, we can expect a gradual increase in the astigmatism with time. LASIK enhancement procedures can continue to perform some degree of correction for this progressive astigmatism, but eventually further procedures will not be possible and the patient will be left with residual astigmatism.

From this example, we can see that forme fruste keratoconus associated with a high degree of astigmatism should be considered a contraindication for LASIK. The other condition that must be considered, which is closely related to keratoconus, is pellucid marginal degeneration. This can also present with irregular topography, however, this condition is associated with inferior corneal thinning (as opposed to the paracentral corneal thinning of keratoconus).

CASE C, LASIK WITH FORME FRUSTE KERATOCONUS

Louis E. Probst, MD, and Jeffery J. Machat, MD

Main Concern: Astigmatism
Patient Age: 54

INITIAL PREOPERATIVE INFORMATION

	OD	OS	COMMENTS
Preoperative Refraction	-8.0 – 2.75 X 92	-7.0 – 3.5 X 120	forme fruste
BCVA	n/a	n/a	keratoconus OS
Topography Details	regular	inferior steepening	
SimK Values	n/a	47.12/42.37	
Pachymetry	540 and 680 μm	520 and 590 μm	

PROCEDURES PERFORMED

	OD	OS	COMMENTS
1. Date/type		1996 M-LASIK	uncomplicated
Laser/keratome/plate		Technolas 116/ACS/160	
2. Date/type		2 months later AK	

CURRENT POSTOPERATIVE INFORMATION

	OD	OS	COMMENTS
Time Postoperative		18 months	progressive
Postoperative Refraction		-4.0 + 7.0 X 22	irregular astigmatism
UCVA		20/300	required PK
BCVA		20/30	
Topography Details		high astigmatism, irregular	
SimK Values		47.0/31.87	
Pachymetry		442 μm	
Visual Complaints		distortion	
Medications		none	
Refractive Correction		hard contact lenses	

(Case and photographs reprinted with permission from Machat JJ, Slade SG, Probst LE. *The Art of Lasik.* 2nd ed. Thorofare, NJ: SLACK Incorporated; 1999.)

A 54-year-old male was originally evaluated for LASIK for high myopia and astigmatism. The preoperative refraction was -8.0 – 2.75 X 92 OD and -7.0 – 3.5 X 120 OS. Corneal topography performed preoperatively indicated forme fruste keratoconus in the left eye (Figure 1C-1). Ocular examination was normal with none of the classic signs of keratoconus (Fleischer's ring, corneal striae, central scarring). Corneal pachymetry found a corneal thickness of 540 and 680 µm centrally and inferiorly respectively OD, and 520 and 590 µm centrally and inferiorly respectively OS. The patient had no past history of hard contact lens use and had stopped his soft contact lens use in the left eye 2 weeks prior to assessment.

The unpredictably of LASIK for the left eye was explained to the patient. The patient was also given the option to try additional contact lenses. After two very detailed consultations, the patient elected to try LASIK in the left eye only.

At the 1 month follow-up, the corneal flap position was excellent, flap and interface were clear, and the flap edge was smooth. The UCVA and BCVA was 20/60 with a refraction of +0.75 + 1.75 X 065.

At the 4 month follow-up, the flap was noted to have healed perfectly. The UCVA was 20/100 and the BCVA had improved to 20/25 with -1.5 + 4.5 X 27. Corneal topography indicated significant inferior steepening of the left cornea with superior flattening from the excimer laser ablation (Figure 1C-2). Corneal pachymetry indicated irregular astigmatism in the same pattern seen preoperatively.

Two months later, the patient was assessed for possible astigmatic surgery. The patient was told that the results would be unpredictable given the irregular nature of the corneal astigmatism. Corneal pachymetry found a central corneal thickness of 436 µm with an inferior thickness of 631 µm. Corneal topography at this time continued to show irregular astigmatism (Figure 1C-3). Two 4 mm straight astigmatic cuts were made at a depth of 550 µm with an 7 mm clear zone.

Three months after the astigmatic keratotomy, UCVA was 20/400 and BCVA was 20/20 with a refraction of -3.0 + 6.0 X 22. Corneal pachymetry found the central thickness to be 438 µm and the inferior thickness to be 685 µm. Corneal topography demonstrated significant irregular astigmatism with more than 15 diopters (D) of cylinder at an axis of 24 (Figure 1C-4).

One year and 6 months following the original LASIK procedure, the patient's UCVA was 20/300 and BCVA was 20/30 with a refraction of -4.0 + 7.0 X 22. The corneal topography continued to indicate significant astigmatism with more than 15 D of astigmatism at axis 22 (Figure 1C-5). Corneal pachymetry at this time found the central corneal thickness was 442 µm and the inferior corneal thickness was 691 µm inferonasally and 502 µm inferotemporally.

Given the visual impairment from the increased astigmatism, a trial with a hard contact lens was attempted in the left eye. This was poorly tolerated. Topography-assisted LASIK was considered, however, the central corneal thickness would not allow for further treatment. Further thinning of the cornea would cause further corneal instability.

After considerable discussion, the patient elected to undergo penetrating keratoplasty (PK) in the left eye. This was performed without complication with a 8.25 mm donor button. The patient is now in the early postoperative recovery phase of the surgery. The BCVA has remained unaffected.

This case illustrates the unpredictability and instability of the corneas of eyes with forme fruste keratoconus identified on preoperative topography. While refractive surgeons have advocated PRK and LASIK with various treatment modifications for these eyes, this case clearly demonstrates that forme fruste keratoconus should be considered a contraindication for refractive surgery and particularly LASIK.

Figure 1C-1. Preoperative corneal topography indicates extensive inferior steepening of the cornea with irregular astigmatism, suggesting forme fruste keratoconus.

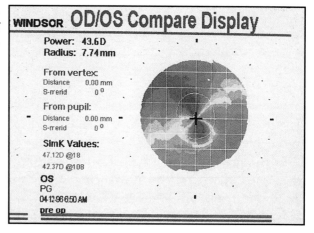

Figure 1C-2. Four-month post-LASIK topography demonstrates the superior flattening from the excimer ablation with the same inferior steepening that was observed preoperatively.

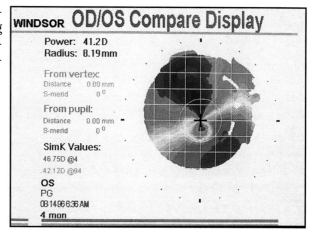

Figure 1C-3. At the 6-month visit, the topography found an increasing amount of irregular astigmatism.

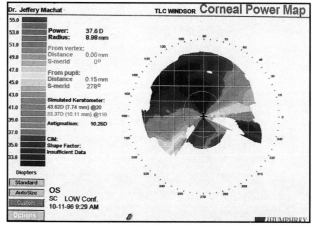

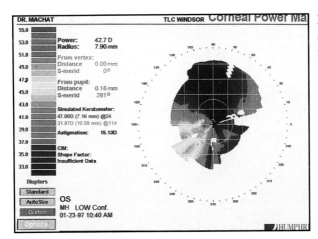

Figure 1C-4. At the 18-month follow-up, the astigmatism has increased to SimK values of more than 15 D.

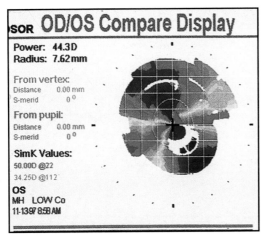

Figure 1C-5. At the 9-month follow-up after astigmatic keratotomy, the topography showed no improvement in the astigmatism.

Editor's Notes

While refractive surgeons have advocated PRK and LASIK with various modifications in the treatment of forme fruste keratoconus, this case clearly demonstrates that forme fruste keratoconus should be considered a contraindication for refractive surgery, particularly LASIK. This case illustrates the unpredictability and instability of the keratoconus cornea. Many eyes will demonstrate mild amounts of inferior steepening. Through the use of different corneal mapping units, such as the Orbscan (Orbtek, Inc., Salt Lake City, Utah), it has been shown that some of this inferior steepening can be an artifact of the topography method itself in some cases.

Several guidelines can be helpful for evaluation of patients with small amounts of inferior steepening. If the difference between the superior and inferior cornea is greater than 3.0 D, this indicates significant steepening (that would contraindicate LASIK). If the central corneal thickness is less than 500 μm, this could suggest slowly progressive keratoconus. Finally, if refractive astigmatism is also present, this confirms some irregularity of the cornea.

Patients with only small amounts of inferior steepening, regular corneal thickness, and no refractive astigmatism, can still achieve excellent results with LASIK.

CASE D, LASIK WITH KERATOCONUS

Michael Lawless, MBBS, FRACO, FRACS, FRCOphth, and Sue Webber, BSc(Hons), FRCOphth

Main Concern: Keratoconus and LASIK
Patient Age: 31

INITIAL PREOPERATIVE INFORMATION

	OD	OS	COMMENTS
Preoperative Refraction	-6.5/-3 X 75	-6.5/-3 X110	keratoconus OU
BCVA	6/7.5	6/7.5	
Topography Details	inferior cones OU		
SimK Values	45.79@127, 44.46	44.94@37, 43.43	
Pachymetry	490 µm	530 µm	

PROCEDURES PERFORMED

	OD	OS	COMMENTS
1. Date/type	7/2/97 LASIK	no surgery	referring center
Laser/keratome/plate	Summit Apex Plus Laser/Chiron ACS/ 160 µm footplate, -7.7 D		
2. Date/type	10/15/97 LASIK		
Laser/keratome/plate	Summit Apex Plus Laser flap lifted pl – 3.5 X 80		

CURRENT POSTOPERATIVE INFORMATION

	OD	OS	COMMENTS
Time Postoperative	6 months after second procedure		progressive keratoconus OD requiring PK
Postoperative Refraction	-8.75/-3.5 X 22		
BCVA	6/45	6/7.5	
Topography Details	cones	cones	
SimK Values	44.46@140, 41.36		
Pachymetry	not performed		
Visual Complaints	poor VA OD		
Medications	none		
Refractive Correction	none	contact lenses	
Other	awaiting right corneal transplant		

There are few indications for excimer laser treatment of keratoconus. Those procedures that have met with some success include small zone PTK to treat the nipple on a cone, or a larger zone to reduce the K values, both with the aim of allowing more satisfactory contact lens fitting. More controversial though, is the refractive correction of eyes that have only topographic evidence of keratoconus or treatment of a clinically normal eye in patients with keratoconus in the fellow eye.

Although not the case here, it has been reported that previously healthy corneas have developed keratoconus after LASIK treatment, although there remains speculation as to whether iatrogenic keratoconus can develop in a totally normal cornea. If this is the case, it should perhaps be referred to as keratoectasia, to differentiate this from eyes that have a preexisting pathological predisposition. It has been suggested that if the residual stromal thickness is too thin, then ectasia can develop in an otherwise normal cornea. A stromal thickness of 250 μm has been proposed as the minimum that should remain to safeguard against ectasia. However, it is unknown whether this would occur in any cornea, or just in those with a predisposition to keratoconus.

There is little doubt that there is a wide range of clinical keratoconus, varying from those patients with an obvious Munson's sign to those with topographic irregularity, minimal signs on clinical examination and normal best spectacle corrected acuity. No one would doubt that both these cases are keratoconic, perhaps qualifying the latter as forme fruste. But what is unknown is whether any lesser degree of keratoconus exists where the patient has the keratoconus genotype, but where this has not been exhibited as a phenotype. Perhaps it is these patients where excimer laser or lamellar keratectomy can unmask the disease.

Clearly, this is not the case with this patient, as she had clear clinical and topographic keratoconus preoperatively (Figure 1D-1). This patient underwent LASIK to her right eye, with both she and the surgeon aware that she had keratoconus. This patient was not treated at our center, and it was not clear from the referral letter what the desired outcome of treatment was. However, we might surmise from the treatment given that the intention was to correct most of her refractive error. She initially appeared to do well, her preoperative refraction was reduced from -6.5/-3 X 75 to +0.25/-2.75 X 65. Presumably this refraction remained stable over the next 3 months, because the surgeon then went on to perform a toric ablation to correct the residual cylinder. Apparently after this second laser treatment with the Summit Apex Plus Laser (Summit Technology, Waltham, Mass), the cornea became unstable and the keratoconus was exacerbated (Figure 1D-2). Whether this was the inevitable outcome following any treatment or it occurred because the treatment extended beyond a crucial depth for this patient is unknown.

This patient was able to wear rigid gas permeable contact lenses in both eyes preoperatively and continues to do so in the left eye. However, despite contact lens fitting by an optometrist experienced with keratoconics, the right eye fails to achieve a satisfactory visual acuity. This patient now requires a right penetrating keratoplasty (PK).

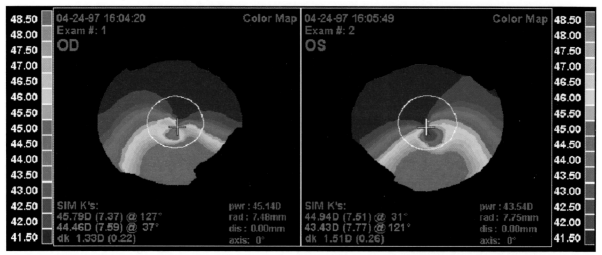

Figure 1D-1. Right and left preoperative corneal topography. Both eyes clearly demonstrate keratoconus.

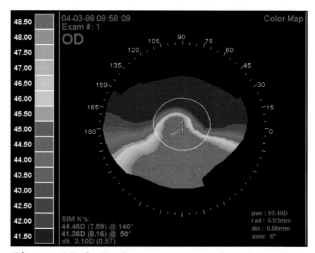

Figure 1D-2. Right eye topography, 6 months after the second procedure. This map is on the same scale as Figure 1D-1 and clearly shows an extension of the inferior steepening.

Editor's Notes

There have been numerous reports in medical literature suggesting that PRK or LASIK can be performed successfully in patients with some degree of keratoconus. It has been my experience that LASIK should not be performed with even moderate degrees of forme fruste keratoconus as this will tend to exacerbate the corneal instability and lead to irregular astigmatism and visual distortions. In this case, the patient actually had keratoconus and LASIK was attempted presumably in an effort to reduce the refractive error temporarily.

Keratoconus is a condition that involves corneal thinning. LASIK is a procedure that thins the central cornea to reduce myopia. Performing a thinning procedure on a cornea that is already undergoing a thinning process is not a logical combination. These two modalities combined will weaken the cornea and hasten the progress of keratoconus.

The only case that can be made for performing LASIK in a keratoconus patient is when the only motivation is to delay the inevitable occurrence of a PK. If the patient already needs a PK, and LASIK is attempted in the effort to delay the inevitable, then LASIK may be successful. This may give the patient 1 or 2 more years of further useful vision for that eye before further decompensation occurs and a PK is required.

CASE E, IRREGULAR ASTIGMATISM

Ted Smith, OD, and Jeffery J. Machat, MD

Main Concern: Poor Initial Preoperative Topography with Unusual Healing
Patient Age: 39

INITIAL PREOPERATIVE INFORMATION

	OD	OS	COMMENTS
Preoperative Refraction	-3.50 – 4.00 X 82	-8.00 D	
UCVA	cf@3 ft	cf	
BCVA	20/20	20/20	
Topography Details	47.50/43.75 X 072	44.50/44.0 X 50	irregular
SimK Values	n/a	n/a	topography OD
Pachymetry	505 µm	520 µm	

PROCEDURES PERFORMED

	OD	OS	COMMENTS
1. Date/type	8/9/96 LASIK OU		
Laser/keratome/plate	Technolas 117/ACS/160		
2. Date/type	12/05/96 AK		
	2 x 3 mm incisions at 162°		
3. Date/type	5/13/99 LASIK		
Laser/keratome/plate	Technolas 217/ACS/200		

CURRENT POSTOPERATIVE INFORMATION

	OD	OS	COMMENTS
Time Postoperative	2 years, 5 months	2 years, 5 months	irregular astigmatism
Postoperative Refraction	+1.25 – 3.75 X 010	pl	and inferior
UCVA	20/100	20/20	steepening
BCVA	20/20	20/20	
Topography Details	43.87/40.50 X 080	n/a	
SimK Values	4.07	n/a	
Pachymetry	457 µm	n/a	
Visual Complaints	blur	none	
Refractive Correction	none	none	

This patient was a 39-year-old white male with an unremarkable medical history. His surgical history consisted of bilateral LASIK on August 9, 1996, for attempted correction of OD -3.50 – 4.00 X 082 and OS -8.00 DS. At that time, topography OD showed the expected astigmatism corresponding with the spectacle *Rx*, however, the topography also showed inferior corneal steepening and poor symmetry. The left topography was essentially spherical with only slight inferior steepening (Figure 1E-1).

The left eye stabilized perfectly within 2 months postoperatively to an UCVA of 20/20+ and a manifest *Rx* of +0.25 D. The right eye stabilized at 4 months postoperatively to UCVA 20/40- and *Rx* OD +1.75 – 2.50 X 077 with BCVA of 20/20. The corneal topography showed K values of 44.00/39.62 X 72 and inferonasal steepening with irregular and asymmetrical astigmatism (Figure 1E-2). Pachymetry readings showed a right corneal thickness of 439 μm. In attempt to reduce the corneal toricity, since the corneal topography contraindicated further laser ablation, AK was performed with two 3 mm incisions at 162° with a clear central zone of 7 mm.

At 2 years and 5 months post AK, the patient presented with an unaided acuity OD of 20/100. The left eye was still successfully stable at 20/20 unaided with a plano *Rx*. The manifesting *Rx* OD showed a dramatic development of with the rule astigmatism at +1.25 – 3.75 X 100. Corneal topography once again showed inferonasal steepening and irregular, asymmetrical astigmatism with K values of 43.87/40.50 X 080 and CIM 4.07 (Figure 1E-3). Pachymetry indicated a central corneal thickness of 457 μm. Biomicroscopy showed clear corneas with a faint incision scar from the primary LASIK and the more prominent incision scars subsequent to the AK (Figure 1E-4). To address the residual refraction OD, LASIK was performed with a target correction of +0.50 – 2.75 X 120. The UCVA OD was 20/20 1 week postoperatively.

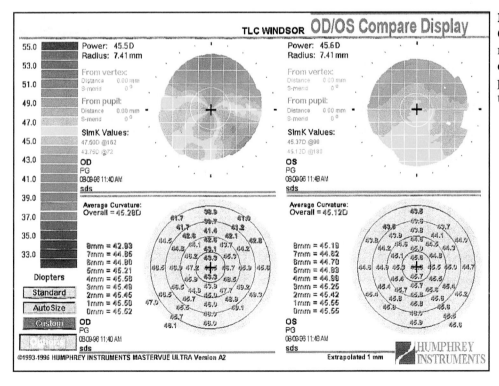

Figure 1E-1. Corneal asymmetry OD was evident on the preoperative topography.

Figure 1E-2. Following LASIK, the right eye continues to demonstrate irregular astigmatism.

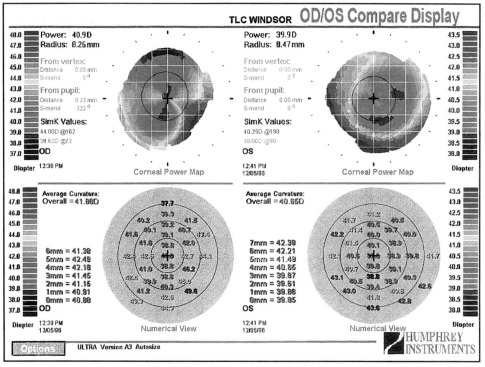

Figure 1E-3. Over 2 years after LASIK and AK, the inferonasal steepening is still present on the right cornea.

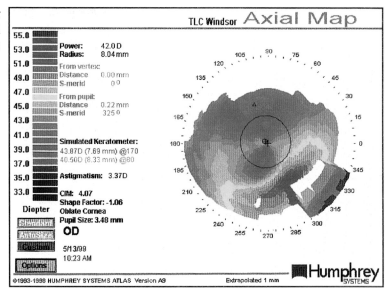

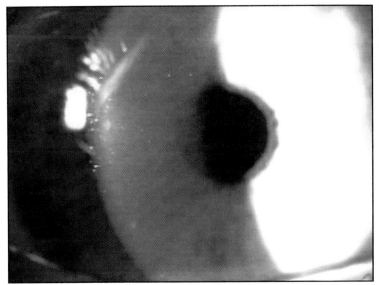

Figure 1E-4. AK cuts are visible along with LASIK keratectomy edge.

Editor's Notes

This patient presented initially with a stable refraction in the right eye, but an irregular topography pattern was identified. While not strictly keratoconic in nature, there was definitely inferior steepening of the cornea. The patient stated that the vision was always poor in the right eye and was quite interested in pursuing refractive surgery. It was explained to the patient that the results would be less predictable OD.

When the LASIK was originally performed in the right eye, the patient achieved an UCVA of 20/40 in the right eye and 20/20 in the left eye. Unfortunately the visual acuity diminished OD, so AK cuts were attempted in an effort to reduce the astigmatism. Two and a half years following the original procedure, the patient returned with over 3 D of astigmatism in the right eye. After explaining to the patient that further instability could be expected in the right eye, a mixed pattern ablation was performed using the Technolas 217 laser. On the first postoperative day the patient was 20/20 in the right eye uncorrected and quite pleased with his vision. Nevertheless, over the long term we do expect further deterioration in his vision and progression of this astigmatism.

This case demonstrates that patients with irregular topographic patterns are poor candidates for LASIK. The irregular topography identified in this patient indicates corneal instability. The current excimer lasers ablate only regular refractive errors and therefore will not effectively treat or eliminate the irregularity. Furthermore, this irregularity of the cornea identified preoperatively may indicate some corneal instability that could be augmented by a corneal thinning procedure.

2

COMPLEX MYOPIC LASIK

COMPLEX MYOPIC LASIK - SUMMARY NOTES

Indications
- up to 12.0 D of myopia
- up to 6.0 D of astigmatism
- pupil size less than 6 mm in dim light

Risks
- overcorrection
- night glare
- microstriae
- decentration
- corneal ectasia

Preoperative
- check for retinal pathology
- BCVA better than 20/40 OU
- stable refraction
- adequate corneal thickness
- regular topography

Operative
- alignment marks placed on cornea
- 160 μm plate selected on ACS or Hansatome
- flap edge retracted minimizing epithelial disruption
- excimer ablation performed
- centering of ablation on pupil
  - eye tracker
  - suction ring on eye with suction off
  - verbal encouragement
- flap refloated into position
- interface irrigation
- alignment marks and gutter checked for alignment
- wait 1 to 5 minutes for adhesion
- blink and/or striae test

Postoperative
- monitor for regression over 1 to 4 months
- pachymetry checked prior to enhancement

CASE A, EXCESSIVELY FLAT CORNEA AFTER MYOPIC LASIK

Jose Güell, MD

Main Concern: Poor Quality of Vision

INITIAL PREOPERATIVE INFORMATION

	OD	OS	COMMENTS
Preoperative Refraction	-14.00	-24.00	extreme myopia OS
BCVA	20/50	20/60	
Topography Details	n/a	slightly irregular	
SimK Values	42/41.45	41.36/41.49	
Pachymetry	n/a	605 μm	

PROCEDURES PERFORMED

	OD	OS	COMMENTS
1. Date/type	no surgery	11/94 M-LASIK	4.6 mm zone
Laser/keratome/plate		Technolas 116/ ACS/160	
2. Date/type		4/95 enhancement	
Laser/keratome/plate		Technolas 116/ACS/160	

CURRENT POSTOPERATIVE INFORMATION

	OD	OS	COMMENTS
Time Postoperative		2½ years	poor qualitative
Postoperative Refraction		-7.75 – 0.50 X 117	vision due to small
BCVA		20/40-	zone and under-
Topography Details		small zone	correction
SimK Values		31.99 X 32.11	
Pachymetry		n/a	
Visual Complaints		poor quality	
Medications		none	

Induced Extremely Flat Cornea After LASIK for Myopia

Figure 2A-1.

		UCVA	Rx	BCVA	Km
Preoperative	OD	cf	-14.00	20/40	42.00 X 41.45
	OS	cf	-24.00	20/40	41.36 X 41.49

November 1994/LASIK OS, 4.6 mm OZ (pachymetry 605 μm)

Figure 2A-2.

		UCVA	Rx	BCVA	Km
March 1995	OS	20/100	-7.75 – 0.50 X 117	20/40-	35.26 X 34.9

April 1995/ReLASIK OS, 4.5 mm OZ

Figure 2A-3 and 2A-4.

		UCVA	Rx	BCVA	Km
March 1997	OS	20/60-		pinhole 20/40-	31.99 X 32.11

(Ophthalmometer < 30 D)

Subjective Analysis

- bad functional vision
- terrible night vision
- vision quality unstable during daytime
- blurring vision with rigid gas permeable contact lenses

Figure 2A-1. Preoperative topography OS with a regular pattern.

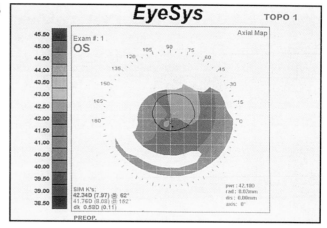

Figure 2A-2. A well-centered but small zone pattern after LASIK for -24.0 OS.

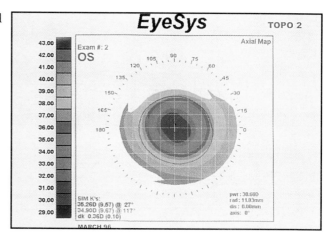

Figure 2A-3. A LASIK enhancement OS lead to further central corneal flattening.

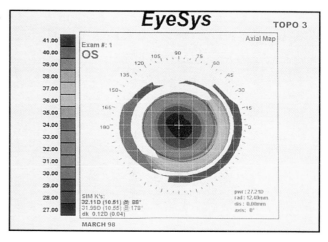

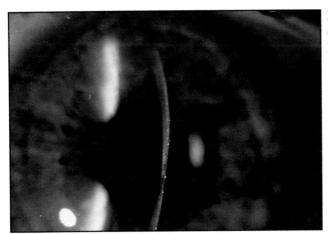

Figure 2A-4. Slit lamp view of cornea demonstrates central thinning after 2 LASIK procedures for extreme myopia.

Editor's Notes

This patient had an extremely high myopic correction of 24.0 D. The patient had preoperative Ks of approximately 41, which was already flatter than the average cornea. The LASIK was originally performed with a small zone of 4.6 mm. The patient was fortunate to have thick corneas with pachymetry reading of 605 µm.

The operation was then performed for another 8 D of correction in the left eye at a 4.5 mm optical zone. The topography shows that the patient did have a well-centered ablation zone, however the small zone and the large correction would clearly cause visual distortion (particularly at night).

It is now known that optical zones should be kept at least in the 5 to 5.5 mm range for the correction of myopia and ideally in the 6 mm range. Depending on the corneal thickness, the maximum myopic correction is now limited to 13.0 D. Small optical zones do make the correction of extremely high myopic refractive errors possible, as this reduces the depth of the ablation. Unfortunately, they also result in a decrease in the quality of vision and an increase in the incidence of visual disturbances, such as poor vision at night and induced astigmatism.

CASE B, HIGH MYOPIA WITH HIGH ASTIGMATISM

Amar Agarwal, MS, FRCS, FRCOphth(Lon), Sunita Agarwal, MS, FSVH(Germ), DO, and Athiya Agarwal, MD, FRSH(Lon), DO

Main Concern: Correction of the High Astigmatism (4 D)
Patient Age: 20

INITIAL PREOPERATIVE INFORMATION

	OD	OS	COMMENTS
Preoperative Refraction		-10.5 – 4.0 X 175	
BCVA		20/20	
SimK Values		43.94/86; 40.77@176	
Pachymetry		542 µm	

PROCEDURES PERFORMED

	OD	OS	COMMENTS
1. Date/type		11/21/98	
Laser/keratome/plate		Chiron 217/	
		Hansatome/180	

CURRENT POSTOPERATIVE INFORMATION

	OD	OS	COMMENTS
Time Postoperative		5 months	well-centered ablation
Postoperative Refraction		-1.0 D sph	
BCVA		20/20	
SimK Values		35.79/90; 34.39@180	
Pachymetry		443 µm	
Visual Complaints		none	
Medications		none	
Refractive Correction		none	

Correction of a patient with high myopia and high astigmatism is a complex situation. This patient came to us with high myopia. The patient also had a high astigmatism of 4 D OS. The problem when treating such cases is to first rule out any keratoconus. Generally if the patient has such high astigmatism they could be suffering from keratoconus. Once this is ruled out, then one can go ahead with LASIK.

The patient had a preoperative refraction of -10.5 – 4.0 X 175 degrees. The preoperative topography (Figure 2B-1) showed a high astigmatism but no keratoconus. The Hansatome microkeratome was used and the excimer laser used was the Chiron 217. The flap was created and the ablation started. When one is performing LASIK on a patient with astigmatism then one should be careful that the eye does not rotate otherwise the axis of the astigmatism which is being ablated will change. Once the laser ablation was completed, the flap was repositioned back.

Postoperatively, the patient was very happy with the result. There was a mild myopia of -1.0 D but the astigmatism had been neutralized. When one sees the postoperative topography (Figure 2B-2), one can see the good ablation. One can also notice in the picture the neutralization of the astigmatism after checking the K value readings.

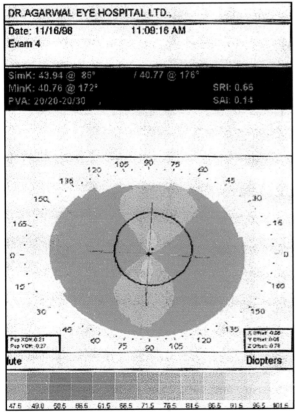

Figure 2B-1. Preoperative topography in which LASIK was done for a patient with high myopia and high astigmatism.

Figure 2B-2. Postoperative topography in which LASIK was done for a patient with high myopia and high astigmatism.

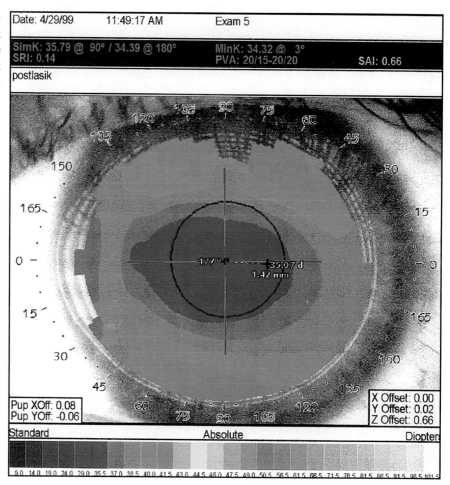

Editor's Notes

When correcting high myopia with high degrees of astigmatism using a scanning laser such as the Technolas 217 laser, there is a large amount of tissue ablated due to the pattern used by the scanning laser to flatten the steep axis for the treatment of minus cylinder. Prior to performing any large myopic ablations on the scanning laser, it is therefore very important to look at the preoperative pachymetry and ensure that at least 400 μm of tissue will be preserved following the end of this procedure. In this case we can see 443 μm were preserved. Therefore the patient could successfully undergo an enhanced procedure in the future if any regression occurs.

CASE C, LASIK ENHANCEMENT

*Amar Agarwal, MS, FRCS, FRCOphth(Lon), Sunita Agarwal, MS, FSVH(Germ), DO,
and Athiya Agarwal, MD, FRSH(Lon), DO*

Main Concern: Performing LASIK Enhancement and Not Tearing the Flap
Patient Age: 24

INITIAL PREOPERATIVE INFORMATION

	OD	OS	COMMENTS
Preoperative Refraction	-18.0 D spherical		extreme myopia
BCVA	20/40		
Topography Details	Figure 2C-1		
SimK Values	44.14/48; 43.06@138		
Pachymetry	568 μm		

PROCEDURES PERFORMED

	OD	OS	COMMENTS
1. Date/type	8/14/97 LASIK		
Laser/keratome/plate	Chiron 217/ACS/160		
2. Date/type	10/15/97 LASIK enhancement		flap lifted OD
Laser/keratome/plate	Chiron 217		

CURRENT POSTOPERATIVE INFORMATION

	OD	OS	COMMENTS
Time Postoperative	13 months		
Postoperative Refraction	-3.50 – 2.50 X 165		
BCVA	20/20		
Topography Details	Figure 2C-2 and 2C-3.		
SimK Values	38.59/37.04@166 after LASIK 35.64/32.62@158 after LASIK enhancement		
Pachymetry	437 μm after LASIK 387 μm after LASIK enhancement		
Visual Complaints	none		
Medications	none		
Refractive Correction	spectacles		

One complex situation is when the refractive power is not neutralized. In such cases, one has to perform LASIK enhancement. If the duration is within 3 months, one need not recut the cornea. One can lift up the previous flap and perform LASIK enhancement. If the patient comes in after that time, then one might have to recut the cornea and create a new flap.

This patient came to the hospital with high myopia. The refraction was -18.0 D with a preoperative BCVA of 20/40. LASIK was done on the patient using the ACS and the Chiron 217. The preoperative topography was normal (Figure 2C-1). The pachymetry was 568 μm. The postoperative topography (Figure 2C-2) showed a good ablation. But one can see in the picture the central area is not dark blue but dark green, showing the flattening was not enough. The postoperative pachymetry was 435 μm. The postoperative refraction was -10.00 with -1.0 cylinder at axis 170° 2 months later.

Then (2 months after the primary LASIK) the decision was made to perform LASIK enhancement. The flap was lifted manually and laser ablation again done with the Chiron 217. The postoperative pachymetry now showed 387 μm. The postoperative topography (Figure 2C-3) showed a good ablation with slight astigmatism. The postoperative refraction was -3.50 D spherical with -2.50 D cylinder at axis 165. The visual acuity was 20/20 with correction. The patient was quite happy, as the preoperative refraction was -18.00 D and it had been explained preoperatively that there would be a bit of residual power left.

This case demonstrates the importance of LASIK enhancement. This can be done depending on the postoperative pachymetry. It is better to do a LASIK enhancement after a few months, rather than wait for too long, as the flap can be lifted manually.

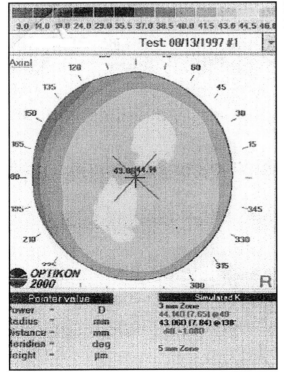

Figure 2C-1. Preoperative topography in which LASIK was done for a patient with high myopia.

Figure 2C-2. Postoperative topography in which LASIK was done for a patient with high myopia. The power had not been neutralized.

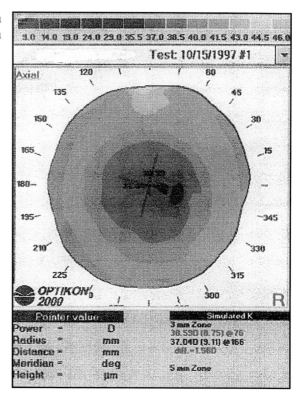

Figure 2C-3. Postoperative topography in which LASIK enhancement was done for a patient with high myopia. Note the ablation is even better than seen in Figure 2C-2.

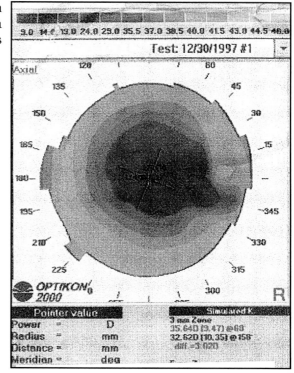

Editor's Notes

This case raises some interesting points in regards to the limitations for the correction of LASIK. It is possible to perform corrections for up to 25 D of myopia with LASIK and corrections to this level have been reported in the literature. It is also important to remember that in order to perform this degree of correction, the ablation zone size must be decreased and therefore the quality of vision and the incidence of decentered ablations will be increased. It is generally recommended that 400 µm of tissue be left following the original LASIK procedure. Since the average corneal thickness is approximately 540 µm, this means that there is 140 µm of tissue available for ablation if we assume that the real flap thickness with a 160 plate is 150 µm and the remaining posterior stromal tissue is 250 µm (540-150-250 = 140). Most excimer lasers ablate between 10 to 15 µm of tissue per diopter. Therefore the maximum ablation possible would be 14.0 D (140/10 = 14). Since this case involved the correction of 18 D, the patient would not be able to be fully corrected using these guidelines. If the patient desired full correction, the other options would be phakic IOL or clear lens extraction.

The patient was fortunate that the pachymetry was 568 µm, giving plenty of thickness to allow this large myopic correction. However, at the end of the procedure, the corneal thickness was 387 µm (which is slightly beyond the minimal thickness that would be acceptable). If we assume that a 160 µm flap was cut with the ACS shaper this would mean that there was approximately 227 µm left in the stromal bed (which is likely adequate in this situation). Ideally we would leave around 250 µm in the stromal bed, which combined with 150 to 160 µm flap would give us a total corneal thickness of 400 µm. Paying close attention to the corneal thickness preoperatively will allow us to preserve adequate corneal tissue postoperatively, and hence avoid long-term problems with corneal ectasia.

3

Complex Hyperopic LASIK

COMPLEX HYPEROPIC LASIK - SUMMARY NOTES

Indications
- up to 5.0 D of spherical hyperopia
- up to 3.0 D of hyperopic astigmatism
- no ABMD

Risks
- undercorrection
- regression
- decentered ablation
- induced astigmatism
- loss of BCVA

Preoperative
- stable refraction
- cycloplegic refraction
- regular topography
- check for ABMD

Operative
- alignment marks placed on cornea
- 180 μm plate for Hansatome (preferred)
- 200 μm plate for ACS if flat K is <42.0 D
- flap edge retracted minimizing epithelial disruption
- excimer ablation performed
- centering of ablation on pupil
  - eye tracker
  - suction ring on eye with suction off
  - verbal encouragement
- flap refloated into position
- interface irrigation
- alignment marks and gutter checked for alignment
- wait 1 to 5 minutes for adhesion
- blink and/or striae test

Postoperative
- monitor for regression over 1 to 4 months
- pachymetry checked prior to enhancement
- topography checked for centration
- enhance selectively as results are less predictable

CASE A, PSEUDOKERATOCONUS AFTER HYPEROPIC LASIK

Jose Güell, MD

Main Concern: Iatrogenic Pseudokeratoconus

INITIAL PREOPERATIVE INFORMATION

	OD	OS	COMMENTS
Preoperative Refraction	+8.00	+6.75 + 1.00 X 140	extreme hyperopia
BCVA	20/25	20/40	
Topography Details	regular	regular	
SimK Values	n/a	n/a	
Pachymetry	n/a	n/a	

PROCEDURES PERFORMED

	OD	OS	COMMENTS
1. Date/type	2/96 H-LASIK	2/96 H-LASIK	small zone
Laser/keratome/plate	117/ACS/160	117/ACS/160	
2. Date/type	7/96 H-LASIK		small zone
Laser/keratome/plate	117		
3. Date/type	8/98 PTK/PRK		pseudokeratoconus
Laser/keratome/plate	217		
4. Date/type	11/98 PK		irregular astigmatism

CURRENT POSTOPERATIVE INFORMATION

	OD	OS	COMMENTS
Time Postoperative	1 month		post-PK
Postoperative Refraction	-1.75 – 4.00 X 85		
BCVA	20/25		
UCVA	20/100		
Topography Details	n/a		
SimK Values	n/a		
Pachymetry	n/a		
Visual Complaints	n/a		
Medications	n/a		

Induced Pseudokeratoconus After LASIK for Hyperopia

Figure 3A-1.

		UCVA	Rx	BCVA	KM
Preoperative	OD	20/400	+8.00	20/25	43.58
	OS	20/400	+6.75 + 1.00 X 140	20/40	41.64

February 1996, LASIK OU, 4.5 optical zone hyperopic ablation

Figure 3A-2.

		UCVA	Rx	BCVA	KM
3 months postoperative	OD	20/40	+3.75	20/25	52.63 centered
June 1996	OS	20/40	+2.00 – 0.75 X 120	20/40	48.31 centered

July 1996, LASIK OD reoperated 4.5 optical zone hyperopic ablation

Figure 3A-3.

		UCVA	Rx	BCVA	KM
3 months after reoperation	OD	20/40	+2.75 – 1.00 X 95	20/30	49.72 centered
September 1996	OS	20/40	+1.75 – 1.00 X 120	20/40	48.52 centered
January 1998	OD	20/60	pinhole	20/50	pseudokerato-conus
	OS	20/50	+1.75 – 0.75 X 120	20/40	

August 1998, transepithelial PRK PTK OD (-6.00 D, 3.5 mm OZ)

Figure 3A-4.

		UCVA	Rx	BCVA	KM
September 1998	OD	20/30	pinhole	20/30	52.83 centered

Figure 3A-5.

		UCVA	Rx	BCVA	KM
October 1998	OD	20/100	pinhole	20/60	severe irregular astigmatism

November 1998, PK OD (8/8.50 mm)

Figure 3A-6.

		UCVA	Rx	BCVA	KM
December 1998	OD	20/100-	-1.75 – 4.00 X 85	20/25	

Figure 3A-1. Preoperative topography OD.

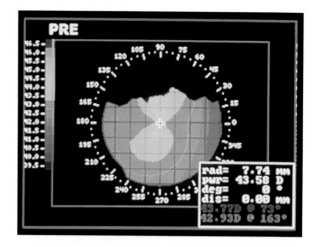

Figure 3A-2. Three-month postoperative topography OD demonstrating a small, steep optical zone.

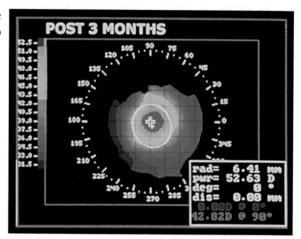

Figure 3A-3. Three months after H-LASIK enhancement OD with a small, steep central zone of cornea-inducing pseudokeratoconus.

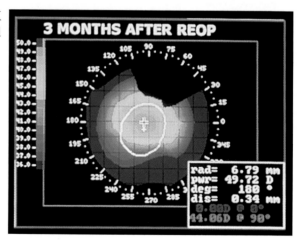

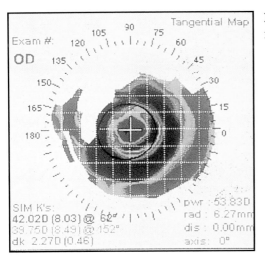

Figure 3A-4. Transepithelial M-PRK/PTK has only moderately reduced the central steepening.

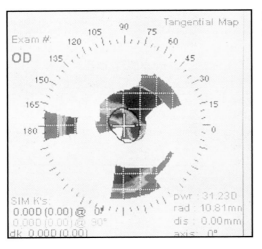

Figure 3A-5. Severe irregular astigmatism 10 months after PRK/PTK for the pseudokeratoconus.

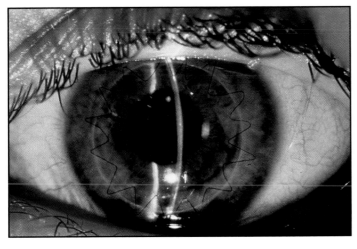

Figure 3A-6. A PK was required to restore the BCVA.

Editor's Notes

This case demonstrates the problems associated with excessive corneal steepening following hyperopic LASIK. This patient had an 8 D hyperopic treatment attempted OD with a 4.5 mm optical zone. We now know that this is an excessive amount of hyperopic treatment, but in February 1996, the parameters of hyperopic LASIK were still being explored. The topography following the original procedure shows a tremendous amount of central corneal steepening. Nevertheless, the patient was left undercorrected in the right eye and therefore an enhancement procedure was performed for another 4 D. This resulted in even more central steepening of the cornea.

Unfortunately, the BCVA had decreased and the patient had developed a pseudokeratoconus configuration to the cornea. In order to reduce some of the central steepening, the patient had transepithelial PRK/PTK over the cone to reduce the degree of steepening in this area. Unfortunately, the cornea remained steep in the central area and the patient was left with severe irregular astigmatism that necessitated a PK.

This case clearly illustrates the limitations of hyperopic LASIK. There is a limit to the amount of steepening the central cornea can endure, which is approximately 50.0 D. The maximum hyperopic correction of the average cornea appears to be about 5 to 6.0 D, but the ideal correction is probably 4.0 D or less. More steepening tends to cause disruption of the tear film interface with the drying of the central steepened cornea, as well as visual distortions in the steepened area. Any decentration of the ablation will also result in an induced astigmatism of up to 3.0 D. These patients with large hyperopic corrections do not tend to be as happy as myopic patients because of the loss of the quality of their vision.

Case B, High Hyperopia Treatment with the Excimer Laser

Michiel S. Kritzinger, MD

Main concern: Poor Quality and Quantity of Vision with High Hyperopia LASIK

Initial Preoperative Information

	OD	OS	Comments
Preoperative Refraction:	+5.25/-0.50 X 165	+5.00/-0.25 X 40	high hyperopia
BCVA	20/20	20/20	
Topography	Figure 3B-1	Figure 3B-2	
SimK values	42.8 X 69/41.5 X 159	42.8 X 89/42.0 X 179	

Procedures Performed

	OD	OS	Comments
1. Date/type	1995 H-LASIK OU		small 4.0 mm zone
Laser/keratome/plate	Technolas 116 20 Hz/ACS/160		
2. Date/type	1995 H-LASIK enhancement OU		small 4.0 mm zone
Laser/keratome/plate	Technolas 116 20 Hz/lift		
3. Date/type	1995 PTK OU		iatrogenic cones OU
Laser/keratome/plate	Technolas 116		
4. Date/type	STAAR ICL OU		iatrogenic
Laser/keratome/plate	phaco and IOL		cataracts OU

Current Postoperative Information

	OD	OS	Comments
Time Postoperative	3 years after first LASIK OU		
Postoperative Refraction	+0.75 – 1.00 X 150	+0.75 – 1.25 X 092	
BCVA	20/50	20/25	iatrogenic anterior
UCVA	20/70	20/30	subcapsular
Topography Details	n/a	n/a	cataract OD
SimK Values	n/a	n/a	
Pachymetry	n/a	n/a	
Visual Complaints	blur	none	
Medications	none	none	

This patient requested information in 1995 regarding surgical refractive procedures available. The patient was a high hyperope with a right exotropia and intermittent diplopia. There was also a recent history of rheumatoid arthritis with no clinical dry eye manifestation. The patient could not wear contact lenses and had severe adaptational problems with bi- and multifocal spectacle lenses.

The patient was willing to have refractive surgery done. In 1995 Technolas released the first planoscan 116 20 Hz software for hyperopia, which I used in this particular case.

First hyperopic treatment: Technolas 116 20 Hz

	OD	OS
Sphere	+6.00	+6.00
Cylinder	-0.50	0
Cylinder Axis	150	0
Zone Diameter	4.0 mm	4.0 mm
Ablation/Total Pulses	3 μm/1376	0 μm/1344

At that time very little, if anything, was known about hyperopic LASIK. The patient regressed quickly postoperatively due to factors that we are only aware of now:
- small zone treatment diameter
- too slow repetition rate of laser
- flap diameter too small
- degree of hyperopia attempted was too high

Four weeks later a second hyperopic treatment was done.

Second Hyperopia treatment: Technolas 116 20Hz

	OD		OS	
	Preoperative	Treatment	Preoperative	Treatment
Sphere	+3.25	+3.50	+2.75	+3.00
Cylinder	-1.75	-1.75	-0.75	-0.75
Cylinder Axis	180	180	140	140
Zone Diameter		4 mm		4 mm
Ablation/Total Pulses		11 μm/941		5 μm/753
Postoperative Topography		Figure 3B-3		Figure 3B-4

Visual outcome was poor with loss of 4 lines of BCVA, which was unacceptable to both patient and doctor. Refractions were:

OD: pl/-0.75 X 60 (20/70)
OS: +1.00/-0.50 X 90 (20/70)

Follow-up visits showed severe regression and fluctuating vision, varying between +3.50 and +8.50 D.

An iatrogenic cone was created in both eyes, more severely in the left. The cone induced tear circulatory deficiencies with resultant severe keratitis sicca (Figure 3B-5). The sicca induced SPK and scarring on the apex of the cone due to chronic scaling of the epithelium. The patient was taken back to the operating room and a PTK was done to flatten the apex of the cone (Figure 3B-6).

The result was higher hyperopia postoperatively, but no epithelial scaling or SPK was noted afterwards, even with the history of rheumatoid arthritis. Lacrimal inferior punctum plugs were inserted.

With hyperopia still at an unacceptable degree after 2 years, I decided to implant the STAAR posterior chamber phakic IOL (Figure 3B-7). A bilateral implant was done. Surgery was uneventful and atraumatic to the crystalline lens.

OD: +3.50/-1.00 X 90 (20/50)
OS: +5.50/-1.00 X 180 (20/60)

Approximately 1 year after the implantable contact lens (ICL) (STAAR Surgical AG, Monrovia, Calif) insertion, the lenses showed anterior subcapsular cataracts (Figure 3B-8). Although there was enough vaulting (Figure 3B-9) of the ICL in the beginning to give +/-100 µm space between the two lenses, cataracts were still induced.

The cataract inducing mechanism of the STAAR Posterior chamber phakic refractive lens (PRL) in this case could be:
- PRL touch to the natural lens (ie, when rubbing the eyes)
- PRL interfered with the aqueous humor flow anterior to the crystalline lens
- PRL interfered with the metabolism of the crystalline lens
- During accommodation the crystalline lens moves forward, touching the PRL
- The haptics of the PRL became more embedded into the ciliary body, resulting in narrowing of the space between the two lenses
- The natural growth of a maturing natural lens can narrow the space between the two lenses

The left PRL was removed and replaced with a 30 D silicon foldable IOL 3 years after the first LASIK was performed. Current refractions are:

OD: PRL – +0.75/-1.00 X 158 (20/50) Cataract still present
OS: IOL – +0.75/-1.25 X 92 (20/25)

Patient satisfaction is good at this stage, especially with the result of the left eye. A phacoemulsification and IOL will be done later for the right eye.

The important lessons to be taken from this case are:
- Do not laser patients with potentially dry eyes (ie, people with immune system deficiencies)
- Do not treat high hyperopes with LASIK, as quality and quantity of vision is reduced (treat to a maximum of +3.00 D)
- IOLs and PRLs give better quality and quantity of vision with less loss of contrast sensitivity, than hyperopic LASIK
- Use phakic anterior chamber refractive lenses if the anterior chamber depth allows it in prepresbyopic patients
- Rather do a clear lens extraction in a presbyopic, or a shallow anterior chamber prepresbyopic patient

Conclusion

Hyperopia is still a major challenge in the refractive arena.

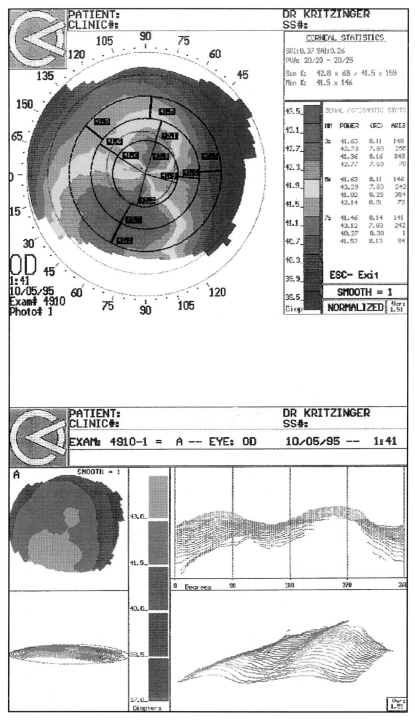

Figure 3B-1. Preoperative topography OD with slightly asymmetrical inferior corneal steepening.

Figure 3B-2. Preoperative topography OS with slightly asymmetrical inferior corneal steepening.

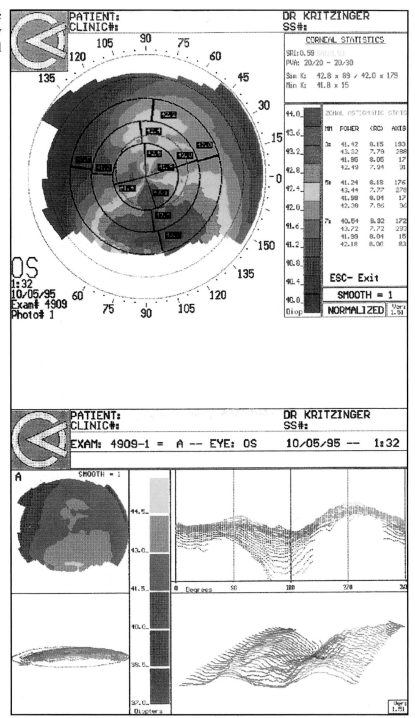

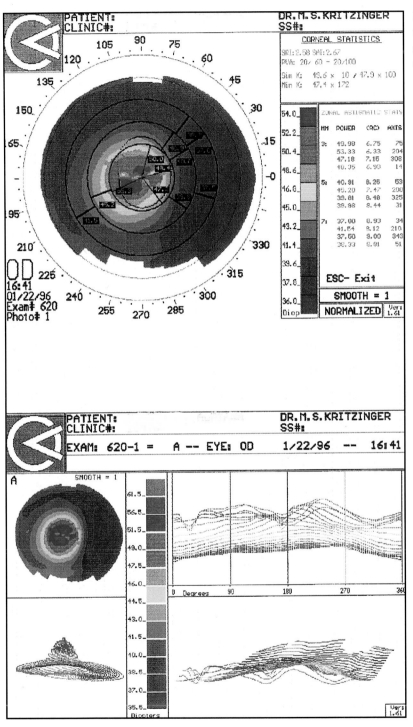

Figure 3B-3. Well-centered, very small optical zone OD after hyperopic LASIK with a 4.0 mm ablation zone.

Figure 3B-4. Well-centered, very small optical zone OS after hyperopic LASIK with a 4.0 mm ablation zone.

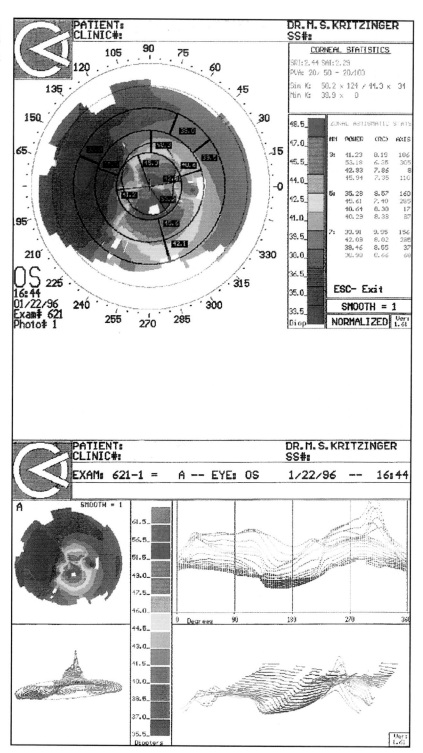

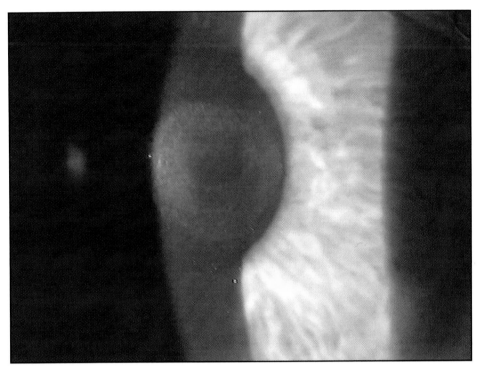

Figure 3B-5. Central corneal staining and haze demonstrating the iatrogenic keratoconus OD.

Figure 3B-6. Central corneal steepening OD, is slightly reduced after PTK.

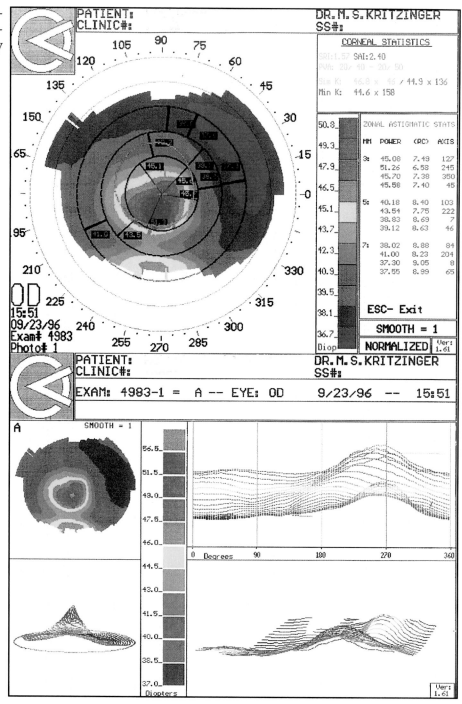

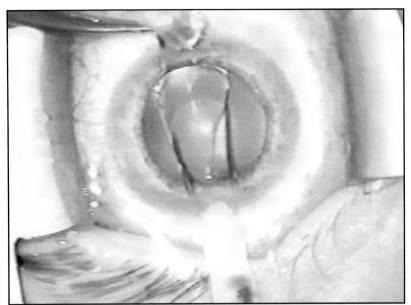

Figure 3B-7. Insertion of the STAAR ICL.

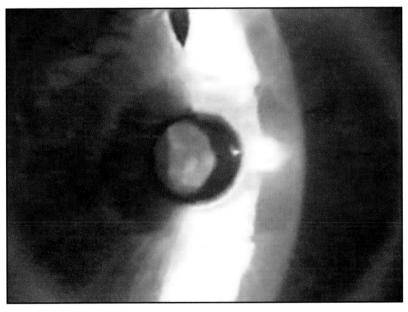

Figure 3B-8. Anterior subcapsular cataract with STAAR ICL. Note large superior iridectomy.

Figure 3B-9. Slit lamp photograph demonstrating anterior vaulting of STAAR ICL away from crystalline lens.

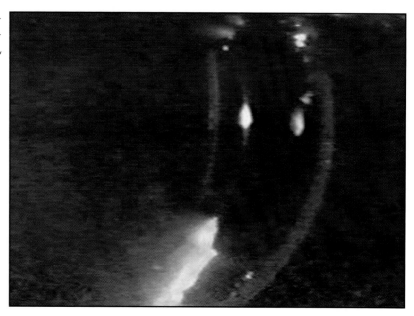

Editor's Notes

While the limitations for myopic LASIK corrections have been fairly well-established over the last 2 years, the limitations for the correction of hyperopia have been less clear. Because we are ablating peripheral corneal tissue, the corneal thickness is not as critical a factor. Peripheral corneal ablations leaving at least 400 µm of total corneal thickness could potentially correct up to 7.0 or 8.0 D of hyperopia in eyes with average corneal thickness. It has become clear, however, that there is a limitation to the amount of the steepening of the cornea that can be induced on the cornea without causing significant alterations in the visual performance as well as alterations in the effectiveness of the cornea tear film/lid interface.

This patient had a large hyperopic correction using a small zone ablation pattern. This resulted in a very small optical zone following the procedure, causing a visual distortion and a loss of BCVA, as well as the induced astigmatism. The enhancement procedure resulted in an even smaller optical zone with a further decentration.

Small optical zones should not be used for hyperopic LASIK, as there is a much greater chance of decentration with induced astigmatism. Enhancement procedures should be very selectively performed in hyperopic patients, as it is very difficult to induce further steepening of the cornea particularly if the original procedure had a slightly decentered ablation. Central corneal K readings in the 50 D range will induce a phenomenon that occurs in patients with keratoconus where the central steepened area of cornea does not achieve an adequate wetting affect from the tear film and develops an abraded and scarred appearance.

There clearly are limitations to the amount of hyperopia we can correct with the LASIK. The optical zones of at least 5 mm should be used and ideally 5.5 to 6.0 mm. We now know that the upper limit of the hyperopic correction is likely 5 D and preferably 4 D. Since there is a higher loss of BCVA in these patients, this issue must be addressed during the preoperative consent process. Finally the centration of the hyperopic ablation is even more important than during myopic ablations, as the decentered hyperopic ablations are difficult to treat and result in significant induced astigmatism. The use of an eye tracker or fixation ring to ensure adequate centration of the hyperopic ablation is helpful to minimize these difficulties.

In this case, a PTK treatment was used to reduce the central corneal steepening causing the central SPK in order to make the patient more comfortable and restore the normal contour to the cornea. Since this patient is also known to have rheumatoid arthritis, any surface ablation procedure should be performed with extreme caution as corneal melts have been reported in patients that are rheumatoid factor positive. The safest option in this case may be to perform the PTK ablation procedure underneath the flap in order to avoid any potential risk of corneal melt.

Case C, Aphakic LASIK

*Amar Agarwal, MS, FRCS, FRCOphth(Lon), Sunita Agarwal, MS, FSVH(Germ), DO,
and Athiya Agarwal, MD, FRSH(Lon), DO*

Main Concern: Extreme Hyperopic LASIK
Patient Age: 69

Initial Preoperative Information

	OD	OS	Comments
Preoperative Refraction	+11.75 − 0.5 X 40		extreme hyperopia
BCVA	20/20		
Topography Details	Figure 3C-1		
SimK Values	45.06/44.29@21		
Pachymetry	518 μm		

Procedures Performed

	OD	OS	Comments
1. Date/type	12/19/96 H-LASIK		5.0 mm zone
Laser/keratome/plate	Chiron 217/ACS/160		

Current Postoperative Information

	OD	OS	Comments
Time Postoperative	26 months		well-centered ablation
Postoperative Refraction	+3.50 + 1.0 X 120		
BCVA	20/20		
Topography Details	Figure 3C-2		
SimK Values	51.85/48.13@55		
Pachymetry	not done		
Visual Complaints	none		
Medications	none		
Refractive Condition	spectacles		

Hyperopic LASIK is not that easy when compared to myopic LASIK. When the case becomes one as complex as an aphakic eye, things get really complicated. This patient was a doctor who was operated in the right eye for cataract in 1982. At that time no IOL was implanted and the patient had an intracapsular cataract extraction done. The preoperative topography (Figure 3C-1) was taken, and showed nothing abnormal. The preoperative refraction was +11.75 D spherical and -0.5 D cylindrical at axis 40 degrees. The pachymetry was 518 µm.

The Chiron 217 the ACS were used to make the keratectomy. No complications occurred during the LASIK. The zone diameter used was 5.0 mm. When one is performing the entry of the refraction in the machine in hyperopic and aphakic cases, always enter the cylinder in the plus sign. If the refraction has been done with a minus cylinder, transpose the value and make it a plus sign. The postoperative refraction was +3.50 + 1.0 X 120. The preoperative and postoperative visual acuity was 6/6 (20/20). The postoperative topography (Figure 3C-2) shows an excellent ablation. The central area has become steep and is denoted in red due to the peripheral flattening. The patient was extremely happy as it was explained preoperatively that the refraction would reduce and not become absolutely zero.

One should be careful when performing aphakic LASIK, as these are complex cases. The points to remember is that one can correct approximately about +8.0 D maximum. Explain to the patient before hand that they will have some residual hyperopia. Another problem in aphakic eyes is that the pupil might be decentered. So, when one is applying the ablation, be careful that the ablation is centered on the pupil. If the case is one of a very badly decentered pupil it is better not to perform LASIK as the results will not be good. In the case discussed the pupil was well-centered. Finally convert the cylinder to the plus value and enter it in the laser machine as a plus cylinder, as this will ablate less tissue.

Figure 3C-1. Preoperative topography in which aphakic LASIK was done.

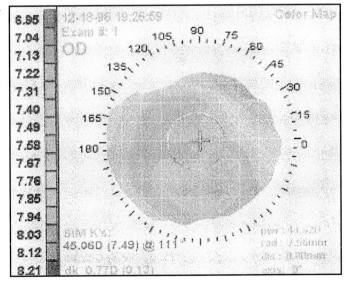

Figure 3C-2. Postoperative topography in which aphakic LASIK was done.

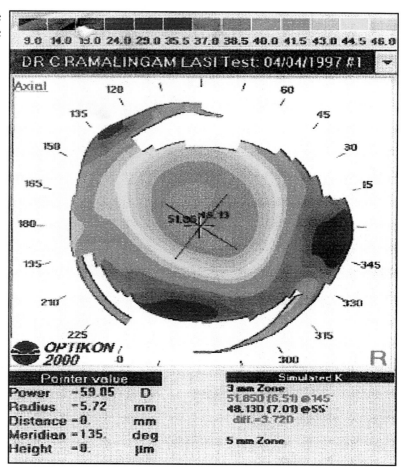

Editor's Notes

This patient is satisfied with the result of approximately 8.0 D of hyperopic correction with H-LASIK for the correction of an aphakic refractive error. Although the result in this case was successful, caution should be exercised when correcting this degree of hyperopia. Hyperopic LASIK corrections are almost always associated with a large amount of regression, resulting in undercorrection or further requests for enhancement procedures that can result in further difficulties. Excessive central corneal steepening can result in disruption of the tear film interface with superficial punctate keratitis at the top of the induced cone with significant discomfort and a reduction in BCVA. Even a small decentration can result in astigmatism.

In general, hyperopic corrections are not recommended for over 4.0 D of hyperopia. A large ablation zone (5.5 to 6.0 mm) can be used for these corrections with minimal risk of decentration and regression.

Case D, High Hyperopia Astigmatism Treated with Cross Cylinder

Ted Smith, OD, and Louis E. Probst, MD

Main Concern: Severe Corneal Cylinder
Patient Age: 30

Initial Preoperative Information

	OD	OS	Comments
Preoperative Refraction	+5.50 − 6.00 X 002		mixed pattern
UCVA	20/150		high cylinder
BCVA	20/20		
Topography Details	49.62/45.25 X 176		
SimK Values	0.82		
Pachymetry	506 µm		

Procedures Performed

	OD	OS	Comments
1. Date/type	5/14/99 LASIK		pl + 3.00 X 092
Laser/keratome/plate	Technolas 117/Hansatome/180		+2.00 − 3.00 X 002

Current Postoperative Information

	OD	OS	Comments
Time Postoperative	2 weeks		
Postoperative Refraction	+2.50 DS		astigmatism (fully cor-
UCVA	20/25-2		rected with cross cy-
BCVA	20/25+		linder technique)
Topography Details	47.62/46.25 X 174		
SimK Values	3.31		
Pachymetry	419 µm		
Visual Complaints	none		
Medications	Inflammase q.i.d.		
Refractive Correction	none		

This patient was a 30-year-old white female with an unremarkable medical history. Her surgical history consisted of LASIK on May 14, 1999, for an attempted correction of OD +5.50 – 6.00 X 002 with BCVA 20/25-. Her left eye was untreated as a precautionary step in case her right eye lost BCVA. Her left eye showed a similar *Rx* of +5.50 – 5.50 X 006 and BCVA 20/25. Topography OD showed the expected severe astigmatism corresponding with the spectacle *Rx*, with K values of 49.62/45.25 X 176 and CIM 0.82 (Figure 3D-1). Pachymetry readings showed a relatively thin cornea OD of 506 μm. The previous approach to treating this level of hyperopic astigmatism would have been to perform AK to reduce the cylinder by approximately a factor of two. After a stabilization period of at least 3 to 6 months, LASIK would be performed to treat the residual *Rx*. In this case, a cross cylinder ablation program was attempted to treat the corneal astigmatism in its entirety, thus alleviating the need for AK. The first ablation was programmed into the Technolas 217 with a treatment of plano + 3.00 X 092. The second treatment consisted of +2.00 – 3.00 X 002. At 1 hour postoperative, the patient had an UCVA of 20/100.

At 3 days postoperatively, the patient presented to her comanaging doctor with an UCVA of 20/70. A refraction of +3.00 – 1.00 X 030 provided a BCVA of 20/30+. Biomicroscopy showed what appeared to be grade 2 NSDIK. The patient was started on Inflammase Forte Q1h. For confirmation of the diagnosis, the patient was referred back to our center 3 days later, at which point UCVA had improved to 20/30 and the manifesting *Rx* had also reduced to +2.00 – 0.75 X 075, giving 20/25. Biomicroscopy showed a resolving grade 1 NSDIK. The Inflammase Forte was continued and the patient was to be followed closely over the next week.

At 2 weeks postoperatively OD, the patient presented for treatment of her fellow eye. The right eye showed an UCVA of 20/25-2 with a manifest *Rx* of +2.50 DS, providing a BCVA of 20/25. Topography showed a markedly reduced corneal cylinder with K values of 47.62/46.25 X 174 and CIM 3.31 (Figure 3D-2). Biomicroscopy showed clear corneas with only traces of observable NSDIK. The regimen of Inflammase Forte was subsequently maintained at Q2h and tapered over the next week.

The result of this cross cylinder approach for high hyperopic astigmatism has been remarkable. It indicates that this technique of treating high astigmats with the scanning laser could vastly reduce the necessity for AK. The patient is currently being followed for stabilization of both eyes.

Figure 3D-1. Severe with-the-rule astigmatism is evident on the preoperative topography.

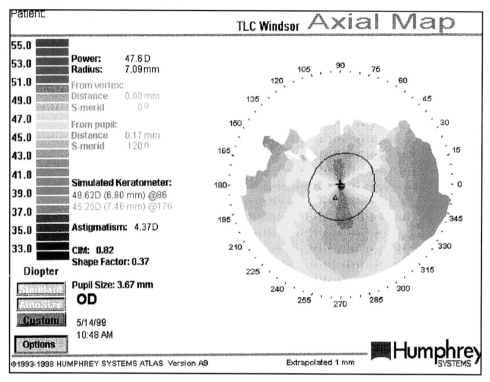

Figure 3D-2. Topography 2 weeks after LASIK with cross cylinder technique demonstrates little residual astigmatism.

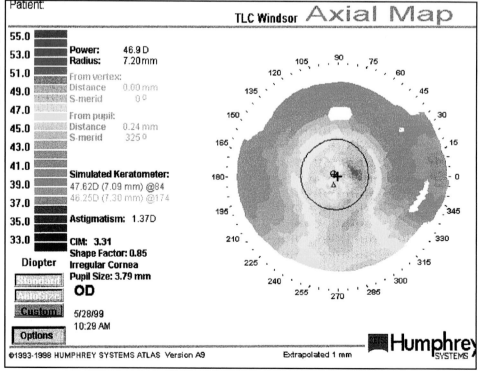

Editor's Notes

This patient was referred to our center for 6 D of bilateral with-the-rule astigmatism. The original plan was to perform AK cuts to reduce the astigmatism to a more manageable range and then perform LASIK in 3 to 6 months. After a long discussion with the patient it was decided that the recently described technique of cross cylinder ablation would be attempted, rather than performing the AK cuts. This procedure involved dividing the astigmatic correction in half. Half the prescription is corrected by steepening the flat axis and the other half of the prescription is corrected by flattening the steep axis. Because this was a new approach for us, we elected to treat one eye at a time.

She underwent the corrective treatment OD first on the Technolas 217 laser. The zone size was adjusted to approximately 5 mm in order to limit the ablation depth so that an enhancement procedure could be performed.

Remarkably, at 2 weeks follow up the patient had absolutely no astigmatic error. This was confirmed on her topography, which showed the central steepening induced by the hyperopic component of the correction. Although the patient is slightly hyperopic, the uncorrected acuity is excellent as she is only 30 years old. She will likely need to undergo a hyperopic LASIK ablation in the future in order to correct the residual hyperopia. These preliminary results suggest that the cross cylinder technique for correcting high astigmatic errors may prove to be very useful. Because this technique involves large amounts of tissue ablation, close attention needs to be paid to the corneal thickness.

Complex Intraoperative Flap Complications

4

Summary Notes

COMPLEX INTRAOPERATIVE FLAP PROBLEMS - SUMMARY NOTES

Clinical

Flap complications include flaps that are too short, too thin, irregular, or free (free cap). Each of these variations can be explained by an alteration of the various forces during the LASIK procedure.

FLAP COMPLICATION	MECHANISM
perforated cornea	absence or incomplete insertion of depth plate
short flap	obstruction of microkeratome path
thin flap	inadequate suction/loss of suction
irregular flap	inadequate suction/loss of suction
buttonhole flap	inadequate suction/loss of suction/Ks>48.0
free flap	Ks< 41.0/no microkeratome stop screw

Management

Any significant flap complication should be managed by aborting the excimer laser correction as this could further alter the irregular stromal bed and effect the final result. The flap should be left in place or replaced as precisely as possible into the stromal bed and left for a least 5 minutes to adhere. The eye should then be monitored weekly for epithelial ingrowth, which is more common after a thin flap. A repeat LASIK procedure could be considered after 3 months using a deeper depth plate (180 or 200 μm). The only exception is a free cap that can still achieve an excellent outcome with laser treatment in the stromal bed and replacement of the cap.

Prevention

The proper assembly and preparation of the microkeratome is fundamental to avoiding flap complications. Training the surgeon and staff is the cornerstone to achieving high quality lamellar incision reproducability. Adequate suction levels should be confirmed by various methods.

Confirmation of Adequate Suction (>65 mmHg)

- dilation of the pupil
- dimming of the patient's vision
- Barraquer tonometer
- Pneumotonometer
- adherence of the suction ring
- level of the suction pressure meter of the base unit

CASE A, FREE CAP INCORRECT REPLACEMENT

Jose Güell, MD

Main Concern: Astigmatism

INITIAL PREOPERATIVE INFORMATION

	OD	OS	COMMENTS
Preoperative Refraction	-4.00 – 1.00 X 65	-4.50 – 2.50 X 120	flat preoperative
BCVA	20/25	20/25	keratometry
Topography Details	regular	regular	
SimK Values	41.1 X 40.41	41.76/40.81	
Pachymetry	n/a	n/a	

PROCEDURES PERFORMED

	OD	OS	COMMENTS
1. Date/type	2/96 LASIK	2/96 LASIK	free cap OD
Laser/keratome/plate	116/ACS/160	116/ACS/160	
2. Date/type	5/96 AK		
Laser/keratome/plate			

CURRENT POSTOPERATIVE INFORMATION

	OD	OS	COMMENTS
Time Postoperative	3 months	6 months	excellent result
Postoperative Refraction	+0.50 – 1.00 X 40	plano	from AK OD
BCVA	20/30	20/25+	
Topography Details	regular	regular	
SimK Values	38.83/37.25	37.21/37.80	
Pachymetry	n/a	n/a	
Visual Complaints	n/a	n/a	
Medications	n/a		

		UCVA	Rx	BCVA	KM
Preoperative	OD	20/400	-4.00 – 1.00 X 65	20/25	41.1 X 40.41
	OS	cf	-4.50 – 2.50 X 120	20/25	41.76 X 40.81

February 1996, LASIK OU (OD free cap, normal size; surgery without other complications)

		UCVA	Rx	BCVA	KM
April 1996	OD	20/80	+2.75 – 5.50 X 25	20/25	39.28 X 37.08
	OS	20/25	-0.50	20/25	37.58 X 38.00

Exam - OU clear cornea: perfect interface, no striae, no folds. Incorrectly replaced free cap with a spherical equivalent refraction near plano.
May 1996, Arcuate Keratotomy OD

		UCVA	Rx	BCVA	KM
August 1996	OD	20/30	+0.50 – 1.00 X 40	20/25	38.83 X 37.25
	OS	20/25	plano		37.21 X 37.80

There were three possible options as a reoperation:
• hyperopic and astigmatic LASIK (standard LASIK enhancement)
• to reposition the flap 180° away
• arcuate keratotomy
We decided to perform option number 3 because it seemed the least aggressive and most predictable.

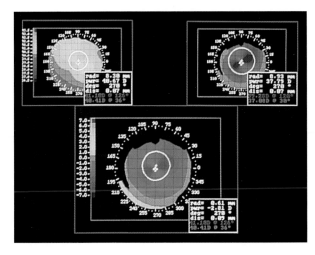

Figure 4A-1. Preoperative and postoperative topography OD after LASIK.

Figure 4A-2. Topography OS after LASIK.

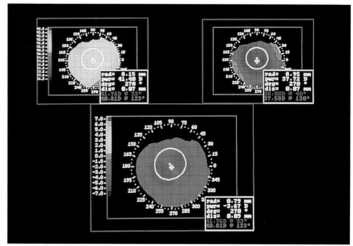

Figure 4A-3. Topography OS after AK over LASIK.

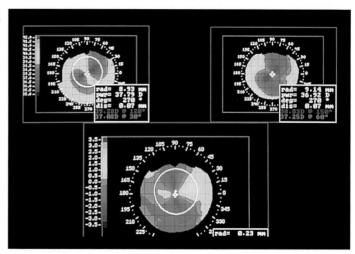

Figure 4A-4. Appearance of OS AK over LASIK.

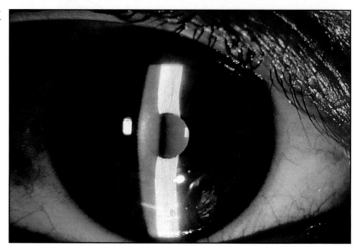

Editor's Notes

The tremendous amount of induced astigmatism after the primary LASIK OD suggests that the laser was incorrectly applied (ie, wrong correction/axis or decentration) or that the flap was incorrectly replaced. This case involved a free flap OD, so this is likely the cause of the astigmatism. Corneal alignment marks are essential to assist with the correct orientation of the flap or cap after LASIK with a free cap.

An excellent result was achieved with AK after LASIK in the case. However, AK should be performed cautiously after LASIK. The astigmatic reduction of AK after LASIK is less predictable than in primary AK. The central corneal thinning from the LASIK means that settling the AK depth at the post LASIK central thicknesses will be too shallow in the peripheral unablated cornea. I generally use 500 to 600 µm for AK following LASIK depending on the pre-LASIK corneal pachymetry.

CASE B, BUTTONHOLE FLAP WITH INGROWTH

Ted Smith, OD, and Jeffery J. Machat, MD

Main Concern: Buttonhole flap with Ingrowth
Patient Age: 36

INITIAL PREOPERATIVE INFORMATION

	OD	OS	COMMENTS
Preoperative Refraction	+5.25	+3.75 – 0.50 X 100	referring center
UCVA	20/80	20/70	
BCVA	20/20	20/20	
Topography Details	n/a	n/a	
SimK Values	n/a		
Pachymetry	n/a		

PROCEDURES PERFORMED

	OD	OS	COMMENTS
1. Date/type	11/11/97 H-LASIK	11/1/97 H-LASIK	buttonhole
Laser/keratome/plate	VISX/Hansatome/200	VISX/Hansatome/200	referring center
2. Date/type	8/26/98 LASIK		
Laser/keratome/plate	Technolas217/ACS/200		
3. Date/type	11/25/98 ingrowth removal		ingrowth/scrape

CURRENT POSTOPERATIVE INFORMATION

	OD	OS	COMMENTS
Time Postoperative	1 day after ingrowth removal	1 year	
Postoperative Refraction	+2.00 – 1.25 X 010	pl	
UCVA	20/30	20/20	
BCVA	20/25	20/20	
Topography Details	48.37/45.87 X 16	n/a	
SimK Values	1.93	n/a	
Pachymetry	593 µm	n/a	
Visual Complaints	blur at near	none	
Medications	Tobradex Q1H	none	
Refractive Correction	none	none	

This 36-year-old white female had an unremarkable medical history. Her surgical history consisted of LASIK performed on her right and left eye on November 11, 1997, for a correction of OD +5.25 D with a BCVA 20/20 and OS +3.75 – 0.50 X 100 with a BCVA 20/20. At that time, the left procedure was uncomplicated, with a postoperative result of UCVA 20/20 and an *Rx* of plano at 1 year postoperative. However, suction was lost with the Hansatome keratome (200 μm flap) and a buttonhole flap was created on the right eye. The incomplete flap was replaced and the procedure was aborted. Over time, there was subsequent central corneal scarring and haze (Figure 4B-1).

Upon stabilization at 10 months postoperative, this patient was referred to our center for management of her right eye. On August 26, 1998, topography indicated irregular astigmatism with K values of 46.75/44.62 X 180 and corresponding CIM value of 1.84 (Figure 4B-2). Refraction OD showed +3.50 + 2.50 X 080, with a surprising BCVA of 20/20-. This patient was treated with LASIK for an attempted correction of +3.50 + 2.00 X 080 using a Chiron ACS keratome and 200 μm flap. There were no surgical complications.

At 3 months postoperative, this patient's topography showed 48.37/45.87 X 016 and a CIM value of 1.93, which was not a significant improvement over the preoperative topography (Figure 4B-3). However, there was substantial refractive improvement to a stable endpoint of +100 +125 X 100 which produced a visual acuity of 20/25-. This patient complained of marked photophobia, and indeed, unexpectedly, this patient had developed a nest of central epithelial ingrowth in the area of the initial buttonhole one year previously (Figure 4B-4). The ingrowth was removed via a diamond blade incision inferior to the ingrowth and using the spreader to scrape the cells (Figure 4B-5). No further progression of ingrowth was noted at 1 week postoperative by the comanaging doctor.

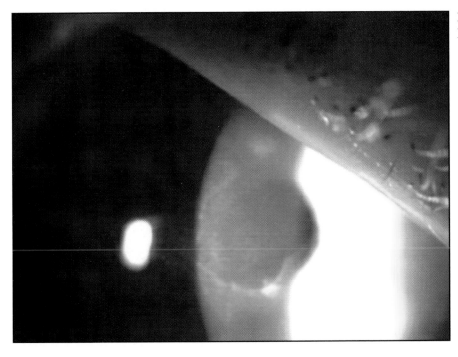

Figure 4B-1. Buttonhole flap OD.

Figure 4B-2. Preoperative topography OD demonstrates an irregular pattern from the buttonhole.

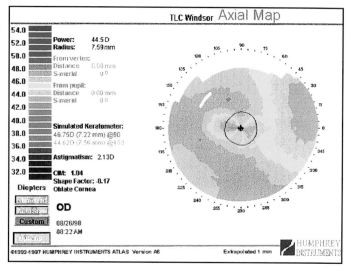

Figure 4B-3. Postoperative topography OS shows a centered hyperopic ablation with some central irregularity.

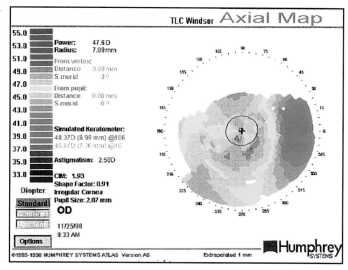

Figure 4B-4. Epithelial ingrowth at the edge of the buttonhole flap.

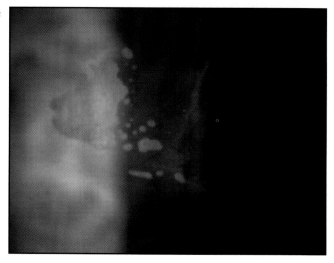

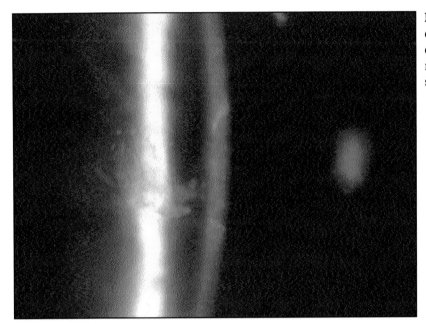

Figure 4B-5. Residual epithelial ingrowth after the epithelial cells have been milked out through the incision.

Editor's Notes

In this case, the flap was recut using 200 m plate, as the original cut was incomplete. It is preferable to use a deeper depth plate when doing an enhancement procedure to ensure that the second lamellar cut is below the first cut, minimizing the risk of creating a free wedge of tissue.

Despite the relative success of the second procedure, epithelial ingrowth still occurred on the edge of the previous buttonhole flap. The ingrowth likely occurs because buttonhole flaps are very thin along the buttonhole edges. This thin edge does not provide a strong barrier against the epithelial cells, which can grow underneath the flap. Since this epithelial ingrowth will be central, and the flap is thin and friable around the buttonhole, it would be very difficult to lift the flap to remove these epithelial cells. However, it is very important to remove this ingrowth because the flap is thin and the release of collagenase from the hypoxic epithelial cells will cause flap melting with central corneal irregularities and a loss of BCVA.

In this case, an innovative technique for removing the epithelial cells was used. A small incision was made adjacent to the epithelial cells through the thin primary flap and the epithelial cells were pushed or milked out through the small incision. This did not necessitate manipulation of the previous thin buttonhole flap and hence did not put the patient at risk for further epithelial ingrowth or flap striae.

CASE C, BUTTONHOLE WITH HAZE

Michiel S. Kritzinger, MD

Main concern: Do Not Hastily Decide on a PKP after a LASIK Procedure

INITIAL PREOPERATIVE INFORMATION

	OD	OS	COMMENTS
Preoperative Refraction		impossible to establish	
BCVA		20/400	
Topography		Figure 4C-1	
SimK Values		38.0 X 104/36.5 X 14	
Pachymetry		500 µm	

PROCEDURES PERFORMED

	OD	OS	COMMENTS
1. Type		LASIK	referring center
		(unknown parameter)	buttonhole
2. Type		transepithelial	
		phototherapeutic	
		keratectomy (TEPTK)	
Laser/keratome/plate		Technolas 217	
3. Type		6 months later PRK	
Laser/keratome/plate		Technolas 217	

CURRENT POSTOPERATIVE INFORMATION

	OD	OS	COMMENTS
Postoperative Refraction		+1.00/-1.00 X 120	
UCVA		20/50	
BCVA		20/30	
Topography Details		Figure 4C-3	
SimK Values		40.3 X 122/38.8 X 32	
Pachymetry		280 µm	
Visual Complaints		n/a	
Medications		n/a	
Refractive Correction		none	

This patient had a LASIK procedure done at another eye center and presented at first consultation with central scarring of the flap due to a buttonhole cut. His ophthalmologist decided to perform a PKP, but the patient was scared of the procedure and consulted me for a second opinion.

I decided to do a transepithelial phototherapeutic keratectomy (TEPTK) on the buttonhole area where most of the scarring was concentrated.

A total of 580 shots of 2 mm spot size was administered during two separate treatments, with the Technolas 217, to flatten the central scarred area.

Postoperatively the patient was treated with Mitomycin 2 mg/10 ml q.i.d. x 2 weekly x 2 times (1 month). The mitomycin can reduce or eliminate haze and fibrosis post PTK/PRK. The mitomycin can be repeated at a later stage for late haze and fibrosis.

A PRK was performed 6 months after the PTK treatment.

Initial PRK preoperative information:

	OS
Refraction	-3.00/-0.75 X 21
BCVA	20/80
UCVA	20/200
Topography	Figure 4C-2
SimK- value	42.5 X 114/41.2 X 24
Pachymetry	445 µm

I decided to perform a PRK and not a new flap LASIK procedure on this patient. I rarely excimer laser a LASIK flap, because it will induce more haze and fibrosis postoperatively. PRK will not only correct this patient's refraction, but will also help to smooth the corneal surface as well as get rid of more haze and fibrosis.

PRK treatment with the Chiron Technolas 217

	OS	
	Preoperative	Treatment
Sphere	-3.00	-2.85
Cylinder	-0.75	-0.82
Cylinder Axis	24	24
Zone diameter		6 mm

Post-PRK information:

	OS
Refraction	+1.00/-1.00 X 120
BCVA	20/30
UCVA	20/50
Topography	Figure 4C-3
SimK value	40.3 X 122/38.8 X 32
Pachymetry	280 µm
Eyewear	none

By first performing a PTK, the patient was saved from the trauma of a corneal transplant. The visual outcome was, under the given circumstances, acceptable to both patient and doctor. Further treatment might include more PRK TopoLink customized ablation, to improve the quantity and quality of vision. The excimer laser PRK procedure will always be followed by a course of mitomycin, to suppress any haze and fibrosis formation.

This case illustrates the importance of considering all your options before doing a PKP. Always remember that PKP surgery has its own refractive problems postoperatively. It is also intraocular surgery with its own risks and problems.

Figure 4C-1. Topography OS after primary LASIK at referring center.

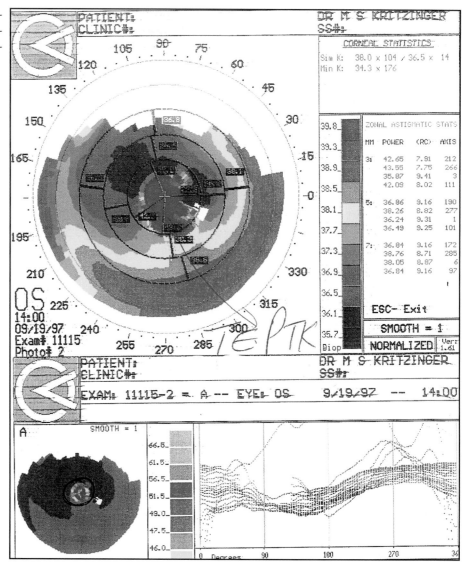

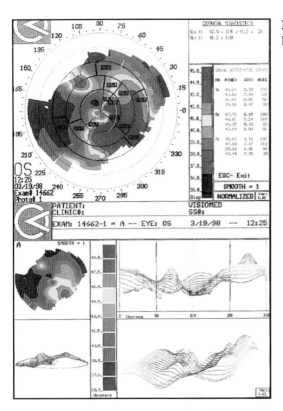

Figure 4C-2. Topography OS 6 months after PTK but before PRK.

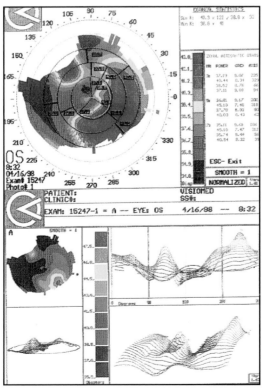

Figure 4C-3. Topography OS following PRK. The UCVA was 20/50.

Editor's Notes

While buttonhole flaps are a relatively uncommon complication of LASIK, they will occur more frequently during the LASIK surgeon's first 500 cases. The appropriate management of a buttonhole flap is to immediately replace the flap and not to perform the excimer ablation.

Although the history is somewhat vague surrounding the original problem in this case, inspection of the initial topography suggests that there is some central cornea flattening surrounding the central island caused by the central corneal scarring. This suggests that the excimer ablation may have in fact been performed. This will increase the chance of developing central corneal scarring following the LASIK procedure. The corneal pachymetry of 500 μm also suggests that previous ablation has been performed.

The PTK performed in this case used a large number of laser shots. Although we are not told the depth of the ablation, generally 50 μm is needed to ablate through the corneal epithelium followed by at least another 10 to 30 μm to remove the central corneal scarring. This procedure is similar to a very large PRK ablation and can therefore result in significant post-PTK haze. It can be controlled with the use of topical mitomycin, as described in this case.

While the final result following the PRK was a vast improvement from the original problem, the topography demonstrates the irregular ablation pattern caused by the buttonhole flap. The central area has been smoothed out by the PTK ablation, however, the irregular pattern will definitely be causing distortion of vision. The corneal thickness is now down to 280 μm, which demonstrates the large amount of tissue that was required to be ablated to remove the central corneal scarring and then to perform the PRK procedure. The general guideline for minimum corneal thickness following PRK/PTK procedure is 300 μm and for LASIK is 400 μm. Therefore, the refractive surgeon must pay very close attention to the corneal thickness whenever any further ablation procedure is considered on a previous LASIK or PRK patient in order to ensure that adequate thickness of the cornea is preserved.

Case D, Incomplete Flap with Haze

Ted Smith, OD, and Jeffery J. Machat, MD

Main Concern: Incomplete LASIK Flap
Patient Age: 50

Initial Preoperative Information

	OD	OS	Comments
Preoperative Refraction	+2.25 – 0.25 X 084		
UCVA	20/200		
BCVA	20/20		
Topography Details	n/a		
SimK Values	n/a		
Pachymetry	n/a		

Procedures Performed

	OD	OS	Comments
1. Date/type	3/17/97 LASIK		referring center
Laser/keratome/plate	VISX/ACS/160		incomplete flap
2. Date/type	6/11/97 PRK		referring center
Laser/keratome/plate	VISX		
3. Date/type	4/24/98 PRK/PTK (6 mm OZ)		severe haze
Laser/keratome/plate	Technolas 217		
4. Date/type	12/11/98 LASIK		residual hyperopia
Laser/keratome/plate	Technolas217/Hansatome/180		

Current Postoperative Information

	OD	OS	Comments
Time Postoperative	day 1 LASIK enhancement		BCVA restored
Postoperative Refraction	-1.25 + 0.75 X 180		to 20/20
UCVA	20/30		
BCVA	20/20		
Topography Details	n/a		
SimK Values	n/a		
Pachymetry	n/a		
Visual Complaints	none		
Medications	none		
Refractive Correction	none		

This patient was a 50-year-old white male with an unremarkable medical history. He was referred to our center following complicated LASIK and PRK surgery involving his right eye. His surgical history consisted of attempted LASIK on his right and left eye on March 17, 1997, using a VISX Star (VISX, Inc., Santa Clara, Calif) with an ACS keratome and 160 μm flap. At that time, *Rx* OD was -2.25 – 0.25 X 084 with BCVA of 20/20, *Rx* OS was -2.50 – 0.50 X 071 with BCVA 20/20. The left LASIK procedure was uncomplicated, with a postoperative UCVA of 20/20 and *Rx* OS +0.25 – 0.50 X 100 at 1 year postoperative. While creating the flap for the right eye however, suction was lost and an incomplete flap was created. The incomplete flap was replaced and the procedure was aborted. Three months later PRK was performed on top of the partial flap for a correction of +0.75 + 2.50 X 034 with BCVA of 20/30. No PTK was performed at that time.

Over the next 9 months, there was subsequent corneal scarring and haze both peripherally and centrally, which prompted his referral to our center (Figures 4D-1 and 4D-2). Topography indicated irregular astigmatism with K values of 44.50/39.50 X 030 with a corresponding CIM value of 3.73. (Figure 4D-3). His *Rx* OD had stabilized at +0.25 + 2.75 X 117, with a surprising BCVA of 20/20. He was subsequently treated with a Chiron Technolas 217 PTK ablation of 80 μm with a 6 mm optic zone to treat the corneal haze, followed by PRK for an attempted correction of +1.25 + 1.50 X 117.

At 8 months postoperative, the patient's topography had improved markedly, showing K values of 41.62/40.37 X 158 and CIM 2.30 (Figure 4D-4). There was a stable refractive endpoint of OD +2.75 + 0.50 X 090 and BCVA 20/20. The corneal haze had been significantly reduced by the PTK. The residual hyperopia was treated by hyperopic LASIK with a target for full correction using the Hansatome and 180 μm flap. There were no intraoperative complications. One day postoperative data showed an *Rx* of OD -1.25 +0.75 X 180 and BCVA 20/20.

Figure 4D-1. Peripheral corneal scarring from the previous LASIK flap.

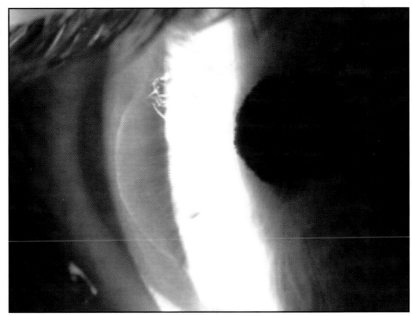

Figure 4D-2. Central cornea scarring from the incomplete flap and the PRK.

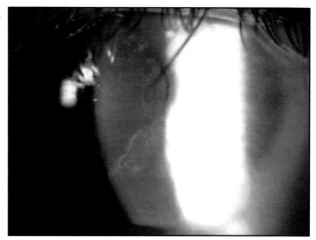

Figure 4D-3. Topography OD demonstrates an irregular pattern centrally following LASIK and PRK.

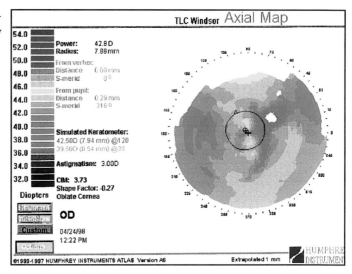

Figure 4D-4. Postoperative topography OD shows a smooth, even pattern with marked improvement after PTK.

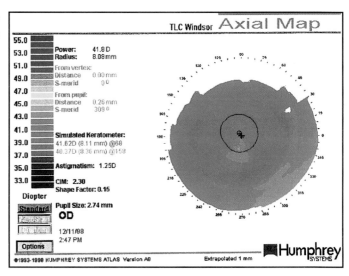

Editor's Notes

In this case, an incomplete LASIK flap was created in the right eye. Since this was performed at the referring center, there is no information as to whether the visual axis was clear. If the visual axis was clear and there is no loss of BCVA, it would have been preferable to perform a repeat LASIK in an effort to reduce the risk of subsequent haze. The PRK procedure that was performed on top of the flap resulted in significant haze with a reduction in BCVA and some induced plus cylinder astigmatism. There is a definite risk of haze formation if PRK is performed on a cornea with any previous surgery including LASIK and RK.

Because of the loss of BCVA and the central corneal haze, PTK was performed to a depth of 80 μm. The 50 μm depth is used to ablate through the epithelial layer of the cornea and an additional 30 μm to ablate through the presumed depth of the corneal haze. Some of the corneal astigmatism would be a result of the haze and the rest would be presumed to be a residual effect from the original refractive error. Approximately half of the astigmatism was treated at the same axis measured by the refraction. The patient also had a hyperopic PRK correction of +1.5. This was done because the PTK of 30 μm could be expected to induce a hyperopic shift of approximately 1.5 to 3 D.

At 8 months postoperatively, this patient did experience a hyperopic shift because of the PTK procedure. The hyperopic PRK correction was not enough and the patient was left +3.0 D spherical equivalent OD. The BCVA had been restored however, and the cornea was now clear. This means that hyperopic LASIK was able to be performed. Although extensive follow-up data is not available, the first day result of a slightly myopic prescription is perfect, as this would be expected to regress and give the patient close to an emmetropic correction within 1 week to 3 months postoperatively.

CASE E, REPEATED BUTTONHOLE

Stephen S. Lane, MD, and Douglas Katz, MD

Main Concern: Buttonhole and Epithelial Ingrowth
Patient Age: 36

INITIAL PREOPERATIVE INFORMATION

	OD	OS	COMMENTS
Preoperative Refraction	-2.50 – 0.50 X 085		
BCVA	20/20		
Topography Details	n/a		
SimK Values	n/a		
Pachymetry	n/a		

PROCEDURES PERFORMED

	OD	OS	COMMENTS
1. Date/type	9/10/98 M-LASIK		buttonhole OD
Laser/keratome/plate	no laser/ACS/160		
2. Date/type	12/31/98		second buttonhole OD
Laser/keratome/plate	no laser/ACS/180		

CURRENT POSTOPERATIVE INFORMATION

	OD	OS	COMMENTS
Time Postoperative	4/20/99		irregular astigmatism
Postoperative Refraction	-2.75 – 0.50 X 100		and loss of BCVA
BCVA	20/40-		
Topography Details	irregular astigmatism		
SimK Values	n/a		
Pachymetry	n/a		
Visual Complaints	blurred vision		
Medications	Pred Forte		
Refractive Correction	original glasses		

A 36-year-old man with an preoperative refraction of -2.50 – 0.50 X 085 OD and -2.00 sphere OS presented requesting bilateral refractive surgery. Preoperative topography was performed, (Figure 4E-1) and revealed mild regular astigmatism. SimK readings were 45.17 X 50 and 45.06 X 130.

After discussion with the patient bilateral simultaneous LASIK was planned. An ACS with a 160 depth plate was used for the procedure. Adequate IOP was confirmed with a Barraquer tonometer, the cornea was moistened, and the keratome was passed. A central buttonhole was evident after the flap was created. The flap was of normal size and thickness, and there was no apparent loss of suction. The flap was carefully repositioned without laser treatment. The flap was allowed to adhere for 5 minutes after which a bandage contact lens was placed for 1 week.

Initially there was edema in the area of the buttonhole that resulted in a BCVA at 1 day postoperatively of 20/40 with the contact lens in place. Topography at 1 week (Figure 4E-2) showed irregular astigmatism which resolved by 1 month. By 1 month postoperatively the buttonhole was well-healed with a paracentral scar evident (Figures 4E-3, 4E-4). BCVA at this time was 20/20. Three months postoperatively the visual acuity was 20/20 with a refraction of -2.50 – 0.75 X 100, almost identical to the preoperative measurements.

Three months postoperatively the procedure was reattempted with an ACS, this time using a 180 μm plate. IOP was measured with a pneumotonometer, and registered it's maximum reading of 81 mm/Hg. The cornea was moistened and the keratome was passed without any apparent loss of suction. Once again a buttonhole was created in the same general area. The flap was repositioned without laser treatment and once again a bandage soft contact lens was placed. Mild irregular astigmatism and subepithelial scarring were noted at 1 week and 1 month with BCVA of 20/40. Two months later, a paracentral scar was present with nests of epithelium present in the interface (Figure 4E-5). Three months postoperatively, the clinical appearance was unchanged and the BCVA was 20/40 with a correction of -2.75 – 0.50 X 100. Topography revealed irregular astigmatism. The last topography reveals some improvement in the corneal contour (Figure 4E-6).

There are many theories regarding why buttonholes occur. Steep corneas have been thought to be a risk factor due to possible bunching of tissue in the keratome as it is passed. Loss of suction has been implicated but it is generally associated with small, incomplete, or irregular flaps. Corneal drying has also been postulated to cause buttonholes particularly in the second eye of a bilateral simultaneous procedure. However, none of these factors seem pertinent in our case involving two consecutive buttonholes. Using a deeper plate in hopes of avoiding the scarred tissue is usually effective in preventing recurrent buttonholes but this was not helpful in this case.

Our current plan is to perform transepithelial PTK to reduce the scar and epithelial nests. Thiotepa with a 1:1000 dilution will be used postoperatively q.i.d. and then tapered over the next month in an attempt to minimize or eliminate postoperative haze. An alternative would be to place intraoperative Mitomycin C 0.2% and taper it from q.i.d. over 4 months. An adjunct to minimize haze is prudent when performing PRK/PTK after prior LASIK surgery as haze is not uncommon. Attempting LASIK with another keratome would be another option, however, with the epithelial nest and irregular astigmatism we feel transeptihelial PTK is the best option for this patient. Calculating the amount of laser necessary to accomplish a -2.50 D correction with a 6 mm optical zone using the Munnerlyn formula (6 mm ablation diameter squared divided by 3) gives a value of 12 per diopter. Therefore 12 D x 2.5 D would require a 30 ablation for a 2.5 D correction. The resumed depth of the epithelium would then be added to obtain the final depth of ablation required.

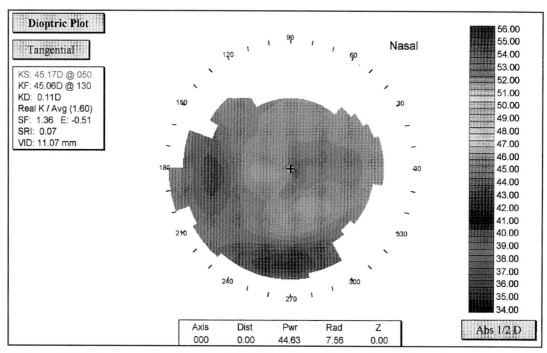

Figure 4E-1. Preoperative topography OD with mild regular astigmatism.

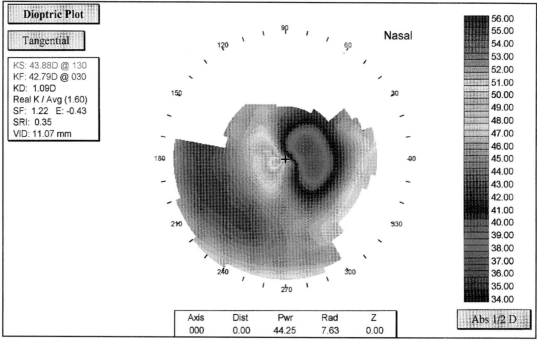

Figure 4E-2. Topography OD 1 week after the first buttonhole with an irregular pattern.

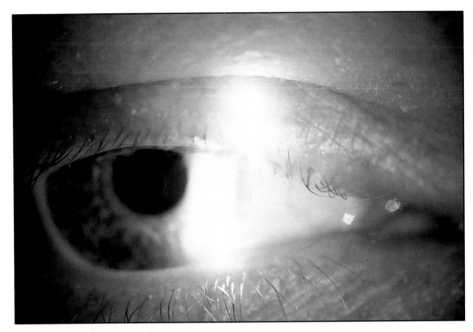

Figure 4E-3. Buttonhole OD 1 month following LASIK.

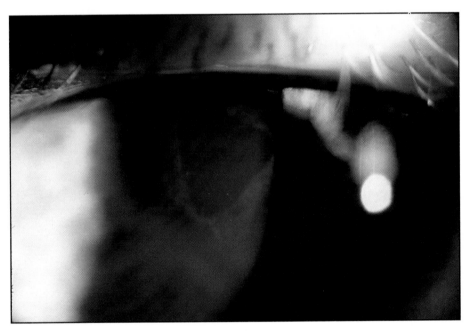

Figure 4E-4. Buttonhole OD 1 month following LASIK.

Figure 4E-5. Two months after the second buttonhole OD with central scar and nests of epithelium.

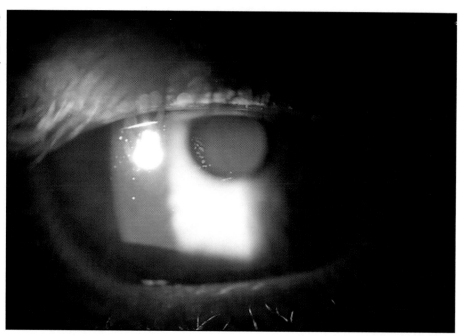

Figure 4E-6. Topography OD 3 months after the second buttonhole demonstrating some residual irregularity.

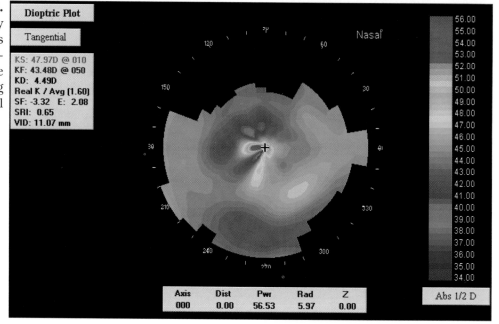

Editor's Notes

It should first be noted that this double buttonhole was treated in the appropriate manner. In both cases, the flap was laid down, a bandage contact lens was placed on the eye and the eye was allowed to stabilize prior to any further procedure. Although there is always pressure in the surgical environment to perform and therefore continue with the ablation despite flap problems, the LASIK surgeons must restrain themselves as this will definitely compromise the postoperative result.

It is interesting to note that in both cases, the pressure was confirmed with tonometry prior to the keratectomy. Despite these confirmations, a buttonhole flap was produced both times. This suggests that the surgical dynamics for this patient were in some way unique. It is possible that the patient's orbit was small and tight, and created pressure of the suction ring. Some eyes may require higher pressures than others to achieve adequate keratectomy cuts.

After the first buttonhole the visual axis was still clear. The initial corneal topography after the first buttonhole was quite irregular, however, this stabilized to a reasonable range which is confirmed by the refraction which returned to the preoperative values. The second procedure was performed using a 180 flap, which should have provided some protection against further buttonhole by making the keratectomy slightly deeper. Unfortunately, the buttonhole did occur again. This suggests that there was some interaction between the suction ring and the microkeratome and the shape of the patient's eye and orbit that resulted in the previous buttonhole. After the second buttonhole, the refraction was once again relatively unchanged. Unfortunately, the patient did have some loss of BCVA with irregular astigmatism and some areas of epithelial ingrowth in the center of the buttonhole flap.

The challenge at this point will be to deal with the irregularly contoured cornea and the central corneal scarring and epithelial ingrowth. A further repeat cut using a 200 μm plate would be possible unfortunately, this would relieve the residual central corneal scarring and irregularity leaving the patient with reduced BCVA and distorted vision. Therefore a PTK through the central part of the cornea in order to remove the scarring and reduce the irregularity would be the most appropriate option. This could be done in a two step procedure where the PTK was initially done approximately 70 to 80 μm to remove the epithelium (50 μm) and corneal scarring (10 to 30 μm). The cornea could be then left to heal. When the refraction stabilized, a repeat procedure could be done with the refractive error. This would result in the maximum smoothing of the cornea. A combined procedure could also be performed, however, some caution must be exercised as a PTK procedure will result in an overall myopic correction of approximately 0.5 D per 10 μm of stromal PTK ablation with a broad beam laser.

Finally, there is high haze risk when performing large PRK or PTK corrections on top of a previous LASIK flap. Therefore the careful use of topical steroids (or mitomycin/thiotepa as the authors have described) are certainly worthwhile considerations to prevent this complication.

CASE F, COMPLETELY TORN FLAP

Amar Agarwal, MS, FRCS, FRCOphth(Lon), Sunita Agarwal, MS, FSVH(Germ), DO, and Athiya Agarwal, MD, FRSH(Lon), DO

Main Concerns: Flap Torn Off
Patient Age: 20

INITIAL PREOPERATIVE INFORMATION

	OD	OS	COMMENTS
Preoperative Refraction	-12.50 – 0.5 X 180		unilateral high myope with amblyopia
BCVA	20/120		
Topography Details	Figure 4-F1		
SimK Values	46.25/44.81@1		
Pachymetry	542 µm		

PROCEDURES PERFORMED

	OD	OS	COMMENTS
1. Date/type	4/28/99 LASIK		Flap tore due to the patient moving abruptly. The laser ablation was done, flap removed from the microkeratome, and aligned with the help of the markers.
Laser/keratome/plate	Chiron 217/ACS/160		

CURRENT POSTOPERATIVE INFORMATION

	OD	OS	COMMENTS
Time Postoperative	1 day		free flap well-positioned
Postoperative Refraction	plano		
BCVA	20/120		
Topography Details	Figure 4F-2		
SimK Values	35.13/33.68@8		
Pachymetry	not taken		
Visual Complaints	none		
Medications	topical steroids and antibiotics for 1 month after LASIK		

This patient was referred to the hospital for LASIK. The patient was a unilateral high myope in the right eye. The preoperative refraction was -12.50 − 0.5 X 180. The left eye was emmetropic. The vision improved to 6/36 (20/120) in the right eye, as it was amblyopic. The pachymetry was 542 μm. The preoperative topography (Figure 4F-1) was subsequently done. The optical zone selected was 4.3 mm. The microkeratome used was the ACS and the excimer machine was the Chiron 217.

Once the suction ring was fixed, the forward movement of the microkeratome was smooth. Then the reverse footswitch was depressed. When the microkeratome came to the end of its movement the patient moved very rapidly and abruptly. This caused the suction ring to come off the eye, and the entire flap got torn off. The flap was now stuck to the microkeratome.

When the complication had occurred, we then finished the laser ablation. Then the flap was taken from the microkeratome. Using the marker on the flap we could make out the epithelial side. The flap was then washed and then placed carefully on the cornea aligning the markers. Once the flap was in position we waited for 5 minutes for the flap to adhere. An eyepad was placed, and the patient was seen as an outpatient the next day.

The postoperative visual acuity was 6/36 (20/120) without glasses. The postoperative topography (Figure 4F-2) showed a very good, well-centered ablation. The flap had adhered very firmly. This case amply demonstrates that such complex situations can be managed very effectively by taking care of aligning the flap correctly even though the flap had been torn completely.

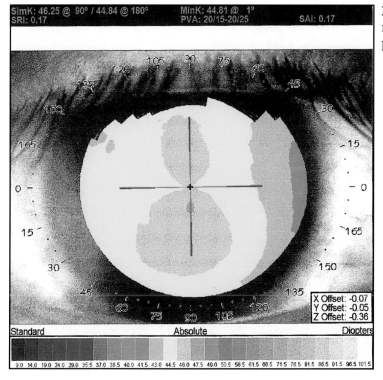

Figure 4F-1. Preoperative topography in which the flap was completely torn off.

Figure 4F-2. Postoperative topography in which the flap was completely torn off.

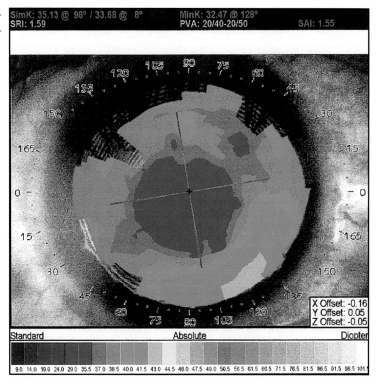

Editor's Notes

This case illustrates several important points of LASIK. The patient was initially monocular when the original LASIK procedure was performed in the amblyopic eye. LASIK was not required in the non-amblyopic eye of the patient. Monocularity could be considered a relative contraindication for LASIK in the good eye. Although the complications of LASIK are infrequent, they obviously can occur. Complications such as flap striae or LASIK interface keratitis can result in a loss of BCVA and therefore a temporary or permanent loss of function in a monocular patient. Because LASIK is an elective procedure, any monocular patient that is being evaluated for LASIK in their good eye should be approached with extreme caution. A clear description of significance of a loss of BCVA should be described, and full informed consent should be obtained. In the litigious North America society, caution is the key factor when dealing with monocular patients.

When a free or torn flap occurs, the procedure can still have an excellent outcome. This emphasizes the importance of putting the corneal epithelial alignment marks on the cornea prior to performing the keratectomy so that the free cap can be replaced with the correct alignment as well as the correct orientation with the epithelial side up. After waiting 5 minutes, the flap should have a good adhesion. In this case, an eyepad was used successfully to secure the eye. However, a bandage contact lens usually can provide a comfortable way of securing the flap in its correct location. The lens will move with the eye so that there will be no trauma to the flap or free cap with eye movement during the healing process.

Case G, Free Cap with Flat K Values

Amar Agarwal, MS, FRCS, FRCOphth(Lon), Sunita Agarwal, MS, FSVH(Germ), DO, and Athiya Agarwal, MD, FRSH(Lon), DO

Main Concern: Flat Cornea with Preoperative Ks Below 40 D
Patient Age: 28

Initial Preoperative Information

	OD	OS	Comments
Preoperative Refraction	-3.0 X 10		note flat
BCVA	20/20		preoperative K values
Topography Details	Figure 4G-1		
SimK Values	40.84/39.74@179		
Pachymetry	482 μm		

Procedures Performed

	OD	OS	Comments
1. Date/type	8/28/97 LASIK		free cap
Laser/keratome/plate	ACS/Chiron 217/160		

Current Postoperative Information

	OD	OS	Comments
Time Postoperative	14 months		free cap in perfect
Postoperative Refraction	pl		position
BCVA	20/20		
Topography Details	Figure 4G-2		
SimK Values	42.40/41.29@166		
Pachymetry	474 μm		
Visual Complaints	none		
Medications	none		

This case will demonstrate how important preoperative topography is when performing LASIK. When the ACS is used, it is important to remember that if the K reading is below 40 there is tendency for the patient to have a free cap. Whenever a patient has a K reading below 40, one should take extra care while performing LASIK.

This patient was referred to the hospital for the treatment of pure astigmatism. The preoperative refraction was -3.0 D cylinder at axis 10 degrees in the right eye. The preoperative topography (Figure 4G-1) shows the reading at 40.84 D@89° and 39.74 D@179°. The microkeratome used was the ACS with a 160 depth plate and the excimer laser was the Chiron 217.

The keratectomy was performed after marking the cornea. A free cap occurred. The flap was still present in the microkeratome. The laser ablation was completed. Then the microkeratome was opened and the flap removed from the microkeratome. The flap was then repositioned back onto the cornea and alignment adjusted using the markers on the cornea. Postoperatively, the vision was 6/6 (20/20) without glasses and the postoperative topography (Figure 4G-2) was normal. The patient was extremely happy and had no complaints.

Figure 4G-1. Preoperative topography in which a free cap occurred.

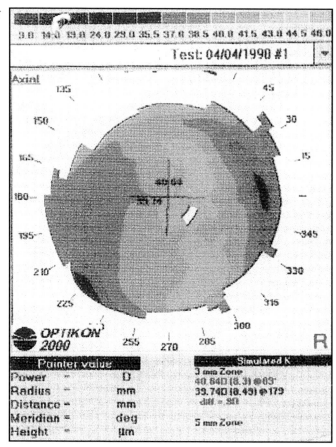

Figure 4G-2. Postoperative topography in which a free cap occurred.

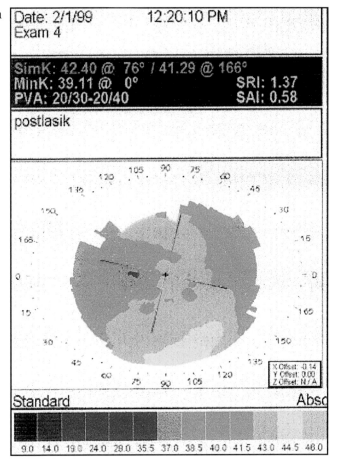

Date: 2/1/99   12:20:10 PM
Exam 4

SimK: 42.40 @ 76° / 41.29 @ 166°
MinK: 39.11 @ 0°   SRI: 1.37
PVA: 20/30-20/40   SAI: 0.58

postlasik

X Offset: -0.14
Y Offset: 0.00
Z Offset: N/A

Standard   Abso

9.0 14.0 19.0 24.0 29.0 35.5 37.0 38.5 40.0 41.5 43.0 44.5 46.0

Editor's Notes

The outcome of a free cap in this case could have been predicted by looking at their preoperative K readings. The flat axis of 39.74 D occurred in the orientation of 179°, which is the same horizontal meridian that the flap was cut. This means that the flattest part of the cornea is exactly where the hinge of the flap should occur when using the ACS. Because the cornea is flattest in this area, the flap will tend to cut short there and create a free cap. Even in cases where the steep K is up to 43 D and the flat K is less than 40 D in the horizontal meridian, a free cap can still occur despite the fact that the average K may be significantly greater than 40 D.

In cases when the K readings are less than 41, it is best not to use the ACS if at all possible. In cases of minor degrees of myopia and astigmatism, PRK could be considered. The results for PRK are excellent for low degrees of myopia and astigmatism, and therefore we must always remember that this is an excellent option for our patients despite our preference for LASIK. Secondly, the Hansatome can be used effectively down to K readings of at least 37 and perhaps 35 D.

Case H, Free Cap with the FLAPmaker Microkeratome

Ioannis G. Pallikaris, MD, Theokliti Papadaki, MD, and Dimitrios S. Siganos, MD

Main Concern: Free Cap
Patient Age: 24

Initial Preoperative Information

	OD	OS	Comments
Preoperative Refraction	-10.5 – 4.75 X 25		high myopia and
BCVA	20/30		astigmatism

Procedures Performed

	OD	OS	Comments
1. Date/type	1995 M-LASIK		free, thin cap
Laser/keratome/plate	FLAPmaker/160		

Current Postoperative Information

	OD	OS	Comments
Time Postoperative	2 days		free cap in excellent
Postoperative Refraction	n/a		position
BCVA	20/30		
Topography Details	regular		

(Case and photographs reprinted with permission from Machat JJ, Slade SG, Probst LE. *The Art of Lasik.* 2nd ed. Thorofare, NJ: SLACK Incorporated; 1999.)

A 24-year-old man with a preoperative OD refraction of -10.5 – 4.75 X 25 and a BCVA of 20/30 was scheduled for LASIK.

The FLAPmaker microkeratome (Refractive Technologies, Inc, Ohio, USA) was used for the operation. This particular device is adjusted to perform flaps of standard width (approximately 10 mm) and thickness (approximately 160 μm). The shaper head has two sites for connection on its lateral side: a superiorly located opening where the motor that oscillates the blade is locked and an inferiorly located groove for connection with a T-shaped motor that advances the blade (Figure 4H-1).

In the present case, the T-shaped motor was inserted but not locked into its site, therefore, as soon as one-third of the actual cut was completed, the motor lost connection to the shaper head and the forward movement of the blade was hindered. This resulted in resection of a corneal meniscus approximately 100 μm thick.

Marking performed prior to the cut helped to properly align the corneal slice. Dry air was used to enhance attachment of the resected corneal tissue and a bandage soft contact lens was fitted. The routine LASIK postoperative treatment regime was administered.

On the first postoperative day, the eye appeared quiet and the flap was still in position (Figure 4H-2). On slit lamp examination, the cornea, when stained with fluorescein, showed a diffuse punctuate epithelial defect and a focal staining at the borders of the free cap (Figures 4H-3 and 4H-4). The contact lens was removed on the second postoperative day when the cornea was completely reepithelialized. Computer-assisted corneal topography revealed almost no alteration of the regular preoperative astigmatic pattern (Figure 4H-5). The patient showed no loss in preoperative BCVA. A second LASIK was scheduled for 6 months later.

Marking is the first, and probably one of the most important, steps in LASIK. Not only does it ensure proper repositioning of the hinged flap at the end of the procedure, but it is also crucial in cases of a free cap, as it allows for better cap alignment and prevents accidental positioning of the cap with the epithelial side down.

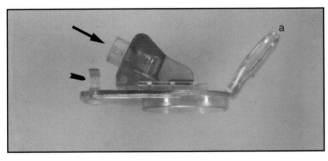

Figure 4H-1. The shaper head of the FLAPmaker, lateral view. The arrow indicates the port where the oscillating motor is connected. The arrowhead shows the site where the T-shaped motor is locked once it is connected to the head. In this instance, the motor was unlocked and consequently disconnected from the head during the cut.

a = the connection site of the suction tube.

Figure 4H-2. On the first postoperative day, the eye, still with the contact lens on, appears white and quiet, and the cornea is clear.

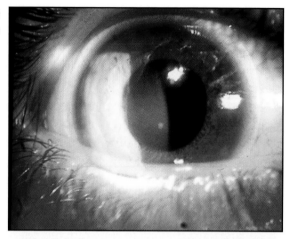

Figure 4H-3. Fluorescein staining after removal of the lens shows a diffuse punctuate epithelial defect and a focal staining at the borders of the half total cap.

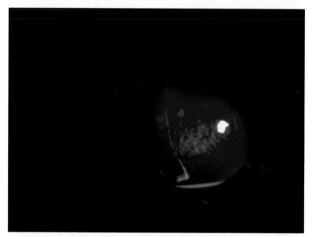

Figure 4H-4. Fluorescein staining after removal of the lens shows a diffuse punctuate epithelial defect and a focal staining at the borders of the half total cap.

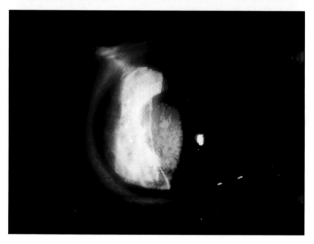

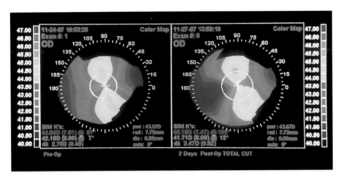

Figure 4H-5. Computerized corneal topography shows a minor flattening at the site of the cut, which does not alter the preoperative regular astigmatic pattern.

Editor's Notes

Free flaps usually occur when there is a loss of suction during the keratectomy or when LASIK is performed on very flat corneas with flat Ks less than 41. In this case, the free cap occurred because the motor of the flap maker was not properly inserted and locked into position.

There are several key points to keep in mind when a free flap occurs. The epithelial markings are extremely helpful in allowing repositioning of the free flap. Not only do they allow correct orientation of the free flap, but they also ensure that the epithelial side will be kept up as this is difficult to evaluate during the procedure. Free flaps generally do not require sutures as they will adhere quite strongly to the stromal bed. However, it may be beneficial to place a bandage contact lens overtop of the free cap to protect it from dislodgement.

When a free flap does occur it should be identified immediately and the free flap obtained from the microkeratome prior to the technicians disassembling and cleaning this instrument. In a busy refractive center, our technicians often take the instrument immediately to be autoclaved for the next procedure. If the free cap is not identified immediately, it could be lost during this process. Once the free cap is obtained, it should be placed epithelial side down in the anti-dessication chamber. No hydration should be applied to the stromal surface as this will induce edema of the free cap and decrease its adherence to the stromal bed once it has been replaced.

Finally, a decision must be made as to whether it is appropriate to perform the excimer ablation. If an inadvertent free cap has occurred which is also irregular, it would be inappropriate to perform the ablation. The flap should be put back down in the correct orientation and a repeat LASIK could be performed in 3 to 6 months. If however, the free cap occurred because of a flat cornea as predicted by the preoperative K readings (Ks <40.0 D) and the free cap appears to be regular and of a reasonable thickness, it may be appropriate to perform the excimer ablation in selected cases. It should be noted that ALK and LASIK were originally performed quite successfully using the free cap technique.

Case I, Thin Cap with the SCMD TurboKeratome

Ioannis G. Pallikaris, MD, Theokliti Papadaki, MD, and Dimitrios S. Siganos, MD

Main Concern: Thin Cap
Patient Age: 31

Initial Preoperative Information

	OD	OS	Comments
Preoperative Refraction	-18.0 – 3.0 X 45		extreme myopia
BCVA	20/40		

Procedures Performed

	OD	OS	Comments
1. Date/type	1995 M-LASIK		thin cap
Laser/keratome/plate	SCMD TurboKeratome		
2. Date/type	postoperative day 1		
	flap repositioning		

Current Postoperative Information

	OD	OS	Comments
Time Postoperative	10 months		some loss of BCVA
Postoperative Refraction	-1.5 – 1.5 X 20		and irregular
BCVA	20/63		astigmatism
Topography Details	irregular		
Visual Complaints	blur		
Medications	none		

(Case and photographs reprinted with permission from Machat JJ, Slade SG, Probst LE. *The Art of Lasik*. 2nd ed. Thorofare, NJ: SLACK Incorporated; 1999.)

A 31-year-old man with a preoperative refraction of -18.0 − 3.0 X 45 OD underwent myopic LASIK. Preoperative BCVA was correctable to only 20/40.

The SCMD LASIK TurboKeratome System (SCMD, Ariz, USA) was used for the operation. The suction achieved during the cut was inadequate, leading to a resection of a very thin (85 μm) flap with a hinge of only 2 mm. Once the ablation was complete, the flap was repositioned using the dry technique. Air through an air pump was used to enhance attachment to the stromal bed and the cornea was additionally exposed to dry air for 3 minutes. A bandage soft contact lens was placed on the eye and the standard postoperative LASIK regime was prescribed.

On the first postoperative day, the patient complained of tearing and mild discomfort. The slit lamp examination revealed that, although the contact lens was in place, the flap was detached from the stromal bed and followed the movement of the lens. The flap was also torn from the rest of the cornea so that no hinge could be detected. An effort was made to suture the total cap back in place, however this was abandoned because the flap was too thin to allow satisfactory alignment. The flap was empirically realigned since the intraoperative markings were no longer visible and the cornea was exposed to dry air for 5 minutes. A bandage soft contact lens was again placed.

The patient was followed up daily for the first postoperative week. On the seventh postoperative day, the contact lens was removed to reveal a firmly attached, yet extremely wrinkled, corneal cup (Figures 41-1 and 41-2). A lubricating agent was administered and the patient continued to be watched.

The condition remained stable throughout the first 2 postoperative months. BCVA was reduced to 20/126 with a manifest refraction of -3.0 − 1.75 X 110. Computer-assisted corneal topography at 2 months postoperatively revealed an irregular induced astigmatism of approximately 7 D oriented at 120° (Figure 41-3).

At the sixth postoperative month visit, the patient reported remarkable improvement in his UCVA (20/80). BCVA had increased to 20/63 (-1.5 − 1.5 X 20) while the central cornea appeared smoother with very few residual wrinkles (Figure 41-4). Comparison of the corneal topography at 6 months to that at 2 months revealed a nasal flattening corresponding to a decrease in irregular astigmatism (Figure 41-5). The cornea became progressively smoother and at 10 months postoperatively a round, well-centered ablation area was detected in the corneal topography, while the patient lost only one line of preoperative BCVA (20/63) with a minor residual myopia of -1.5 − 1.5 X 20. The slit lamp appearance of the cornea at 10 months postoperatively is presented in Figures 41-6 and 41-7. Nevertheless, analysis of the Holladay Diagnostic Summary at 10 months postoperatively (Figure 41-8) revealed that distortions ranging from 20/16 to 20/200 are visible within the 3 mm pupil zone (distortion map), indicating a significantly detrimental effect on vision. CU Index = 0%, indicated that the optical quality of the cornea was not uniform throughout the 3 mm pupil zone. Predicted visual acuity was evaluated as 20/160, which, although not correlating with the patient's actual BCVA, indicated a severely distorted cornea within the 3 mm pupil zone.

Adequate suction must be confirmed prior to the creation of the cut. The cut must not be made unless the suction IOP exceeds the border level of 65 mm Hg, otherwise the flap created will have a variable and suboptimal thickness because an inadequate amount of tissue will have passed through the suction ring opening.

Flap thickness should ideally range from 130 to 170 μm. Thicker flaps may not leave enough residual stroma for ablation, while thinner ones are difficult to manipulate.

Figure 4I-1. Slit lamp view of the fluorescein-stained cornea 1 week after the operation.

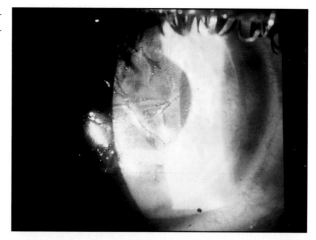

Figure 4I-2. One week postoperatively: the wrinkles become more prominent when the cobalt blue filter was used.

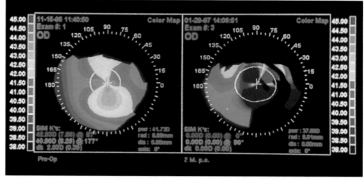

Figure 4I-3. Early postoperative topographic appearance of the corneal surface revealed an asymmetrical ablation pattern with nasal steepening of the cornea inducing irregular astigmatism of approximately 7 D oriented at the 120° axis.

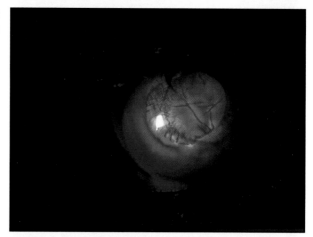

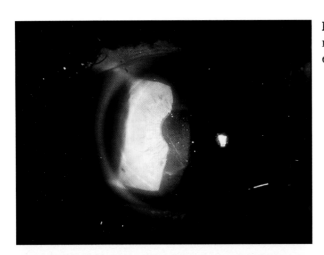

Figure 4I-4. Six months postoperatively, a noticeable smoothing of the cornea is detected on slit lamp examination.

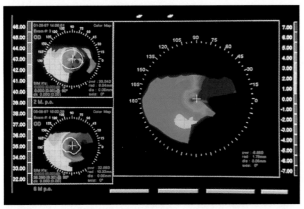

Figure 4I-5. The difference map comparing 2 to 6 months postoperatively reveals a shifting of the ablation zone towards the pupil center together with a nasal flattening corresponding to a decrease in induced astigmatism.

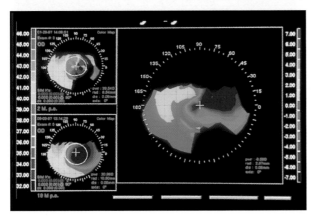

Figure 4I-6. Improvement becomes more obvious when the difference between the topographic maps of 2 and 10 months postoperatively is examined. The ablation area becomes more centered and oval, while induced irregular astigmatism can hardly be detected (at least with this scale).

Figure 4I-7. At 10 months postoperatively the center of the cornea shows only minor residual wrinkles which, unfortunately, interfere with the visual axis.

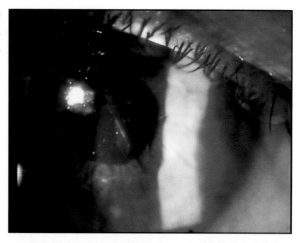

Figure 4I-8. The Holladay diagnostic summary at 10 months postoperatively. See text for a detailed analysis.

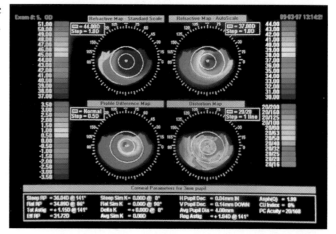

Editor's Notes

This case demonstrates the problems that can occur when a thin flap occurs. This is perhaps one of the most difficult problems to solve during LASIK. The thin flap will be difficult to realign. Because there is very little stromal tissue and mostly epithelial tissue composing the flap, it will be prone to developing striae. The thin flap will not adhere well to the stromal bed as it becomes edematous. In some cases they will not adhere well at all and they will have to be removed which result in an irregular cornea surface and a loss of BCVA.

Prevention is key in these situations. Suction should be verified in all situations to ensure that an adequate thickness will be cut. In cases with flatter corneas, a thicker depth plate should be set to decrease the chance of developing a thinner flap.

There are two options for the management of this case. It would be possible to perform a second LASIK cut for the residual refractive error. Unfortunately, the patient does have an irregular corneal surface and a small loss of BCVA. This would not be eliminated by performing a second LASIK cut, and the patient would continue to have visual distortions from the central corneal area. The second option is to perform a PTK ablation through the epithelium in the center cornea to smooth out the irregularities caused by the initial thin flap. This would remove the irregularities and the central corneal scarring. Unfortunately, this large PTK ablation would be similar to a large PRK treatment so there would be a high risk of developing haze and further altering the refractive correction. The development of haze could be modulated with the use of postoperative steroids, thiotepa, or mitomycin.

CASE J, FREE CAP SOAKED IN ALCOHOL

Ioannis G. Pallikaris, MD, Theokliti Papadaki, MD, and Dimitrios S. Siganos, MD

Main Concern: Damaged Flap
Patient Age: 30

INITIAL PREOPERATIVE INFORMATION

	OD	OS	COMMENTS
Preoperative Refraction	-14.50		high myopia
BCVA	20/32		

PROCEDURES PERFORMED

	OD	OS	COMMENTS
1. Date/type	1995 M-LASIK		free cap soaked in
Laser/keratome/plate	ACS/160		alcohol

CURRENT POSTOPERATIVE INFORMATION

	OD	OS	COMMENTS
Time Postoperative	1 year		clouded central
Postoperative Refraction	n/a		cornea
BCVA	20/63		
Topography Details	central steepening		
SimK Values	n/a		
Pachymetry	n/a		
Visual Complaints	blur		
Medications	none		

(Case and photographs reprinted with permission from Machat JJ, Slade SG, Probst LE. *The Art of Lasik.* 2nd ed. Thorofare, NJ: SLACK Incorporated; 1999.)

A 30-year-old woman with a preoperative OD refraction of -14.5 D sph and a BCVA of 20/32 was scheduled for LASIK.

The ACS was used to create an 8 mm wide, 100 μm thick total free cap. The cap was left in the microkeratome slit during the ablation. A member of the operating team, unaware of this, soaked the shaper head into absolute (90°) ethyl alcohol for sterilization purposes. Accidental splash of absolute or nearly absolute ethyl alcohol causes necrosis and opacification of the cornea by inducing protein coagulation and cell death due to abstraction of water.

Although the cap was immediately removed from the alcohol and thoroughly irrigated with BSS, severe opacification of the tissue, together with complete epithelial defect, were immediately evident. After the ablation was complete, the damaged corneal tissue was sutured back in place and a bandage soft contact lens was fitted. A lubricating agent was administered along with the routine LASIK postoperative medication, but at a more frequent rate.

The appearance of the cornea on the first postoperative day is shown in Figures 4J-1 and 4J-2. Two intermittent sutures were visible at 12 and 6 o'clock, respectively. The sutures were removed at 2 months postoperatively. A noticeable change in corneal topography was detected at 5 months (Figure 4J-3) and a steepening of the whole central corneal part of approximately 9 D was detected. This change probably reflects the healing activity in the area of the burned tissue. One year after the operation, the patient still complained of blurred vision. The eye experienced a loss of three lines in BCVA, and slit lamp examination revealed a cloudy central cornea with full thickness opacification of the corneal cap (Figures 4J-4, 4J-5 and 4J-6). Analysis of the Holladay Diagnostic Summary at 12 months postoperatively (Figure 4J-7) revealed a perfectly centered ovoid 5 mm ablation zone with no irregular astigmatism present. The optical quality of the corneal surface within the 3 mm pupil zone appeared to be excellent (distortion map). Within the 6 mm ablation zone, however, distortions ranging from 20/16 to 20/125 were visible. The CU Index was 40%, indicative that the cornea was not uniform throughout the 3 mm pupil zone, while predicted corneal acuity is evaluated as 20/63, which corresponds exactly to the patient's actual BCVA in this eye.

Prior to proceeding to more radical and invasive procedures, such as PK, and since the opacification was limited to the anterior 100 μm of the stroma, we suggest that a PRK over a photoablatable lenticular module as a masking agent should be tried in order to restore corneal clarity. Homoplastic lamellar grafting is another option.

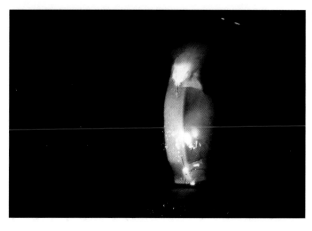

Figure 4J-1. Day 1 postoperative: the total cap is held in place by two sutures located at 12 and 6 o'clock. Mucin concentration on the side of the suture is evident.

Figure 4J-2. On retroillumination, the central corneal surface corresponding to the cap area appears rough due to a total epithelial defect induced by the chemical burn.

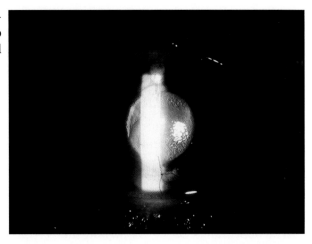

Figure 4J-3. The healing process induces a remarkable change in the topographic appearance of the cornea from 1 to 5 months.

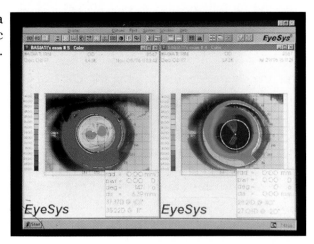

Figure 4J-4. One year postoperative: slit lamp view of the cornea with direct diffuse illumination barely detects a mild central clouding of the cornea.

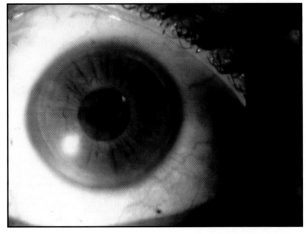

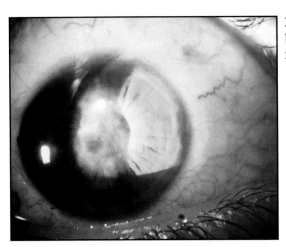

Figure 4J-5. One year postoperative: a broad slit beam directed obliquely towards the corneal surface helped identify a severe corneal opacification.

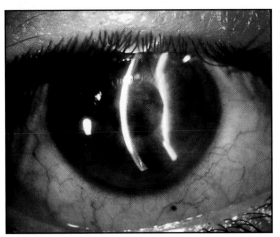

Figure 4J-6. One year postoperative: a narrow slit beam revealed that the opacification was limited to the anterior stroma (ie, was not extending deeper than the interface).

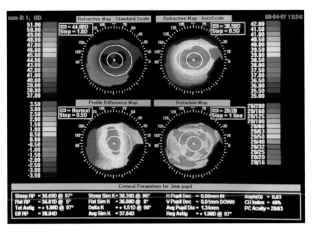

Figure 4J-7. The Holladay Diagnostic Summary at 1 year postoperative.

Editor's Notes

In the busy environment of a refractive surgery center, there is a tendency for technicians to clean and autoclave the microkeratome immediately after use, so it is ready for the next procedure. With the tremendous demand for LASIK, this efficiency is often necessary. However, if the free cap is not immediately identified it could be lost because of this efficiency.

It is helpful to warn the technicians if a free cap is predicted such as when the ACS is used and the flat Ks are less than 41.0 D. The technicians should be told that they should hold off cleaning the instruments until they are given permission to proceed.

This case presents some difficult options with regards to the management. A homoplastic lamellar graft could work well since the scarring is confined to the anterior third of the cornea where the damaged flap was replaced. While this procedure can be successful, it is a transplant procedure with a small risk of graft rejection. This would be a two-step procedure, with the second enhancement procedure used to correct the residual refractive error after the graft had stabilized.

Performing a PTK ablation through the scarred flap could remove some of the scarring, but it would leave some residual cornea astigmatism and could be followed by recurrence of the haze. Postoperative drops after the PTK treatment such as topical steroids, thiotepa, or mitomycin drops may reduce this risk.

CASE K, CORNEAL CAP TORN IN HALF

Ioannis G. Pallikaris, MD, Theokliti Papadaki, MD, and Dimitrios S. Siganos, MD

Main Concern: Torn Cap
Patient Age: 22

INITIAL PREOPERATIVE INFORMATION

	OD	OS	COMMENTS
Preoperative Refraction		-13.75 – 0.75 X 30	high myopia
BCVA		20/63	

PROCEDURES PERFORMED

	OD	OS	COMMENTS
1. Date/type		1995 M-LASIK	free cap torn in half
Laser/keratome/plate		unknown laser/ACS/180	

CURRENT POSTOPERATIVE INFORMATION

	OD	OS	COMMENTS
Time Postoperative		n/a	no follow-up data
Postoperative Refraction		n/a	

A 22-year-old man with a preoperative refraction of -13.75 – 0.75 X 30 and a BCVA of only 20/63 underwent myopic LASIK in OS.

The ACS microkeratome was used to resect a total cap 7.5 mm wide and 180 µm thick. To avoid excessive handling and dehydration, the flap was left in the microkeratome slit during ablation. At the end of the ablation, an effort was made to pull the corneal cap out of the slit without hydrating the cap with BSS or disassembling the microkeratome. During this manipulation, the partially dehydrated flap was rubbed against the blade and cut in two.

The operation was completed without any further complications. Proper marking, which was performed prior to the cut, allowed the satisfactory mounting and alignment of the chopped corneal disk. A bandage soft contact lens was placed on the eye and the standard postoperative LASIK treatment regime was prescribed (Figures 4K-1 through 4K-3).

The most appropriate action is to wait until the refraction is stable. It is only then, and never earlier than the third postoperative month, that one should consider reoperation. We propose a second LASIK with an intended flap thickness of 200 µm. A superiorly hinged flap may prove safer than a nasally based one in order to not accidentally detach the primary cap.

The patient's fellow eye had been operated on 1 year earlier. This operation was also complicated with a small total cap. It is important to notice in the preoperative topography (Figure 4K-4) if the cornea is very flat (steepest K reading: 39.3 D). In the case of a very flat cornea, it is advisable to preestimate the diameter of the flap to be resected using applanator lenses. This allows for adjustment of the hinge position so that the risk of a total cap is diminished.

Excessive handling of a total cap should be avoided. In addition to the defects that excessive handling can produce and the potential of overhydration or dehydration, differentiation of the epithelial and stromal surfaces can become extremely difficult.

The best action when facing a total cap is to leave the cap undisturbed in the microkeratome slit during the laser ablation and have an assistant instill one drop of BSS every 5 seconds in order to prevent dehydration. Careful inspection of the microkeratome head after every cut and immediately informing the surgical team in cases of a total cap should prevent accidental cap loss or inappropriate handling of the corneal cap.

Applanator lenses used to preestimate the diameter of the flap to be resected may diminish the risk of a total cap, especially in eyes with very flat corneas.

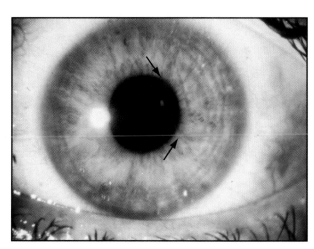

Figure 4K-1. On direct diffuse illumination, linear scarring is just visible at the upper temporal corneal quadrant (see arrows).

Figure 4K-2. The two pieces of the cap are viewed more easily from the lateral side (arrows demarcating the smaller piece).

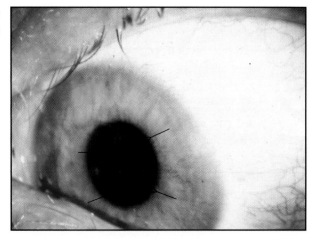

Figure 4K-3. Narrow beam slit lamp view of the area corresponding to the junction between the two corneal pieces indicates no significant alteration in corneal thickness.

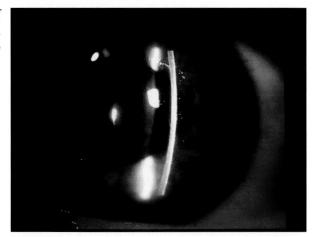

Figure 4K-4. The differential topographic map comparing the preoperative pattern to that obtained at 1 month postoperatively.

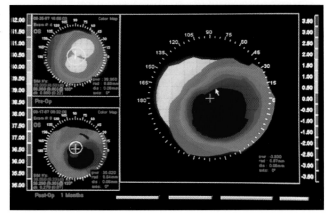

Editor's Notes

When a free flap occurs, it must be immediately identified so that the cap can be preserved in the microkeratome. The authors describe the method of leaving the cap in the microkeratome and using frequent hydration with BSS in order to prevent cap dehydration. This will also assist in smooth removal of the cap from the microkeratome head. However, this irrigation of the free cap will also cause hydration and edema of the cap, which will reduce the adherence of the cap to the stromal bed.

When a free cap is identified, our preferred method of treatment is to immediately notify the technician so that the microkeratome is not cleaned and disassembled. Careful disassembly of the microkeratome by the surgeon with removal of the ACS depth plate will allow the cap to be removed from the keratome gently without the risk of tearing the flap in half by catching it on the microkeratome blade. The cap is then placed epithelial side down on a drop of BSS in the antidessication chamber. This will prevent corneal edema, but also continue to hydrate the epithelial side so the flap does not come excessively dehydrated.

A judgement call must always be made in the case of a free cap as to whether it is appropriate to perform the excimer ablation. If the free cap is performed intentionally or it appears to be symmetrical and regular, then ablation can be performed and the cap replaced successfully. Generally sutures are not required. If the flap is irregular, torn, or damaged in any way, it is best not to perform the excimer ablation, but replace the flap and follow the patient until the refraction has stabilized.

Case L, Second Cut Following an Incomplete Flap

Ioannis G. Pallikaris, MD, Theokliti Papadaki, MD, and Dimitrios S. Siganos, MD

Main Concern:
Patient Age: 24

Initial Preoperative Information

	OD	OS	Comments
Preoperative Refraction	-13.5 – 0.50 X 165		previous incomplete
BCVA	20/20		flap
Topography Details	regular		
SimK Values	n/a		
Pachymetry	n/a		

Procedures Performed

	OD	OS	Comments
1. Date/type	1995 M-LASIK		
Laser/keratome/plate	FLAPmaker/160		

Current Postoperative Information

	OD	OS	Comments
Time Postoperative	n/a		no follow-up data
Postoperative Refraction	n/a		

(Case and photographs reprinted with permission from Machat JJ, Slade SG, Probst LE. *The Art of Lasik*. 2nd ed. Thorofare, NJ: SLACK Incorporated; 1999.)

A 24-year-old woman was referred for a second myopic LASIK OD 1 year after the first attempt, which resulted in an incomplete flap. Preoperative BCVA was 20/20 with a correction of -13.5 – 0.5 X 165. On slit lamp examination, the borders of a 5 mm wide flap with a broad hinge approximately 7 mm long could be detected on the temporal half of the cornea. A few interface particles that did not interfere with the visual axis were also visible (Figure 4L-1). The preoperative topography indicated a normal non-astigmatic cornea (Figure 4L-2).

A second LASIK procedure was planned. The aim was to create a wider and thicker flap in order to avoid disposition or partial resection of the primary half cut. The FLAPmaker microkeratome was used for the reoperation. This microkeratome can be adjusted to create flaps approximately 10 mm in diameter and 160 μm thick. In the present case, a 9.8 mm wide, 136 μm thick flap was created. The operation was successfully completed. The eye was left unpatched and the standard LASIK postoperative regime was prescribed.

On the first postoperative day, the patient was comfortable and the eye showed no signs of inflammation. On slit lamp examination, no epithelial defect was detected (Figure 4L-3). The postoperative corneal topography is presented in Figure 4L-4. At the corneal periphery, three concentric lines were visible. These were, laterally to medially, the linear cut at the borders of the second flap, the linear scarring at the borders of the smaller half flap, and the borders of the 6 mm ablation zone (Figures 4L-5 and 4L-6).

A well-aligned and healed incomplete flap affects neither the topographic appearance of the cornea nor the quality of vision. Firm reattachment of the incomplete flap should be confirmed in order to proceed to a second cut. We suggest that the second cut be postponed for at least 3 months. The area of the second cut should ideally include the first one in order to avoid undesired lamellar corneal resection. Therefore, the second flap should be thicker and, if possible, wider than the first one, especially if it is performed earlier than the sixth postoperative month.

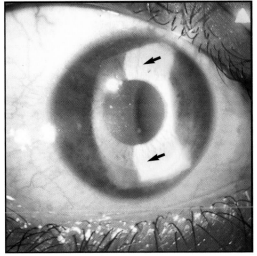

Figure 4L-1. Preoperative appearance of the eye on slit lamp examination. The hinge of the incomplete flap (see arrows) demarcates the clear nasal half of the cornea from the area of the flap temporally where minor interface remnants can be detected.

Figure 4L-2. Preoperative computer-assisted corneal topography reveals a normal cornea with a regular with-the-rule astigmatism of only 0.5 D.

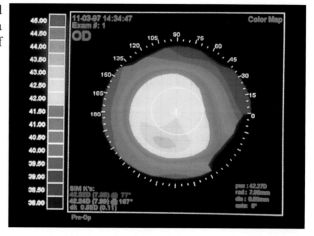

Figure 4L-3. Appearance of the same eye on slit lamp evaluation on the first postoperative day.

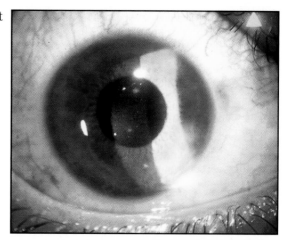

Figure 4L-4. Day 1 postoperative corneal topography reveals a well-centered 6 mm ablation zone.

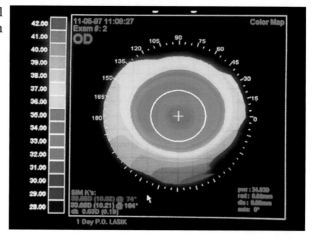

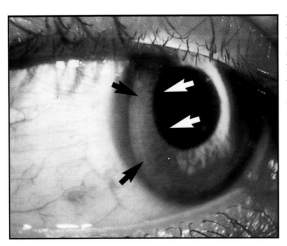

Figure 4L-5. Lateral view of the corneal periphery at 1 day postoperatively. Two concentric lines can be distinguished: the linear scarring at the borders of the half flap (see black arrows) and the borders of the 6 mm ablation zone (see white arrows).

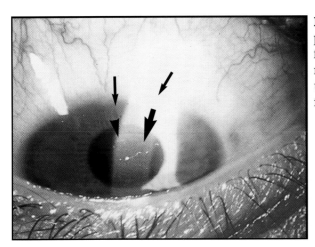

Figure 4L-6. Superior view of the corneal periphery. Apart from the borders of the half flap (see big arrow) and the borders of the 6 mm ablation zone (see arrowhead), the cut at the borders of the wider second flap is just indicated near the limbus (see small arrows).

Editor's Notes

Incomplete cuts can occur during LASIK due to obstruction of the microkeratome or occasionally because of mechanical difficulties with the microkeratome itself causing it to fail to advance. If the incomplete cut does not extend significantly through the visual axis, it is not appropriate to perform the excimer ablation. It is best not to try to surgically extend the flap further as this will result in an irregular stromal bed and in an unpredictable refractive result. In the event of an incomplete flap it is best to put the flap down, let it heal for 3 months, and then return to recut the flap using a deeper depth plate.

When recutting a flap, it is important to wait at least 3 months after the original LASIK procedure. Otherwise a free wedge of tissue may be created because the previously cut flap has not healed completely. It is also helpful to change the location of the second cut. If the original flap was decentered nasally for a nasal hinge, the second cut could be centered on the pupil so that the microkeratome would engage at a more peripheral point. The cut can be made slightly deeper (180 or 200 μm) to ensure that the second cut is beneath the first cut, thereby reducing the risk of the creation of free wedges of tissue.

CASE M, FREE CAP AND EPITHELIAL INGROWTH

Jonathan Woolfson, MD

Main Concern: Free Cap
Patient Age: 45

INITIAL PREOPERATIVE INFORMATION

	OD	OS	COMMENTS
Preoperative Refraction	-8.5 + 0.5 X 90	-9.0 + 0.5 X 87	
BCVA	20/25	20/25	
Topography Details	flat K 41.5 D	flat K 41.5 D	flat Ks
SimK Values	n/a	n/a	
Pachymetry	n/a	n/a	

PROCEDURES PERFORMED

	OD	OS	COMMENTS
1. Date/type	1996 M-LASIK	1996 M-LASIK	free cap OS
Laser/keratome/plate	VISX Star/ACS/160	VISX Star/ACS/160	
2. Date/type		1997 LASIK enhancement	
Laser/keratome/plate		VISX Star/ACS/200	
3. Date/type		1997 LASIK enhancement	
Laser/keratome/plate		VISX Star/lift	

CURRENT POSTOPERATIVE INFORMATION

	OD	OS	COMMENTS
Time Postoperative		6 months post-lift	slight loss of BCVA
Postoperative Refraction		-0.25 – 0.25 X 160	
BCVA		20/30	
Topography Details		irregular	
SimK Values		n/a	
Pachymetry		n/a	
Visual Complaints		none	
Medications		none	

(Case and photographs reprinted with permission from Machat JJ, Slade SG, Probst LE. *The Art of Lasik.* 2nd ed. Thorofare, NJ: SLACK Incorporated; 1999.)

A 45-year-old female was evaluated for LASIK. The preoperative refraction was -8.5 – 0.5 X 90 for a BCVA of 20/25 OD and -9.0 – 0.5 X 87 for a BCVA of 20/25 OS. The corneal pachymetry indicated adequate corneal thickness, and the corneal topography found regular astigmatism with a curvature flat K value of 41.5 D. LASIK was performed with the Chiron ACS and a 160 depth plate.

When LASIK was performed in the left eye, a free cap occurred. The free cap was left on the cornea when the microkeratome was reversed rather than left inside the microkeratome. The cap was torn nasally suggesting that adhesion to the microkeratome had occurred. The cut was insufficient for laser to be performed, as the edge of the flap overlapped more than 1 mm into the ablation zone. The cap was carefully replaced and smoothed onto the stromal bed with interface irrigation. The correct orientation was verified with the preplaced corneal alignment marks. The free cap was then allowed to seal into place for 10 minutes without sutures. Thirty minutes following the procedure, the cap eye was examined and found to be stable. On the first postoperative day, the flap was healing well, the eye was comfortable, and the BCVA was unchanged.

One month later, the patient had significant epithelial ingrowth nasally in the region of the torn hinge. The patient was taken back to the laser room and the complete cap was lifted. The bed and underside of the cap were scraped. The free cap was replaced. The patient was examined each week and no further epithelial ingrowth was noted in that area.

Over the next month, the patient developed significant epithelial ingrowth in the temporal region of the cap (Figure 4M-1). The cap was again removed, the cap and bed scraped of epithelium, and the cap replaced without complications. The eye was followed closely after surgery and no further epithelial ingrowth was identified.

One year after the original procedure, the preoperative refraction had not significantly changed. LASIK was repeated in the left eye with a 200 μm plate, and this time the procedure was uncomplicated. The patient was followed for an additional 8 months. The last UCVA OS was 20/100 with an unchanged BCVA of 20/25 with refraction of -2.5 – 0.75 X 150 = 20/25, indicating some regression of the correction. Corneal topography indicated a small central island. Despite the multiple procedures and the central island, there has been no loss of BCVA. Enhancement LASIK was performed by lifting the second successful flap, rather than risking another flap complication. She is now 6 months out with UCVA OS 20/30 and BCVA 20/25 with -0.25 – 0.25 X 160.

In this case, the free cap could have occurred for many reasons. The corneal topography had found that the cornea was relatively flat. This increases the risk of a free cap and guarantees that the flap will be smaller with a narrower hinge. The flap may have been thin due to inadequate suction, which might explain why it detached nasally so easily. The flap may have become adherent to the microkeratome head due to a prolonged procedure or inadequate lubrication. Small flaps and free caps can be avoided in flat corneas by using a 200 μm depth plate.

Unfortunately, thin flaps are also more prone to the postoperative problems of striae and epithelial ingrowth. Flap melts are also more common since the flap is already thin. In this case, epithelial ingrowth was removed twice. A second lamellar cut can be performed without difficulty after a previous cut, however at least 3 months should pass after the first procedure and a deeper (200 μm) plate should be used. In the case of a free flap, it is controversial whether the refractive ablation should be performed. Since the free cap was not planned, the occurrence of this complication suggests that there was a problem during the surgery that may include a loss of suction or inappropriate technique. If the free cap is abnormal in any manner, it should be replaced without treatment. If the free cap is of an adequate size and thickness, the decision to treat can be based on the surgeon's evaluation of the case.

Figure 4M-1. The epithelial ingrowth can be seen extending under the small irregular free cap edge.

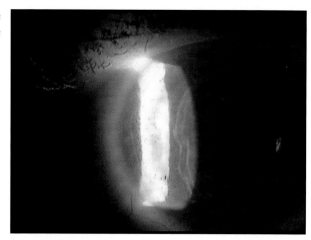

Editor's Notes

Patients with free caps need to be monitored closely for both the development of striae and epithelial ingrowth (which occurs with a much higher frequency as the free caps are also generally thin). Therefore, when a thin free cap is replaced it should be carefully smoothed into place and then protected with a contact lens to ensure that no striae develop. The patient should be examined after the procedure and on the following day to ensure that striae are not present. It is more difficult to manipulate a free cap as it does not have a hinge. Epithelial ingrowth is also more difficult to treat, as the thin cap is more difficult to lift and can easily be torn because it is more friable. Since the free cap has no hinge, the surgeon must be careful not to completely dislodge the cap and increase the risk of a loss of the cap.

CASE N, FREE CAP AND IRREGULAR ASTIGMATISM WITH LASIK

Jonathan Woolfson, MD

Main Concern: Free Cap

INITIAL PREOPERATIVE INFORMATION

	OD	OS	COMMENTS
Preoperative Refraction	-4.75 – 1.25 X 25	-5.0 – 0.50 X 165	
BCVA	20/20	20/20	
Topography Details	normal	normal	
SimK Values	n/a	n/a	
Pachymetry	n/a	n/a	

PROCEDURES PERFORMED

	OD	OS	COMMENTS
1. Date/type	1996 M-LASIK	1996 M-LASIK	free cap OD
Laser/keratome/plate	VISX Star/ACS/160	VISX Star/ACS/160	
2. Date/type		1 week postoperative removal of epithelial ingrowth	
3. Date/type		3 weeks postoperative removal of epithelial ingrowth	

CURRENT POSTOPERATIVE INFORMATION

	OD	OS	COMMENTS
Time Postoperative		1 year	slow improvement
Postoperative Refraction		n/a	in vision
BCVA		20/25	
Topography Details		irregular	
SimK Values		n/a	
Pachymetry		n/a	
Visual Complaints		distortion	
Medications		none	

(Case and photographs reprinted with permission from Machat JJ, Slade SG, Probst LE. *The Art of Lasik.* 2nd ed. Thorofare, NJ: SLACK Incorporated; 1999.)

This patient was assessed for LASIK with a refraction of -4.75 – 1.25 X 0.25, 20/20 OD, and -5.0 – 0.5 X 165, 20/20 OS. During LASIK OD, a free cap occurred. We elected to continue with the full refractive correction. The cap was carefully replaced making use of the corneal alignment marks to ensure that the orientation was correct. Thirty minutes later, the cap was stable and smooth. Unfortunately, in the immediate postoperative period, the patient rubbed his eye and dislodged the cap, which was identified on the patient's cheek. The patient was returned to the laser bed and the free cap was repositioned and refloated onto the stromal bed after the interface had been vigorously cleaned. The cap was repositioned and secured without the use of sutures.

On the first postoperative day, the patient had a moderate epithelial abrasion that healed over the next several days. The free cap was stable and smooth in the stromal bed. The UCVA slowly improved. By the third postoperative week, the UCVA was 20/40 with a refraction of plano, the cap was clear, and no complications were noted (Figure 4N-1 and 4N-2). Significant epithelial ingrowth was noted on the fifth postoperative week and was subsequently treated by lifting the cap and scraping on the base and underside of the cap.

On the third postoperative month, the UCVA was 20/60. A correction of +3.5 – 2.5 X 160 improved vision to 20/25. Irregular astigmatism was evident on the corneal topography (Figure 4N-3 and 4N-4). Epithelial ingrowth was again identified and removed. In the immediate postoperative period, the UCVA was 20/60. Over the course of the following several weeks, the UCVA vision was 20/150.

On the fifth postoperative month, the UCVA was 20/150 and improved to 20/25 with pinhole and best correction. Although he could see well, the patient was not happy with the spectacle or contact lens correction. The corneal topography suggests irregular astigmatism. After one year, his UCVA is 20/70 and BCVA is 20/25.

While the free cap has remained clear, the irregular cornea has resulted in a large amount of induced astigmatism. Since the patient feels the vision is slowly improving, no immediate treatment is planned. Future considerations include topography-assisted LASIK. Similar cases may be treated with homoplastic lamellar grafts.

This case clearly demonstrates the problems that can occur following a thin, free cap. The decision to proceed with the refraction ablation with a free cap produced a very poor result. While LASIK and ALK were originally performed with free caps on a routine basis, this was a planned aspect of the surgery. When an inadvertent free cap occurs during LASIK, this suggests that there has been an intraoperative problem, which could have compromised the quality of the cap. If this cap is replaced without the refractive ablation, it will sit perfectly into the stromal bed and probably heal well. If the ablation is performed, another variable has been added that may cause the already compromised cap to heal in an irregular manner. The refractive ablation should not be performed in the case of a free cap unless the surgeon is confident the cap has adequate integrity. Epithelial ingrowth seems to occur more commonly with thin flaps—possibly because of a poorly defined flap edge.

Figure 4N-1. Corneal topography after the second enhancement procedure demonstrates a well-centered ablation with a small central island.

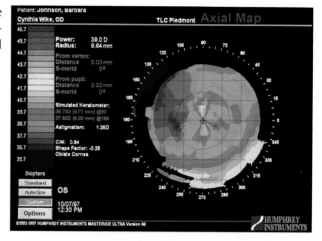

Figure 4N-2. Slit lamp view demonstrates the small, well-healed free cap.

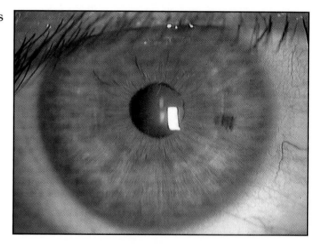

Figure 4N-3. Corneal topography indicates an irregular decentered ablation.

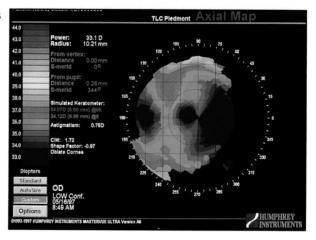

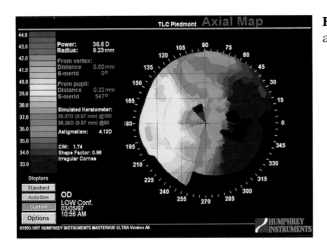

Figure 4N-4. Corneal topography indicates an irregular decentered ablation.

Editor's Notes

The irregular topography in this case demonstrated the difficulties that can occur when the parameters are altered during LASIK. Although the epithelial ingrowth has stabilized, the patient has ended up with a poor outcome, which will be difficult to correct except with a hard contact lens. Most patients who undergo refractive surgery are not interested in wearing contact lenses, particularly uncomfortable hard contact lenses.

The best option for this patient at this time would be topography-assisted LASIK. A conventional laser could not adequately treat this irregular cornea. While topography-assisted LASIK is still in its development stages, the ability to use the irregular topography to plan a customized ablation to smooth the corneal contour is the best potential option.

CASE O, BLADE DEFECT

Charlotte Burns, OD, MS, and Louis E. Probst, MD

Main Concern: Blade Defect with Flap Irregularity
Patient Age: 21

INITIAL PREOPERATIVE INFORMATION

	OD	OS	COMMENTS
Preoperative Refraction	-2.50 − 1.00 X 135	-2.00 − 1.00 X 030	
BCVA	20/20	20/20	
Topography Details	normal	normal	
SimK Values	46.87/48.25 X 170	45.62/47.75 X 016	
Pachymetry	521 µm	539 µm	

PROCEDURES PERFORMED

	OD	OS	COMMENTS
1. Date/type	1/28/99 LASIK	no surgery	blade defect
Laser/keratome/plate	VISX Star/ACS/180		
2. Date/type	5/26/99/LASIK	5/26/99	
Laser/keratome/plate	VISX Star/ACS/200	VISX Star/ACS/200	

CURRENT POSTOPERATIVE INFORMATION

	OD	OS	COMMENTS
Time Postoperative	1 day	1 day	excellent results OU
Postoperative Refraction	+0.50 DS	+0.50 DS	
BCVA	20/20	20/20	

A 21-year-old white male presented for LASIK on January 28, 1999. His ocular history was unremarkable, systemic history was positive for epilepsy. Entering refraction was -2.50 – 1.00 X 135 OD, and -2.00 – 1.00 X 025 OS. The BCVA was 20/20 OU. Topography showed slightly irregular astigmatism (Figure 40-1), pachymetry readings were 521 μm OD, and 539 μm OS.

After the flap was made OD, it was determined that there was a flap defect inferior to the visual axis. A horizontal linear defect was present in the flap that was about 2 mm in length and less than 0.5 mm in thickness. The procedure was aborted. The flap was carefully replaced. Upon closer inspection of the blade, it was determined that the blade had a defect area on the cutting edge.

Four months later the patient returned for LASIK, with refraction of -3.00 – 1.50 X 155 OD, and -2.25 – 1.50 X 020 OS, and both eye's BCVA is 20/20 (Figure 40-2). The right cornea showed a scar about 3 mm inferior to the visual axis (Figure 40-3). LASIK was performed with the 200 μm depth plate to ensure that the new keratectomy would be below the original flap defect.

One day later the patient was 20/20 OU uncorrected with a refraction of +0.50 OU.

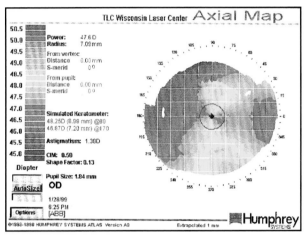

Figure 40-1. Preoperative topography OD demonstrates a regular astigmatic pattern.

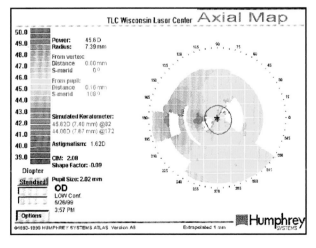

Figure 40-2. Postoperative topography OD shows some irregularity centrally but it is otherwise unchanged from the preoperative map.

Figure 40-3. A horizontal linear cornea scar is visible about 3 mm inferior to the visual axis OD.

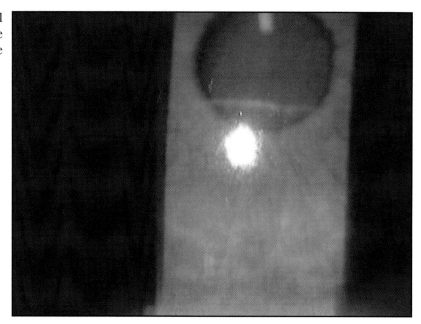

Editor's Notes

With the increasing demand for LASIK, the microkeratome manufacturers and the blade manufacturers have become overwhelmed with the demand for their services. This has resulted in a decrease in the quality of their product. We have noticed a tremendous increase in the number of blade defects, although our technicians carefully screen these prior to every surgical day and the blades are checked prior to each procedure, it can be difficult to identify blade defects that occur at the very tip of the blade. Flap problems from blade defects can be recognized as they create a horizontal linear defect along the flap in the direction that the microkeratome travels. While relatively uncommon, these can be quite devastating particularly if they travel through the visual axis.

In this case, the patient had a horizontal line blade defect that was several millimeters below the visual axis. The flap was replaced without any laser treatment being performed. The eye was left to stabilize. The postoperative refraction changed only slightly from the preoperative values. The topography indicated some irregularity but indicated a reasonably symmetrical pattern. The second procedure was performed in the right eye followed by the primary procedure in the left eye, both of which achieved excellent results, demonstrating that patients with flap defects can still have an excellent outcome.

CASE P, BUTTONHOLE
Charlotte Burns, OD, MS

Main Concern: Frustrated Patient
Patient Age: 41

INITIAL PREOPERATIVE INFORMATION

	OD	OS	COMMENTS
Preoperative Refraction	-2.00 DS	-3.00 – 0.25 X 025	
BCVA	20/20	20/20	
Topography Details	normal	normal	
SimK Values	42.62/42.62	42.50/42.62 X 180	
Pachymetry	551 μm	543 μm	

PROCEDURES PERFORMED

	OD	OS	COMMENTS
1. Date/type	12/30/98 LASIK		buttonhole OD
Laser/keratome/plate	VISX Star/ACS/200		(referring doctor)

CURRENT POSTOPERATIVE INFORMATION

	OD	OS	COMMENTS
Time Postoperative	3 months		loss of BCVA
Postoperative Refraction	-2.00 – 0.50 X 135		and regression
BCVA	20/30		
Topography Details	irregular astigmatism (see map)		
SimK Values	38.75/42.12 X 090		
Pachymetry	n/a		
Visual Complaints	distorted vision		
Medications	none		
Refractive Correction	spectacles		

A 41-year-old white male presented for LASIK OU on December 30, 1998. His systemic and ocular histories were unremarkable. Presenting refraction was -2.00 DS OD, and -3.00 – 0.25 X 025 OS, with BCVA of 20/20 OU. Topography was normal OU (Figure 4P-1) and pachymetry readings were 551 μm OD and 543 μm OS. During the pass on the OD with the ACS microkeratome, suction was lost and the blade skimmed across the middle of the cornea. The referring surgeon aborted the procedure after discovering the buttonhole flap.

The following day the UCVA OD was 20/150, and with -2.00 – 0.50 X 078 the BCVA was 20/25. At 1 month, the BCVA vision had decreased to 20/40+2 with -2.75 – 0.50 X 060. There was central scarring noted with haze (Figure 4P-2). By the second month, the BCVA had improved to 20/30 with -2.00 – 0.25 X 090. The findings have remained constant and stable to the present except for a shift in the axis of the astigmatism. The topography showed an irregular pattern centrally OD (Figure 4P-3).

The patient was angry and confused as to what action he needed to take, and obtained several opinions on the appropriate treatment for his right eye. He was assured by several doctors that the appropriate course of action had been followed by the surgeon in handling the complication by not proceeding with applying the laser. He has elected to have PTK/PRK performed on the OD in the future.

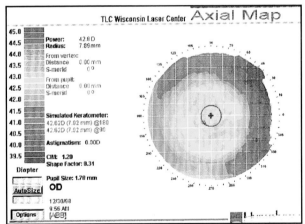

Figure 4P-1. Preoperative topography OD demonstrates a regular pattern.

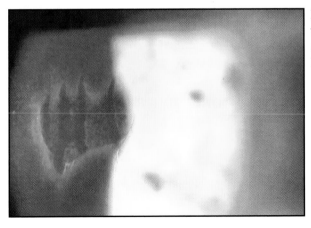

Figure 4P-2. A distinct central cornea scar was caused by the microkeratome skipping across the central cornea causing the irregular marks and the buttonhole.

Figure 4P-3. Postoperative topography OD shows central corneal irregularity from the buttonhole.

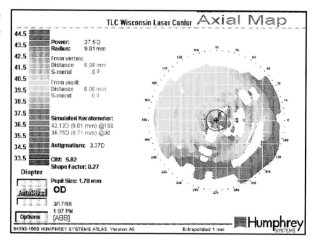

Editor's Notes

This fellow experienced a buttonhole flap that unfortunately skipped through the visual axis leaving multiple scars and reducing the BCVA. The surgeon correctly aborted the procedure and put the flap back into place. This patient will likely need a PTK procedure to ablate through the corneal scarring. This would need to be followed by a PRK type of procedure to deal with the residual refractive error. The fact that he is still myopic makes this easier to accomplish, as the PTK can often result in a hyperopic shift. In this case after 80 μm of PTK, the patient would likely be left approximately 1 to 2 D myopic. This residual correction could be easily treated with PRK. There is a significant risk of haze when performing an ablation through the flap. Additional topical therapy to reduce the risk of haze such as thiotepa or topical mitomycin along with topical steroids will be necessary for several months postoperatively in order to reduce this risk.

CASE Q, BUTTONHOLE FLAP WITH LASER AND STRIAE

Charlotte Burns, OD, MS

Main Concern: Laser Applied with Buttonhole
Patient Age: 33

INITIAL PREOPERATIVE INFORMATION

	OD	OS	COMMENTS
Preoperative Refraction	-9.50 – 1.50 X 010	-9.00 – 1.25 X 165	referral doctor
BCVA	20/20	20/20	
Topography Details	regular bow-tie pattern OU		
SimK Values	43.75 mean K	44.00 mean K	
Pachymetry	560 µm	565 µm	

PROCEDURES PERFORMED

	OD	OS	COMMENTS
1. Date/type	4/3/97 LASIK	4/3/97 LASIK	buttonhole OS lasered
Laser/keratome/plate	VISX Star/ACS/180	VISX Star/ACS/180	(referral doctor)
2. Date/type		4/16/97	removal of striae
Laser/keratome/plate		lifted flap	and epithelial plaque
3. Date/type		6/10/97 PTK	
Laser/keratome/plate		removed flap	
4. Date/type	10/17/97 LASIK enhancement		
Laser/keratome/plate	VISX Star/lifted flap		
5. Date/type		3/6/98 PTK	
Laser/keratome/plate			

CURRENT POSTOPERATIVE INFORMATION

	OD	OS	COMMENTS
Time Postoperative	15 months	10 months	loss of BCVA OS
Postoperative Refraction	pl – 0.75 X 115	+1.50 – 1.00 X 045	
BCVA	20/15-1	20/40	
Topography Details	n/a	central island	
SimK Values	n/a	n/a	
Pachymetry	n/a	n/a	
Visual Complaints	n/a	c/o triple image	
Refractive Correction	n/a	rigid gas permeable contact lens	

A 32-year old male presented for LASIK on April 3, 1997. His systemic and ocular histories were unremarkable. His BCVA was 20/20 OU, with refraction of -9.50 – 1.50 X 010 OD, and -9.00 – 1.25 X 165 OS. Topography was normal (Figure 4Q-1), and pachymetry readings were 560 μm OD, and 565 μm OS. The VISX Star laser was used, and a Chiron ACS unit with a 180 μm plate OU.

The surgery was uneventful OD. When the microkeratome made its pass on the OS, suction was lost and a buttonhole flap was created. The referring surgeon elected to perform the laser ablation despite the buttonhole flap. The following day, the patient was 20/200 OD and 20/50-1 OS uncorrected. A refraction was not done because the patient was emotional and difficult to refract. Biomicroscopy showed epithelial disruption OU with striae, edema, and rolled edges of the flap OS.

The patient was sent back to the laser clinic to lift the flap and "iron" out the striae 1 week later (Figure 4Q-2). One month later, the patient was 20/80 uncorrected OS, with a refraction of +2.25 – 2.25 X 175, giving no improvement in acuity. The BCVA OD was 20/20, with a refraction of -1.75 DS. Biomicroscopy showed striae, and 2-3+ haze centrally OS, and the inferior part of the flap was rolled at the edge (Figure 4Q-3). The haze continued to worsen, and the patient came in for another consultation at 2 months postoperative.

The patient now refracted at +4.00 – 1.25 X 075 with BCVA of 20/60 OS. Topography was unobtainable. Pachymetry measured 490 μm. Since the patient had developed central scarring and increased irregularity associated with central flap melting, the flap was considered non-viable and removed. The stromal bed and margins were blended with PTK. PTK was performed to 50 μm.

It took an incredible 34 days for the cornea to reepithelialize (Figure 4Q-4). Patching was alternated with bandage contact lenses. The patient also became a steroid responder, and Betagan 0.5% (Allergan Pharmaceuticals, Irvine, Calif) was added. Since he was a truck driver, the patient was unable to work for several months. The patient became very depressed, and was started on an antidepressant. He was kept on Fluorop (Solopak Pharmaceuticals, Elk Grove Village, Ill) for 5 months, using a very slow taper.

Since the OD was undercorrected, an enhancement was performed 6 months from the original procedure (Figure 4Q-5). Five months after the flap removal OS, (1 month postoperative OD enhancement) the patient had a UVCA of 20/25-2 OD and OS. The OD refracted to pl – 0.75 X 085, and the OS refracted to +0.50 DS, neither improving the BCVA. The patient was diplopic OS.

At 3 months postoperative OD enhancement the patient was 20/20-2 uncorrected, and refracted to -0.25 – 0.75 X 085. The OS was 20/30-1 uncorrected, and refracted to +1.50 – 1.50 X 135, with great variability and only one letter improvement in visual acuity with refraction. He had developed moderate confluent haze OS, and was scheduled for a PTK.

Two months later he presented to the clinic for the PTK OS. The topography indicated a well-centered ablation OD with an irregular central island pattern OS (Figure 4Q-6). The total laser treatment applied was 70 μm. This time the patient reepithelialized in 4 days. At the 10 day follow-up, UCVA was 20/70 OS, with diplopia. At 1 month, the uncorrected vision had improved to 20/50 OS, and +1.00 DS was corrected to 20/40-1. The patient reported seeing triple images OS.

At 15 months S/P OD enhancement (10 months S/P PTK OS), UCVAs were 20/20-2 OD, and 20/40-1 OS. The refraction for the OD was stable at pl – 0.75 X 115, and was at +1.50 – 1.00 X 045 OS, correcting the OD to 20/15-3, and the OS to 20/40. The corneal surface, OS, appeared very irregular with biomicroscopy. The patient still reported seeing triple images.

The patient currently wears a rigid gas permeable lens to take care of the triplopia OS. The contact lens corrects the OS to 20/15. He is coping much better and had stopped taking the antidepressant 6 months prior. His internet research has given him some hope that topography-assisted LASIK will help his condition in the future.

Figure 4Q-1. Preoperative topography demonstrating regular astigmatism.

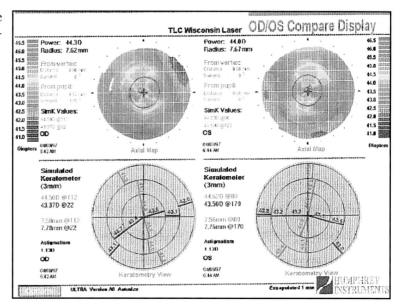

Figure 4Q-2. One week postoperative topography with bilateral irregularities.

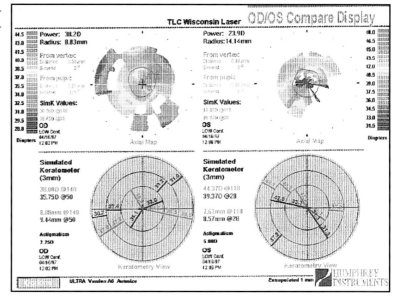

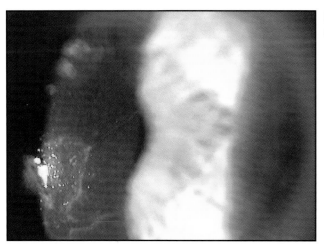

Figure 4Q-3. Central buttonhole with central corneal haze and striae.

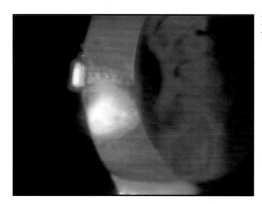

Figure 4Q-4. Slow reepithelialization of the stromal bed following removal of the flap.

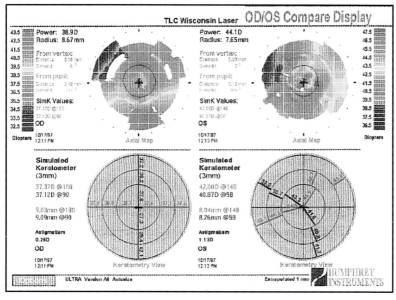

Figure 4Q-5. Six month postoperative topography demonstrates smooth, well-centered ablation OD and a central island pattern OS.

Figure 40-6. Topography OD following enhancement shows a well-centered ablation. Topography OS demonstrates irregular central island pattern.

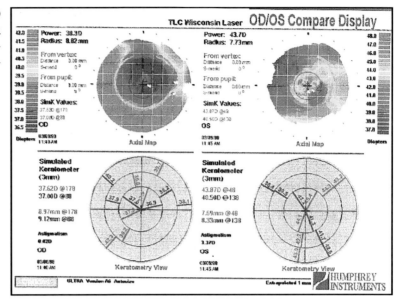

Editor's Notes

This case demonstrates the problems that occur when a buttonhole flap is lasered. When there is a flap complication, the flap should be replaced in the stromal bed so that it can heal as uneventfully as possible. Jeff Machat, MD, has described the lock and key concept for irregular flaps. The irregular flap fits back into the irregular stromal bed like a key into a lock. When the laser is applied to the stromal bed the flap does not fit perfectly into the altered stromal surface, so the lock and key relationship is lost. This results in irregular healing and many subsequent problems that can be seen in this case including a reduction in BCVA, flap striae, and confluent haze.

This case also demonstrates the difficulties with reepithelialization once the flap is removed. Because there is a distinct edge produced by the removal of the flap, the cornea has difficulty with reepithelialization. Generally, these cases can take up to 10 days to reepithelialize. In this case, the reepithelialization took over 34 days. This placed the patient at a significant risk for infection and haze and is also difficult for the patient as the vision is poor and the eye is uncomfortable for this entire period. In this case, once epithelization had occurred, the result was originally good. However, recurrent haze formation required additional PTK treatment. Now that the visual axis is clear and the BCVA is 20/15, the eye is at least stable, however the patient continues to complain of multiple images from the left eye which is a very significant problem because he is a truck driver. Of course these multiple images are created by the irregular corneal surface that was originally caused by the buttonhole flap and the laser application.

Clearly this case illustrates that laser should not be performed when a buttonhole flap occurs. While some irregularity could be expected in the cornea following the buttonhole, much of this problem could have been avoided. The patient's options at this point include continued use of the hard contact lens, topography-assisted LASIK, a homoplastic graft with replacement of the anterior third of his cornea, or a PK.

CASE R, BUTTONHOLE FLAP WITH LASER AND HAZE

Charlotte Burns, OD, MS, and Louis E. Probst, MD

Main Concern: Laser Applied
Patient Age: 37

INITIAL PREOPERATIVE INFORMATION

	OD	OS	COMMENTS
Preoperative Refraction	-9.50 – 0.75 X 057	-10.50 – 1.50 X 164	
BCVA	20/20	20/20	
Topography Details	normal	normal	
SimK Values	45.50/45.62@180	45.37/46.75@164	
Pachymetry	508 μm	518 μm	

PROCEDURES PERFORMED

	OD	OS	COMMENTS
1. Date/type	8/24/98 LASIK	8/24/98 LASIK	buttonhole OD
Laser/keratome/plate	VISX Star/ACS/160	VISX Star/ACS/160	with laser (referral
2. Date/type	2/26/99 PTK/PRK		doctor)
Laser/keratome/plate	VISX Star		

CURRENT POSTOPERATIVE INFORMATION

	OD	OS	COMMENTS
Time Postoperative	3 months	9 months	recurrent haze OD
Postoperative Refraction	+1.75 – 0.75 X 100	plano	
BCVA	20/15	20/15	

A 37-year-old white male presented on August 24, 1998, for LASIK. His systemic and ocular histories were unremarkable. His preoperative refraction was -9.50 – 0.75 X 057 OD, and -10.50 – 1.50 X 160 OS with BCVA of 20/20 OU. The patient was a long-term rigid gas permeable contact lens wearer and had discontinued contact lens wear for 8 weeks prior to the surgery date. Topography was normal OU. Pachymetry readings were 508 µm OD, and 518 µm OS. The patient chose to have LASIK, and the VISX Star laser was used, along with the Chiron ACS microkeratome. A 160 µm plate was used on the left eye with uneventful surgery.

When the microkeratome made its pass on the right eye suction was lost, which produced a doughnut-shaped flap. The referring surgeon proceeded to apply the laser despite the flap problem (Figures 4R-1 and 4R-2). Results initially were good, with postoperative findings of 20/20+2 UCVA OD, refraction of +1.75 – 1.00 X 170 at 1 week, and 20/20 UCVA OS with +2.00 – 0.50 X 110. At 1 month postoperative the patient was 20/15-1 uncorrected OD with plano refraction, and 20/15 uncorrected OS with +0.50 – 0.50 X 090 refraction. The cornea showed striae at day 1, then started to show trace haze at the 1 week follow-up. The doctor noted epithelial ingrowth centrally for the first time at 8 weeks, although visual acuity was still good at this time. Corneal haze had increased also at this time, so the patient was placed on Pred Forte (Allergan Pharmaceuticals, Irvine, Calif) drops 4 times a day and these were tapered over a 1 month period.

The patient's refraction started regressing after being taken off the steroid drops, and at 1 month after discontinuing drops, UCVA was 20/50-2 OD, with refraction of -1.50 – 0.25 X 015 best corrected to 20/25. Corneal haze had worsened at this point to the 2+ grade in the middle of the buttonhole (Figure 4R-3). At 9 weeks after discontinuing the drops the patient's UCVA had dropped to 20/400 and the refraction was -2.50 – 0.75 X 015 correcting the eye to 20/40-. The corneal haze had worsened to the 3+ grade. Three weeks later the visual findings showed no appreciable change.

At 14 weeks after discontinuing the steroid drops, the patient presented to the clinic for an evaluation and possible treatment. Findings at that time were counting fingers at 4 feet UCVA OD, and with a refraction of -3.00 – 0.75 X 015 the patient's BCVA was 20/200. The K reading was 42.75/44.00 at 178. Topography showed an irregular central pattern from the central haze. The pachymetry OD was 476 µm. Biomicroscopy showed dense central corneal haze.

The planned treatment for the eye was 80 µm of PTK, and then a -2.00 PRK that left trace haze. The patient took 48 hours to reepithelialize. At the 2 week postoperative visit, the patient was 20/30-1 uncorrected. The refraction of +1.75 – 1.00 X 100 improved visual acuity to 20/25-2. Biomicroscopy revealed mild, focal reticular haze. One month postoperatively the patient saw 20/20-2 uncorrected, and with +1.25 – 0.25 X 045 was correctable to 20/15. The cornea still showed mild, reticular haze. At the 2 month follow-up visit, the UCVA was 20/25-2, and the refraction of +1.75 – 1.25 X 080 yielded BCVA of 20/20-1. Biomicroscopy, however, showed moderate confluent haze in a circular pattern, with the central cornea clear.

At 3 months postoperative, findings included refraction of +1.75 – 0.75 X 100, correcting the OD to 20/15. Biomicroscopy showed haze distributed in a different pattern than had been seen at 2 months postoperative. The haze was only centrally located, about 3 to 4 mm in diameter, and the peripheral haze had disappeared. The patient was much happier at this time. He had been quite hostile and litiginous since the initial treatment.

Figure 4R-1. Still capture from the operative videotape of the LASIK procedure OD demonstrating the forceps passing through the hole in the center of the flap as the flap is retracted.

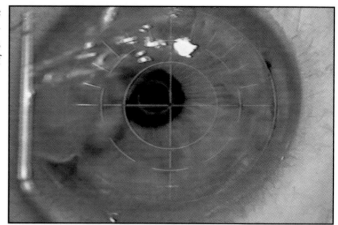

Figure 4R-2. Still capture from the operative videotape of the LASIK procedure OD demonstrating the cannula passing through the hole in the center of the flap during the interface irrigation after the excimer ablation.

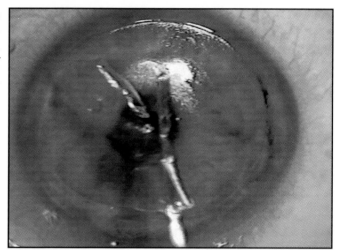

Figure 4R-3. Central buttonhole with haze developing centrally.

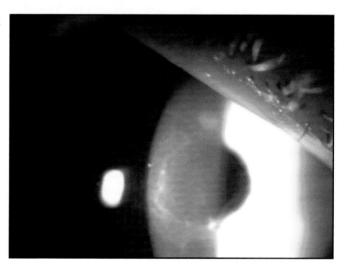

Editor's Notes

This is an example of the problems that occur with a buttonhole flap when the surgeon decides to laser. Surprisingly, this patient had an excellent result initially with a UCVA of 20/20 in the right eye. Unfortunately, this was complicated by a small amount of epithelial ingrowth along the buttonhole edges at 8 weeks, and was followed by regression and extensive central corneal scarring. The extent of the corneal scarring in this case was rather remarkable approaching the level of grade 3 haze (which is now rare since PRK is rarely performed for extremely high myopic corrections).

Fortunately, the PTK procedure was successful in removing most of the haze, however there was some recurrent haze following the procedure. Should another PTK procedure be required, postoperative thiotepa or mitomycin may be required in order to prevent recurrence of the haze.

CASE S, BUTTONHOLE FLAP AND OVERCORRECTION

Charlotte Burns, OD, MS

Main Concern: Laser Applied
Patient Age: 47

INITIAL PREOPERATIVE INFORMATION

	OD	OS	COMMENTS
Preoperative Refraction	-5.25 – 1.00 X 075	-6.75 – 1.00 X 093	
BCVA	20/20	20/20	
Topography Details	normal	normal	
SimK Values	42.37/43.00@166	42.37/43.12@016	
Pachymetry	588 μm	601 μm	

PROCEDURES PERFORMED

	OD	OS	COMMENTS
1. Date/type	1/7/99 LASIK	1/7/99 LASIK	buttonhole OS
Laser/keratome/plate	VISX Star/ACS/200	VISX Star/ACS/200	(referral doctor)

CURRENT POSTOPERATIVE INFORMATION

	OD	OS	COMMENTS
Time Postoperative	3 months	3 months	overcorrection OS
Postoperative Refraction	pl – 0.50 X 135	+1.75 – 0.25 X 030	
BCVA	20/20	20/50-1	
Topography Details	central flattening	central flattening	
SimK Values	38.00/38.12 X 090	37.75/38.25 X 036	
Visual Complaints	none	poor vision, blur	
Refractive Correction	none	none	

A 47-year-old white male presented for LASIK on January 7, 1999. His systemic and ocular histories were unremarkable. His preoperative refraction showed -5.25 – 1.00 X 075 OD, and -6.75 – 1.00 X 093 OS with BCVA of 20/20 OU. Topography was normal OU (Figure 4S-1). Pachymetry readings were 588 μm OD and 601 μm OS. The patient chose to have LASIK, and the VISX Star was used, along with the Chiron ACS microkeratome. A 200 μm plate was used on the OD first, with an uneventful procedure.

When the microkeratome made its pass on the OS, a doughnut-shaped flap was created. The referring surgeon elected to perform the laser ablation despite the buttonhole. Results on day 1 looked good for the OD with UCVA of 20/20. The OS was 20/100 uncorrected, and biomicroscopy showed a central epithelial defect, and haze.

At month 1, UCVAs were 20/30 OD and 20/70 OS. Refraction gave pl – 0.50 X 135 OD, and +1.75 – 0.25 X 030 OS, with the OD best corrected to 20/20, and OS 20/50-1. Topography showed a well-centered ablation (Figure 4S-2). Biomicroscopy revealed two fine striae centrally, and trace diffuse haze with a central oval scar OS. The findings on the cornea were subtle, however, a small central buttonhole was barely visible (4S-3). The patient is currently awaiting treatment, as we wanted to wait at least 6 months after the original LASIK before treating.

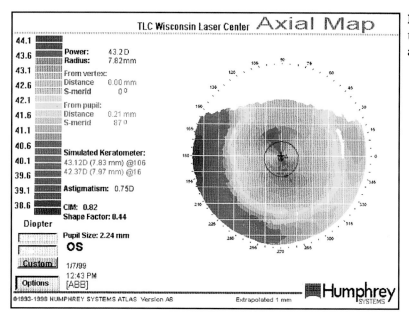

Figure 4S-1. Preoperative topography OS demonstrates a regular pattern.

Figure 4S-2. Postoperative topography OS shows a well-centered ablation with little irregularity.

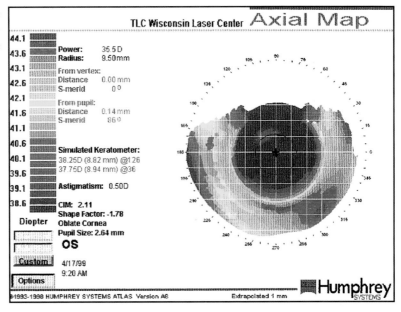

Figure 4S-3. A small central buttonhole was barely visible on the left cornea.

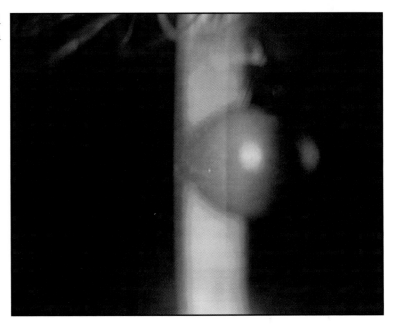

Editor's Notes

This case describes a buttonhole with a poor outcome. On the clinical photograph a fairly subtle buttonhole is visible, but the small degree of irregular astigmatism and striae in the central cornea have resulted in a drop in the BCVA. This once again demonstrates that LASIK should not be performed when a buttonhole occurs.

During the preoperative consent process it is important to inform patients of microkeratome complications. In my preoperative consent for LASIK, I state that the flap may be thin, small or irregular. If it is not perfect, I tell the patient that I will put it back, let it heal and have them come back in 3 months. I inform them that this is the safe thing to do and will result in the best outcome for them. I also tell them that this is relatively rare and occurs in approximately 1/500 to 1/1,000 cases in my hands. I also state that any problems following the procedure including wrinkles in the flap, debris underneath the flap, infection, or problems with the vision will be evaluated and we will get them sorted out as soon as possible. Finally, I tell the patient that the worst problem that could occur is that the microkeratome could perforate their eye and that they could go blind. I let them know that this could occur only if the microkeratome was set up incorrectly and that I check it personally every time before performing LASIK. This direct and honest approach tends to be appreciated. Complications are presented along with the solutions so the patient understands that these problems are generally correctable and we are fully committed to helping them.

CASE T, PARTIAL BUTTONHOLE FLAP WITH LASER

Charlotte Burns, OD, MS, and Louis E. Probst, MD

Main Concern: Laser Applied
Patient Age: 47

INITIAL PREOPERATIVE INFORMATION

	OD	OS	COMMENTS
Preoperative Refraction	-4.00 DS	-4.25 – 1.00 X 001	
BCVA	20/20	20/20	
Topography Details	normal OU		
SimK Values	44.12/44.12	44.12/44.87 X 088	
Pachymetry	549 μm	546 μm	

PROCEDURES PERFORMED

	OD	OS	COMMENTS
1. Date/type	8/20/98 LASIK	8/20/98 LASIK	buttonhole OD
Laser/keratome/plate	VISX Star/ACS/180	VISX Star/ACS/180	(referral doctor)
2. Date/type	1/7/99 LASIK enhancement (aborted)		
Laser/keratome/plate	lifted flap		
3. Date/type	3/31/99 LASIK enhancement		
Laser/keratome/plate	VISX Star/ACS/200		

CURRENT POSTOPERATIVE INFORMATION

	OD	OS	COMMENTS
Time Postoperative	1 month	9 months	excellent outcome OD
Postoperative Refraction	pl – 0.25 X 090	-1.25 DS	
BCVA	20/20	20/20	
Topography Details	central flattening	central flattening	
Pachymetry	482 μm		
SimK Values	41.62/41.75 X 180		
Refractive Correction	none		

A 47-year-old white male physician presented for LASIK on August 8, 1998. His systemic and ocular histories were unremarkable. His preoperative refraction was -4.00 D OD and -4.25 – 1.00 X 001 OS, with BCVAs of 20/20 OU. Topography was normal (Figure 4T-1) and pachymetry readings were 549 µm OD and 546 µm OS. The VISX Star laser was used, with the Chiron ACS microkeratome. A 180 µm plate was used on the left eye first, with a successful procedure performed.

The right flap was very thin, but the referring surgeon elected to continue with the laser treatment. On day 1 postoperative, the patient could see 20/20 uncorrected OU. Biomicroscopy revealed what appeared to be a large drop of oil in the interface OD. The refraction was +0.50 – 0.50 X 096 OD, and +1.00 DS OS. At 1 week, the uncorrected vision had improved to 20/15 OD and OS. The right cornea showed no changes by slit lamp. Topography indicated well-centered ablations with some superior extension (Figure 4T-2).

Two months later the patient was 20/20-1 uncorrected OD and 20/15 OS, with refraction showing -0.50 – 0.25 X 088 OD, and -0.25 DS OS. The noted biomicroscopy examination read "interface opacity." By 4 months postoperative, the patient had regressed to -1.00 DS OD 20/15-2, and -0.75 – 0.25 X 100 OS 20/15. The UCVA was 20/40- OD and a very blurry 20/20 OS. The patient decided he wanted an enhancement only on the OD, since he was dominant in that eye, and would leave the OS for slight monovision. The patient chose to wear spectacles at this time for distance only.

An enhancement was scheduled for 5 months postoperative, and on that day the patient's uncorrected vision was still 20/40 with -1.25 DS OD, with a BCVA of 20/20. The pachymeter read 485 µm and the topography was regular. Since it was less than 6 months postoperative, the surgeon decided to lift the flap rather than recut (we had not been notified about the previous buttonhole flap). When the flap was lifted, it was apparent that the flap was actually a buttonhole flap (Figure 4T-3). Only the outer edge lifted, so the surgeon laid the flap back down and decided to recut in 3 months.

At the 1 day follow-up visit, the patient could see 20/20 uncorrected, even though no treatment had been done, and was correctable with -0.50 – 0.25 X 120 to 20/15-1. There were two small interface opacities seen by biomicroscopy. One week later he could still see 20/20-1 uncorrected, and the BCVA was 20/15 with -0.75 – 0.25 X 098.

When he returned in 3 months for his enhancement, the OD had regressed back to 20/40-2 uncorrected, and was corrected to 20/20 with -0.75 – 0.25 X 090. The edge of the buttonhole was barely visible on slit lamp examination (Figure 4T-4). The topography was regular showing a well-centered ablation with some superior extension (Figure 4T-5). The laser was programmed subtracting our usual 9%. The flap was recut with a 200 µm depth plate and the ASC microkeratome.

On day 1, the patient could see 20/15-1 uncorrected, and refracted at +0.75 DS. The flap looked no different than it had from the very beginning, except for the new edge, as the surgeon had decentered the flap slightly temporal to the first flap. One week later the patient was 20/20 uncorrected, and refracted to +0.50 – 0.25 X0 90. At one month, the patient was seeing 20/15-2, and the refraction was pl – 0.25 X 090. The topography showed a well-centered ablation with no central irregularities from the buttonhole (Figure 4T-6). The patient is now quite happy with his vision.

Figure 4T-1. Preoperative topography indicated a reasonably regular pattern OU.

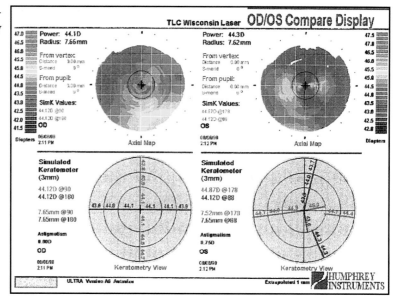

Figure 4T-2. Two weeks postoperative, topography showed well-centered ablations with some flattening extending superiorly OU.

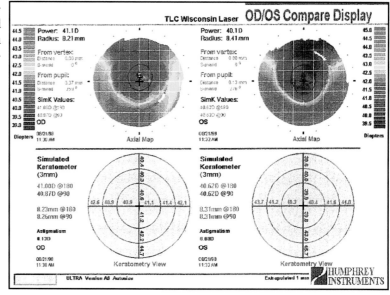

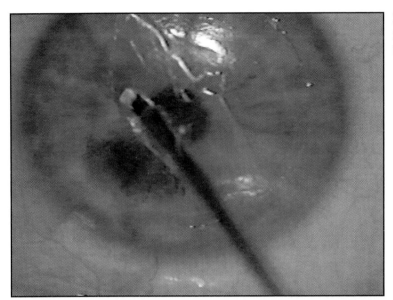

Figure 4T-3. Lifting the original flap at 5 months uncovers the buttonhole flap.

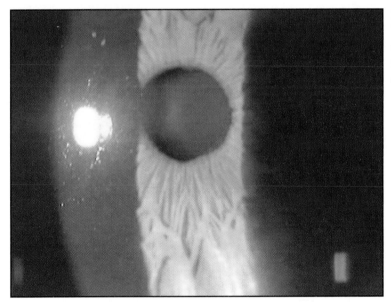

Figure 4T-4. Replacement of the buttonhole flap results in a clear cornea except for a very slight irregularity inferior to the visual axis.

Figure 4T-5. Topography prior to enhancement OD.

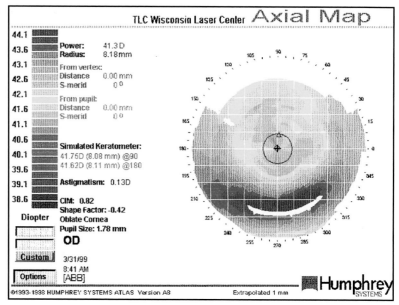

Figure 4T-6. Topography following enhancement OD showing a well-centered ablation with some superior extension.

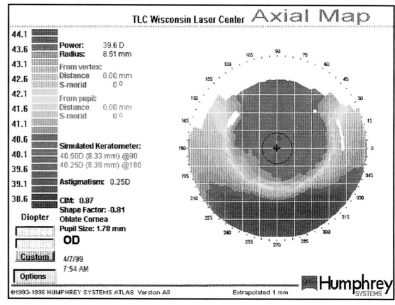

Editor's Notes

This case seemed to progress in a fairly normal manner in the right eye except for a small amount of interface debris and haze. There was some regression in the right eye that necessitated an enhancement. At the time of enhancement, it was evident that the center of the flap was very thin. It was also found that the flap was very thin and friable.

This is an example of an incomplete buttonhole flap. The flap was thin overall and even thinner in the central area of the cornea, however, the microkeratome did not perforate the central corneal epithelium. The center of the flap was likely composed of only the epithelial layer. Therefore the flap was still intact. When it was laid down, the eye healed in a fairly normal manner. Nevertheless, some debris and scarring resulted from the central thin area of the flap. When the flap was lifted, only the central epithelial layer existed in the middle and therefore this stayed adherent to the stroma resulting in the creation of the buttonhole.

The flap was immediately laid down without any further laser treatment and left to heal for 3 months. The patient's BCVA was restored completely to the previous refraction. The patient had the enhancement procedure repeated with another keratectomy at 200 μm and has achieved an excellent result. This case demonstrates that with appropriate management, buttonhole flaps can still achieve an excellent outcome.

Case U, Half Flap
Charlotte Burns, OD, MS

Main Concern: Laser Applied
Patient Age: 52

Initial Preoperative Information

	OD	OS	Comments
Preoperative Refraction	-7.00 – 1.25 X 165	-5.50 – 3.25 X 007	
BCVA	20/20	20/20	
Topography Details	regular bow-tie pattern OU		
SimK Values	45.63/45.50 X 168	43.25/46.37 X 004	
Pachymetry	514 µm	504 µm	

Procedures Performed

	OD	OS	Comments
1. Date/type	10/29/98 LASIK	10/29/98 LASIK	partial flap OD
Laser/keratome/plate	VISX Star/ACS/10	VISX Star/ACS/180	with laser
			(referral doctor)

Current Postoperative Information

	OD	OS	Comments
Time Postoperative	6 months	6 months	reduced BCVA OD
Postoperative Refraction	+3.00 – 2.50 X 165	pl – 1.00 X 172	with irregular
BCVA	20/40	20/20	astigmatism and scar
Topography Details	included		
SimK Values	36.25/39.12 X 158	39.87/41.87 X 004	
Pachymetry	460 µm	470 µm	
Visual Complaints	diplopia, poor vision		
Refractive Correction	spectacles		

A 52-year-old white female presented for LASIK on October 29, 1998. Her systemic and ocular histories were unremarkable. Her refraction was -7.00 – 1.25 X 165 OD, and -5.50 – 3.25 X 007 OS, with BCVA of 20/20 OD and OS. Topography showed a normal bow-tie pattern (Figure 4U-1), and pachymetry readings were 514 μm OD, and 504 μm OS. The VISX Star laser was used, as well as the Chiron ACS microkeratome. A 180 μm plate was used on the OS first, and the surgery proceeded normally. The laser was programmed to leave the OS for monovision.

When the microkeratome made the pass on the OD, it only made a partial flap, which appeared to be a three-fourths flap. The surgeon proceeded with the surgery despite the incomplete flap, and did not cover the tissue remaining in the ablation zone.

On the first day after surgery, the patient was 20/150 uncorrected OD, and 20/25 OS. A refraction was not performed. Biomicroscopy showed irregular epithelium, and haze OD.

One week later the patient was 20/70-1 OD, and 20/20 OS uncorrected. Refraction revealed +2.00 – 1.00 X 164 OD and pl – 0.50 OS with BCVA of 20/60-2 OD. Biomicroscopy showed a corneal ridge at the temporal edge of the pupil, and striae OD. The patient was having difficulty working, as she is a dental hygienist and needs to see fine detail.

At 6 months postoperative the patient was 20/50 uncorrected OD, and 20/25 OS. The refraction showed +3.00 – 2.50 X 165 OD, and pl – 1.00 OS, with BCVA of 20/40 OD, and 20/20 OS. Biomicroscopy was unchanged with a vertical linear cornea scar about 2 mm nasal to the visual axis OD (Figure 4U-2 and 4U-3). Topography indicated a slightly decentered ablation with irregularities nasal in the region of the cornea scar (Figure 4U-4). The patient is unhappy with the result and wishes an enhancement. It was suggested to her that her comanaging doctor could fit her with a contact lens for the OD. She wanted to wait for enhancement when hyperopic astigmatism is approved in the US, rather than travel to Canada.

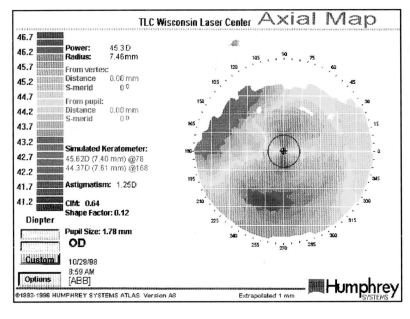

Figure 4U-1. Preoperative topography OD demonstrates a regular pattern.

Figure 4U-2. A vertical linear cornea scar is visible about 2 mm nasal to the visual axis OD.

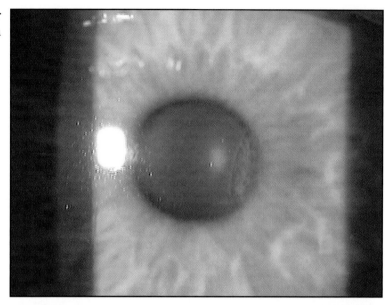

Figure 4U-3. The vertical linear cornea scar is more visible with tangential illumination.

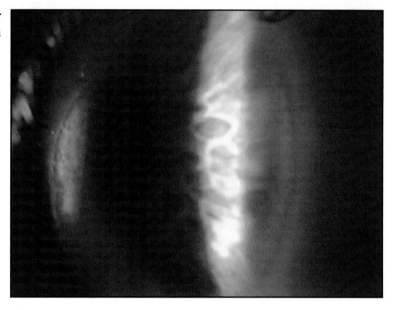

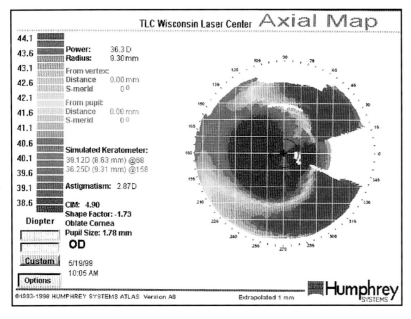

Figure 4U-4. Postoperative topography OD shows a decentered ablation with irregularity nasally from the corneal scar.

Editor's Notes

This case represents a difficult situation with an imperfect flap that received laser treatment. A corneal scar had developed just nasal to the visual axis in the right eye. While the UCVA has maintained a reasonably good level, the patient is disturbed by blurred images and what she describes as a hazy line just off the center of her vision.

The treatment decisions in this case are quite difficult. She certainly could have hyperopic LASIK to correct her residual hyperopic refractive error, however, this would not remove the scar. She could have the scar removed with a PTK but this would not treat the hyperopia. In fact, this would tend to induce the hyperopia. A further refractive procedure would be required after the PTK and this could lead to haze and an actual reduction in the quality of her vision. At the present time we have elected to continue with the contact lens wear in the right eye and monitor for further improvement prior to considering further treatment options.

CASE V, INCOMPLETE FLAP

Charlotte Burns, OD, MS, and Louis E. Probst, MD

Main Concern: Laser Applied
Patient Age: 52

INITIAL PREOPERATIVE INFORMATION

	OD	OS	COMMENTS
Preoperative Refraction	-8.75 – 0.25 X 050	-7.75 – 0.50 X 030	
BCVA	20/20	20/20	
Topography Details	normal	normal	
SimK Values	44.50/45.12@090	44.75/45.00@135	
Pachymetry	540 µm	530 µm	

PROCEDURES PERFORMED

	OD	OS	COMMENTS
1. Date/type	10/29/98 LASIK	10/29/98 LASIK	incomplete flap OD
Laser/keratome/plate	VISX Star/ACS/180	VISX Star/ACS/180	(referral doctor)
2. Date/type		1/20/99 LASIK	overcorrection OS
		enhancement	
Laser/keratome/plate		VISX Star/lifted flap	

CURRENT POSTOPERATIVE INFORMATION

	OD	OS	COMMENTS
Time Postoperative	7 months	4 months	
Postoperative Refraction	+3.00 DS	pl – 0.50 X 042	
BCVA	20/40	20/20	
Topography Details	n/a		
Refractive Correction	contact lenses		

A 52-year-old female attorney presented for laser vision correction on October 29, 1998. Systemic and ocular histories were unremarkable. Her BCVAs were 20/20 OD and OS with refraction of -8.75 – 0.25 X 050 OD, and -7.75 – 0.50 X 030 OS. Topography was normal, and pachymetry showed 540 μm OD, and 530 μm OS. The VISX Star laser was used, as was the Chiron ACS. A 180 μm plate was used on the OS first, with surgery proceeding uneventfully.

When the microkeratome made its pass on the OD, it made an incomplete flap and bisected the pupil. The referring surgeon proceeded to apply the laser, without covering the flap. On the first day following the procedure, the patient was 20/60 uncorrected OD. With a refraction of +1.25 DS, she could see 20/30. The left eye was 20/100 uncorrected, and with a refraction of +3.00 DS, she could see 20/25. There was a "ridge" bisecting the right pupil, and a large central epithelial defect by biomicroscopy (Figure 4V-1).

Six days later, the patient could see 20/40 BCVA OD, with +3.00 DS. The OS was 20/25 with +2.50 DS. The slit lamp showed the same central corneal irregularity OD, and the patient complained of diplopia OD.

At 3 months postoperative, the patient came in for a hyperopic enhancement on the OS only. She refracted to +3.00 DS OD and +2.50 DS OS, and BCVAs were still 20/40 OD, and 20/20 OS. The full +2.50 was programmed into the laser for the OS. The result at 4 months postoperative for the OS was pl – 0.50 X 042, with 20/20 UCVA.

What to do with the OD is still a question. A PTK may be planned in an attempt to improve acuity first. The patient has calmed down somewhat after the improvement of the OS, however, she is still not happy. She is currently wearing a soft contact lens OD.

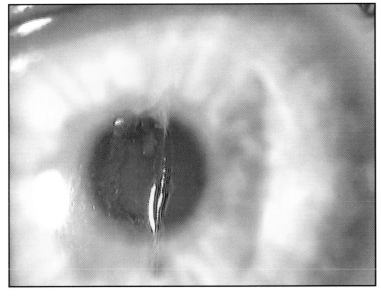

Figure 4V-1. Incomplete thin flap with a ridge bisecting the pupil 1 day after LASIK.

Editor's Notes

This represents another example of an inappropriate excimer ablation with an irregular LASIK flap. There has been a loss of BCVA due to the interface haze in the central cornea. The patient is complaining of double vision in the right eye. Clearly the laser procedure should not have been performed in this case.

It is interesting to note that many of these cases of thin flaps are associated with hyperopic outcomes. It may be that the superficial stroma has less hydration as compared to the mid-stroma where the usual LASIK ablation is performed. Perhaps this less-hydrated tissue has more response to the excimer laser, causing overcorrections. Whatever the cause, these hyperopic overcorrections are difficult to treat as hyperopia is difficult to treat with PRK, and hyperopic LASIK will not remove the central corneal scarring.

LASER-RELATED COMPLICATIONS

5

SUMMARY NOTES

LASER-RELATED COMPLICATIONS - SUMMARY NOTES

ERRORS IN REFRACTIVE OUTCOME

Clinical

Any significant error in the refractive outcome results in some disappointment from the patient, as they are still dependent on refractive correction. Even a -12.00 D myopia will return for a -0.50 D enhancement, despite a remarkable improvement in the uncorrected vision. While the excimer laser ablation can be accurately programmed and the keratectomy technique can be perfected, the unknown variable with LASIK is the healing response of the cornea. While some patients will regress up to 3.0 D, others will not regress at all. Younger patients (<25 years) tend to regress and experience undercorrections, while older patients (>45 years) regress less and can experience overcorrections.

Management

Any refraction can initially be managed with a contact lens as early as 1 week following LASIK and the patient can then return to full activities. Topical steroids have little effect on the refractive result following LASIK. Once refractive stability has been achieved an enhancement procedure can be performed. The greater the primary LASIK correction, the greater the amount of postoperative time required to achieve full refractive stability. PRK should not be performed over a LASIK flap, as this can induce corneal haze.

Errors in Refractive Outcome

ERROR	COMMENT	TREATMENT
Hyperopia	normal cornea	hyperopic LASIK at 4 months
	thin cornea	laser thermokeratoplasty at 6 months
Myopia	1 to 3 D preoperatively	myopic LASIK enhancement at 1 month
	3 to 6 D preoperatively	myopic LASIK enhancement at 2 months
	>6 D preoperatively	myopic LASIK enhancement at 3 to 4 months
Regression	wait for stability	myopic or hyperopic LASIK
Astigmatism	wait for stability	LASIK at 3 to 4 months

Prevention

The first step in improving the results of LASIK is to ensure the accuracy and stability of the preoperative refraction. A consistent LASIK technique with control of stromal hydration/drying is also essential. Nomograms have been developed for LASIK that account for the degree of correction and the age of the patient to minimize errors in the refractive predictability. Most myopia nomograms error towards undercorrection, as it is generally less difficult to treat myopia. Hyperopes treated with hyperopic LASIK should be overcorrected by 10 to 20% as they will tend to regress back to emmetropia over 1 to 3 months. Each surgeon must carefully evaluate their own technique, location, and results to determine the best nomogram.

Probst LASIK Nomogram for VISX SmoothScan Laser

	<25 YEARS	25 TO 45 YEARS	>45 YEARS
<2.0 D myopia	90%	90%	90%
>2.0 D myopia	84%	82%	80%

CENTRAL ISLANDS

Clinical

Central islands occur from the central accumulation of fluid when using a broad beam excimer laser. Central islands present with a loss of UCVA, BCVA, irregular astigmatism, monocular diplopia, and undercorrection. While central islands often resolve after PRK, they do not resolve after LASIK.

Management

Central islands should be identified and monitored on topography until they are stable in size and severity. The refraction should not be used as an indicator of stability as it will often vary considerably with each refraction. The size and the height of the islands are then measured on corneal topography and the Munnerlyn formula is used to calculate the height of the islands.

Munnerlyn Formula

height in microns = diameter^2 X diopter height/3

The exact number of microns and the diameter size of the island can then be corrected using the PTK mode on the VISX (Star or Smooth Scan) or the Chiron 116 excimer laser. An alternative approach involves treating the refractive myopia in the PRK mode of the VISX laser but only performing the first 50% of the ablation. The Chiron 217 is poor at treating central islands as the blending effects of the scanning laser does not allow the beam to be focused into the central area alone. A conservative approach is essential as an over treatment will result in a central divot which will almost impossible to correct.

Prevention

The central islands factor (CIF) software has been incorporated into the VISX laser to provide extra treatment for the central cornea to compensate for the central island effect of the broad-beam laser. Scanning excimer lasers eliminate the risk of central islands, as there is no central accumulation of fluid. Any central accumulation of fluid can be removed by wiping the stromal bed during LASIK, however this maneuver will alter the overall stromal hydration and therefore effect the final refractive outcome.

NIGHT GLARE

Clinical

Night glare occurs when the pupil dilates greater than the optical zone of the refractive correction, resulting in glare for the edge of the ablation zone. Night glare is more common both preoperatively and postoperatively in high myopes. Patients experience halos, starbursts, and reduction in the quality of vision. While manageable in most patients, it can be disabling in some.

Management

Fortunately, most symptoms of night glare reduce for up to 1 year following LASIK. The refinements in the ablation profiles have resulted in a large reduction in the complaints of night glare following LASIK.

Treatment of Night Glare
- Conservative
  - LASIK for other eye
  - eliminate monovision
  - night driving glasses (-1.00)
  - night light in car while night driving
  - diluted pilocarpine
- Surgical
  - retreatment with larger zone
  - topography-assisted LASIK

Prevention

Patient should be screened preoperatively for pupil size. Patients with a pupil over 6 mm in dim illumination should be counseled about the potential risk of postoperative night glare. Patients with large pupils can be treated with a scanning excimer laser with ablation zones up to 9 mm. However, these lasers ablate significantly greater amounts of stroma so the stromal thickness is critical when determining candidacy.

DECENTERED ECCENTRIC ABLATIONS

Clinical

Decentration of the ablation results in a residual refractive error associated with visual distortions or ghosting, particularly at night. The patient's concerns are often more significant than would be expected from the small refractive error. There may be a loss of BCVA. (The decentration is obvious when postoperative topography is performed.)

Etiology of Decentered Ablations
- pharmacological pupillary dilation
- pharmacological pupillary constriction
- large kappa angle
- poor patient fixation
- wide flap hinge encroaching on ablation zone
- eccentric fixation

Management

Because the decentered ablation creates an irregular ablation pattern, treatment of the decentration is difficult with a broad-beam laser. While the refractive error can be treated and the flap replaced, this does not treat the edge glare effect from the sort edge of the ablation zone. A second ablation in the opposite direction of the original decentration has also been suggested, but this could result in a more irregular pattern. The most promise for decentered ablation is topography-assisted LASIK, which can treat the untreated area of the ablation zone.

Prevention

Excimer ablations should be centered on the pupil in all cases in order to minimize decentrations. Pharmacological alteration should be avoided several days prior to LASIK. Patients often have difficulty fixating on the fixation beam once the flap has been cut, as the stroma does not provide a clear interface. In order to ensure centration on the pupil the suction ring can be left on the eye (with the suction off) to control the position of the ablation completely. An eye tracker that has been locked onto the center of the pupil can also be used.

CASE A, CENTRAL ISLAND

Stephen S. Lane, MD, and Douglas Katz, MD

Main Concern: Central Island
Patient Age: 59

INITIAL PREOPERATIVE INFORMATION

	OD	OS	COMMENTS
Preoperative Refraction	-8.25 – 1.50 X 175	-8.25 – 1.75 X 180	
BCVA	20/20	20/20	
Topography Details	regular astigmatism	regular astigmatism	
SimK Values	46.72 X 180	49.18 X 090	

PROCEDURES PERFORMED

	OD	OS	COMMENTS
1. Date/type	1/14/99 M-LASIK	11/14/99 M-LASIK	uncomplicated
Laser/keratome/plate	VISX S2/ACS/160	VISX S2/ACS/160	

CURRENT POSTOPERATIVE INFORMATION

	OD	OS	COMMENTS
Time Postoperative	1 week	3/1/99	
Postoperative Refraction	-1.00 – 1.00 X 140	pl	central island OD
BCVA	20/40	20/20	with loss of BCVA
Topography Details	central island	normal	
SimK Values	40.67 X 150	n/a	
Visual Complaints	distortion of vision	none	
Medications	timoptic b.i.d	timoptic b.i.d	
Refractive Correction	none	glasses	

A 59-year-old man with a history of primary open angle glaucoma controlled with medications presented for bilateral refractive surgery. His preoperative medications consisted of timolol maleate (Merck and Company, Inc., West Point, Pa) 0.25% b.i.d. OU. His manifest refractions were: -6.50 – 3.00 X 177 OD and -8.25 – 1.75 X 180 OS. Topography shows regular bow-tie astigmatism in each eye with simulated keratometry readings of 45.83 D X 180/ 48.74 D X 90 OD and 46.72 X 180/ 49.18 X 090 OS (Figure 5A-1).

Bilateral LASIK was performed without incident using the Automated Corneal Shaper and a 160 μm depth plate. A VISX S2 laser was used for the ablation. Both procedures were performed in an identical fashion that included mild drying of the bed with a damp spear prior to ablation. There was no pooling of fluid noted during the ablation of either eye.

The postoperative course was unremarkable in the left eye with 20/20 UCVA being achieved. The right eye on postoperative day 1 had a UCVA of 20/100 with a clear interface and intact epithelium. There was minimal improvement at 1 week. BCVA at this time was 20/50 with a correction of -1.50 – 1.00 X 150. Topography was performed and it revealed a central island (Figure 5A-2). Postoperative refractions remained relatively stable over the next 2 months with -1.00 – 1.00 X 140 giving a BCVA of 20/40. There was no significant change of the central island on the topography throughout this time (Figure 5A-3).

Central pooling of fluid has been implicated as a possible etiologic agent in the development of central islands, particularly in the higher levels of myopia. In this case no pooling of fluid was observed in either eye. However, the eye that developed the central island was more myopic and theoretically more prone to fluid accumulation. Modern software has significantly decreased the frequency of central islands. However, while central islands are uncommon they do still occur and can be challenging to deal with. For this case, once we are assured of the stability of the refraction, we plan to lift the flap and perform a PTK with a narrow beam. The diopteric power or height of the central island can be determined with modern topography. The Munnerlyn formula states that the diameter in millimeters of the proposed ablation squared divided by 3 equals the depth of ablation per diopter. The appropriate depth of ablation pulses of the laser can be calculated based on the height or power of the central island. In our case, the central island measures approximately 5 D, therefore, with a 3 mm PTK approximately 15 μm would need to be ablated to correct the central island. Alternatively, several topographic instruments are now available that can measure the elevation directly to determine the amount of ablation needed. A modulating agent may be used to provide a more uniform and localized ablation of the central island. While this is not an exact science, good results can still be obtained, although it may take more than one treatment to achieve.

Figure 5A-1. Regular bow-tie astigmatism on preoperative topography.

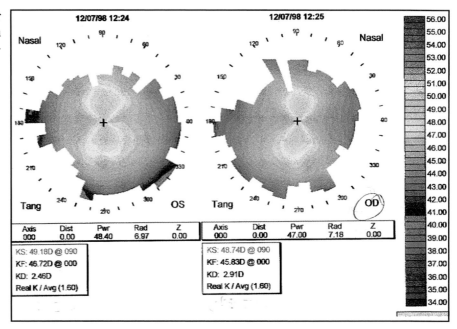

Figure 5A-2. Topography 1 week postoperatively OD revealed a central island.

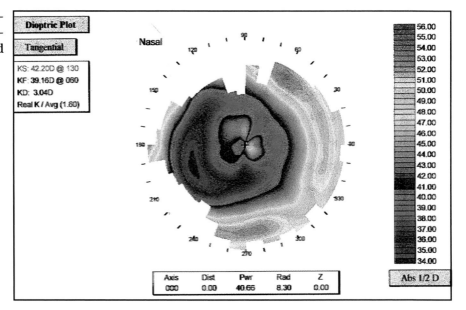

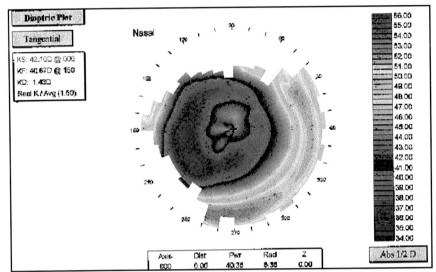

Figure 5A-3. Topography 2 months postoperatively OD demonstrates a persistent island pattern.

Editor's Notes

This case raises a number of important concepts for LASIK. Preoperatively the patient had primary open-angle glaucoma that was controlled on topical beta-blockers. Opinions vary as to whether this patient would be an appropriate surgical candidate for LASIK. Certainly if the optic nerves were healthy and the visual fields appear stable, there is no reason to expect this patient not to achieve the same results as a patient with a normal eye. However, during LASIK, the suction required during the keratectomy does increase the IOP to at least 80 mmHg. It is possible this could attenuate the nerve fibers of the optic nerve. However, there have been no reports of nerve fiber layer loss and the associated visual field defects after LASIK, suggesting that this risk may be more theoretical. LASIK surgeons should still exercise caution with glaucoma patients if there are any signs of optic nerve damage.

The steeper central keratometry in this case will result in a larger flap with a bigger hinge, which tends to provide a more stable flap. It has been proposed that very steep corneas with Ks in the 49 to 50 range can be prone to buttonholes during the keratectomy because of a central buckling of the cornea as the keratome traverses the cornea. My experience with steep corneas using copious lubrication and a greater depth plate has shown that buttonholes can be avoided in virtually 100% of cases.

The VISX laser has CIF software that provides pretreatment to prevent the occurrence of central islands. Unfortunately, they do still occur in approximately 1 in 200 cases. The treatment of central islands involves a PTK treatment in the center of the cornea with use of the Munnerlyn formula. The depth of the ablation should be calculated conservatively, as a second treatment for the central island is always possible. However, however a deep central corneal divot from excessive PTK can be very difficult if not impossible to correct. It should also be noted that any central application of excimer laser for the treatment of central islands would result in a hyperopic shift in the refractive error. Generally this is in the range of 2 to 3 D. Following the successful treatment of a central island it may be necessary to perform a hyperopic LASIK enhancement procedure to deal with this hyperopic shift.

Fortunately, the next generation of excimer lasers that use scanning spot or slit systems are not associated with the development of central islands because there is no overall central accumulation of fluid during the excimer ablation.

CASE B, WRONG AXIS

Stephen S. Lane, MD, Douglas Katz, MD, and Louis E. Probst, MD

Main Concern: Ablation of Axis 90° from Intended Axis
Patient Age: 51

INITIAL PREOPERATIVE INFORMATION

	OD	OS	COMMENTS
Preoperative Refraction	-0.25 – 3.00 X 108		
BCVA	20/20		
Topography Details	regular astigmatism		
SimK Values	41.87 X 120		

PROCEDURES PERFORMED

	OD	OS	COMMENTS
1. Date/type	12/17/98		wrong axis
Laser/keratome/plate	VISX S2/ACS/160		
2. Date/type	3 month postoperative		mixed astigmatism
Laser/keratome/plate	Technolas 217/flap lifted		treated

CURRENT POSTOPERATIVE INFORMATION

	OD	OS	COMMENTS
Time Postoperative	4/19/99		excellent outcome OD
Postoperative Refraction	-1.00 – 1.00 X 170		
BCVA	20/20		
Topography Details	regular		
SimK Values	40.97 X 180		

A 51-year-old man with a preoperative refraction of -0.25 – 3.00 X 180 OD and -0.75 – 2.50 X 068 OS presented requesting refractive surgery. Preoperative topography revealed regular bow-tie astigmatism in both eyes. Simulated keratometry measured 41.87 Dx 120 and 43.54 Dx 030 in the right eye.

An ACS with a 160 µm plate was used to make the corneal flap. Ablation with the VISX S2 Laser was carried out at the incorrect meridian of 018 degrees. This incorrect meridian had been transcribed consistently throughout the preoperative worksheet including both the manifest and cycloplegic refractions. The UCVA 30 minutes postoperatively was <20/200. Careful examination of the data at that time revealed that an error in the treatment meridian had occurred.

The postoperative refractive error stabilized at +2.00 – 5.00 X 108. The additional 2.5 D of cylinder at an axis of 120 can be seen on topography (Figure 5B-1). Three months postoperatively the flap was lifted and a mixed hyperopic astigmatism ablation was performed using the Technolas 217. Additionally, uncomplicated LASIK was performed on the left eye at this time. The UCVA at 1 month measured 20/50 OD and 20/20 OS (Figure 5B-2). The visual acuity improved to 20/20 OD with a refraction of -1.00 – 1.00 X 170. Once the refraction has been allowed to stabilize we will discuss the options with the patient and decide if further enhancement would be advisable if he is happy with his newly attained monovision.

The most important point to be gleaned from this case is the necessity of paying close attention to the preoperative refraction. Particular emphasis should be placed on the meridian of the cylinder. Errors can easily be made when converting from plus to minus cylinder in both the meridian and the sphere. It is imperative to be certain that the meridian of the proposed correction correlates with the topography and keratometry values. If there is a discrepancy, the measurements should be carefully reviewed or repeated. In this case a quick preoperative check of the topography could have averted this outcome. This case also illustrates that a reasonable outcome can be achieved with a mixed hyperopic astigmatism correction after an inadvertent wrong axis ablation.

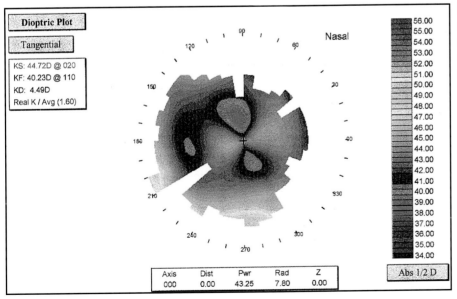

Figure 5B-1. Postoperative topography demonstrates 2.5 D of induced cylinder at 120°.

Figure 5B-2. Post-operative topography OU after mixed pattern LASIK OD and M-LASIK OS.

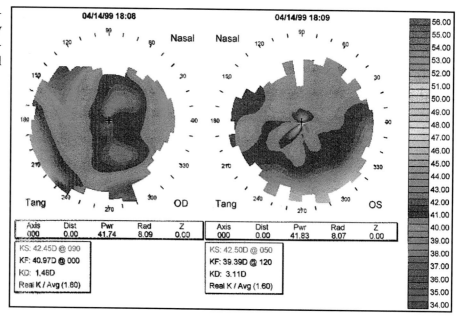

Editor's Notes

With the rapid increase in the popularity of LASIK, many refractive centers have become extremely busy. While this repetition certainly leads to consistency and improved results, it also can lead to errors in the programming of the laser. In order to avoid these situations, it is essential that a system be set-up so that information is checked on multiple occasions.

At my centers all patients are given a name-tag so there is absolutely no confusion about either their first or their last name. Patients are always addressed by their full name so that those with similar first names do not have a chance of getting mixed up. On our surgical planning sheets, we have the referral refraction, the spectacle refraction, the refraction, and the topography axes all aligned up to ensure that they are consistent and similar. The cylinder axis is checked by the center optometrist, the surgeon, and the laser room technician. Everyone checks that the axis of the refraction, topography, and the programmed correction are all the same and none have been "flipped". Because of these, we have had very few problems in this regard.

Nevertheless, errors of this nature will occur on occasion. It is comforting to know that using the scanning lasers, such as the Technolas 217 laser, we are able to treat mixed astigmatism patterns and get excellent results. The patient in this case ended up slightly myopic, however, this could be easily corrected with a myopic LASIK enhancement using any broad-beam laser system. When correcting mixed astigmatism patterns with the scanning excimer laser, the patient should be switched into plus cylinder format to minimize the amount of tissue ablated and therefore preserve stromal tissue.

Case C, Eccentric Ablation and Undercorrection

Ioannis G. Pallikaris, MD, Theokliti Papadaki, MD, and Dimitrios S. Siganos, MD

Patient Age: 25

Initial Preoperative Information

	OD	OS	Comments
Preoperative Refraction	-14.5 – 2.25 X 40		high myopia
BCVA	20/40		

Procedures Performed

	OD	OS	Comments
1. Date/type	1995 M-LASIK		decentered ablation
Laser/keratome/plate	ACS/150		
2. Date/type	1996 LASIK		
	enhancement and AK		
Laser/keratome/plate	ACS/160		

Current Postoperative Information

	OD	OS	Comments
Time Postoperative	6 months		loss in BCVA
Postoperative Refraction	+3.00 – 1.5 X 145		
BCVA	20/40		
Topography Details	irregular		
SimK Values	n/a		

(Case and photographs reprinted with permission from Machat JJ, Slade SG, Probst LE. *The Art of Lasik.* 2nd ed. Thorofare, NJ: SLACK Incorporated; 1999.)

A 25-year-old woman underwent LASIK in OD for the correction of -14.5 – 2.25 X 40. BCVA was 20/40. Preoperative appearance of the eye is presented in Figure 5C-1. The ACS microkeratome was used to create a 8.5 mm wide and 150 µm thick flap. Immediately prior to the ablation, the patient became very anxious and burst into tears. Instead of interrupting the procedure until the patient's composure was restored, the surgeon chose to immediately proceed with the ablation. Ablation was interrupted, and the ablation mask was removed and recentered twice in order to dry the stromal surface with microsponges.

Nineteen months postoperatively, the eye presented an undercorrection of -5.5 – 4.75 X 165 with no loss in BCVA (Figures 5C-2 and 5C-3). Furthermore, the patient experienced glare and halos, especially in dim light, and asthenopic symptoms even when corrected with glasses. Computer-assisted corneal topography revealed an eccentricity pattern in which the center of the map was situated outside the area of mean refractive power (middle green) and one quadrant of the 3 mm pupil zone was out of the green encircled area (Figure 5C-4). These characteristics correspond to category E2A of Pallikaris' classification.

A second thicker flap (160 µm) was created using the ACS microkeratome. Subsequently, diagonal ablation was applied for correction of the eccentricity. Attempted correction was -6 D with a 6 mm optical zone. The center of the diagonal ablation was placed on the decentration axis 2 mm superiorly from the pupil. A supplementary arcuate cut of 90° radius centered along the decentration axis but situated at 180° opposite the direction of decentration was performed at the borders of the new flap in order to enhance the ablation zone. A bandage soft contact lens was fitted and the routine LASIK postoperative regime was administered.

On the first postoperative day, the eye was quiet (see Figure 5C-3). A noticeable change was detected in corneal topography (see Figure 5C-4) in that a new ablation zone 6 D deeper, but perfectly centered, could be seen. The slight shifting of the borders of the zone at the upper temporal quadrant corresponded exactly to the area of the arcuate cut.

At 6 months postoperatively, the patient reported marked improvement in vision. UCVA was 20/50, while BCVA was 20/40 with a correction of +3.00 – 1.5 X 145. On slit lamp examination, the cornea showed mild interface opacities and pigment deposits that did not interfere with the visual axis (Figure 5C-5), while on narrow slit beam, a cornea of even thickness was detected (Figure 5C-6). At the upper temporal corneal periphery, three concentric lines can be seen. Superiorly to inferiorly, these are: the linear scarring of the cut, the borders of the second flap, the borders of the diagonal ablation (Figures 5C-7 and 5C-8).

Corneal topography at the sixth postoperative month showed a slight inferior shifting (Figure 5C-9). This alteration represents the expected partial reversal of the relaxing effect of the arcuate cut with time due to healing of the epithelium and scarring within the area of the cut.

Excessive lacrimation and inability of the patient to follow the surgeon's directions and fixate properly are reasons for interrupting the procedure in order to diminish the risk of undercorrection due to excessive hydration or decentration. In these cases, the most appropriate action is to replace the flap to its original position and proceed as soon as the patient is able to cooperate. With the flap in place, the cornea can be irrigated without affecting stromal hydration.

The same management is also recommended in cases in which there is a time lapse between creation of the flap and laser ablation (ie, temporary laser failure) in order to avoid stromal dehydration, which could result in overcorrection.

Figure 5C-1. Preoperative appearance of the eye.

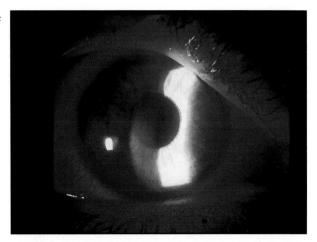

Figure 5C-2. Slip lamp view of the eye prior to retreatment.

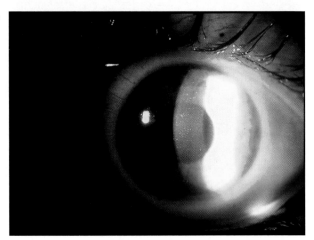

Figure 5C-3. Slip lamp view of the eye on the first day after retreatment. A thin, perfectly arcuate line (see arrows) just indicates the area of the cut.

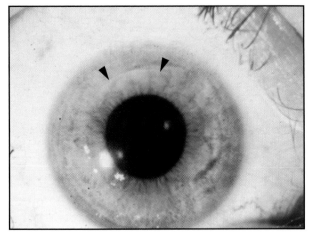

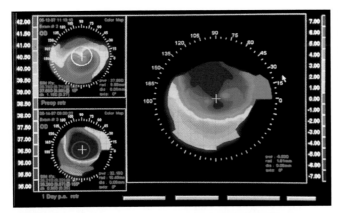

Figure 5C-4. Corneal topographic difference map comparing the topographic map prior to retreatment to that obtained at the immediate post-retreatment interval.

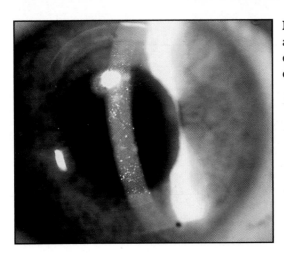

Figure 5C-5. Slit lamp view of the eye 6 months after retreatment. Mild opacities and pigment deposits are detected in the interface though they do not interfere with the visual axis.

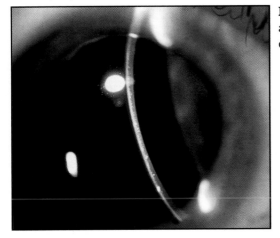

Figure 5C-6. Narrow slit view of the eye 6 months after retreatment. No noticeable corneal thinning is detected.

Figure 5C-7. At the upper temporal corneal periphery, three concentric lines can be detected. Superiorly to inferiorly, these are: the linear scarring at the site of the cut (see small arrow), the borders of the second flap (see big arrow), the borders of the diagonal ablation (see arrowheads).

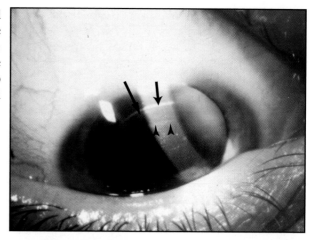

Figure 5C-8. View of the upper temporal periphery of the corneal surface on retroillumination. The same three zones can be easily distinguished. Additionally, a few striae radiating from the hinge can be detected (see small arrow).

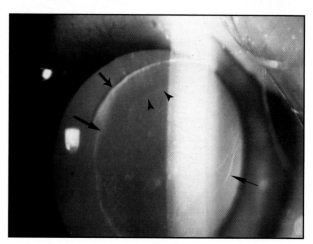

Figure 5C-9. Corneal topography at the sixth postoperative month shows a slight shifting of the ablation zone inferiorly. This alteration corresponds with the partial reverse of the relaxing effect of the arcuate cut with time. The latter is caused by the normal healing process that results in sealing the cut.

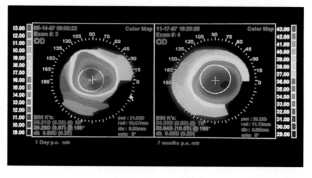

Editor's Notes

It is important to remember that LASIK is a very frightening and anxiety provoking experience for the patients. They are undergoing a bilateral procedure that will change their vision for life. They have just completed a consent form, which outlines the various complications that can occur. Many of these patients are young and therefore they have very high energy levels. They have spent a considerable amount of money on LASIK. Finally, many of the patients have decided to have LASIK because they are contact lens intolerant so their eyes are sensitive, and therefore difficult eyes to work with. It is no wonder that some patients are anxious before LASIK!

While approximately 1 in 10 patients will be quite nervous and tense, about 1 in 50 patients will be so anxious that this should result in some type of adjustment in the actual procedure. If a patient is so nervous that they are having difficulty controlling their head position and the position of their body, I generally elect to stop the procedure and discuss the situation with the patient with additional reassurances to provide a calming effect. I will also give them a little more sedation. Finally, I will arrange for a family member to come in to the laser room and hold the patient's hand during LASIK so that they will have additional support.

If a patient becomes emotional during the procedure, it is best to stop at that point. The most convenient time to stop is in between the right and the left eye. While most patients find the first eye reassuring and therefore the second eye is much easier, some patients find that the prolonged experience of having both eyes done is a little too much for one sitting. In this rare situation it is best to stop, allow the right eye to settle down and allow the patient to relax. Usually within an hour they are calm enough to come back and have the left eye done.

It is crucial in these situations that the patient understands that they are in control. This is an elective procedure, not an emergency, therefore it does not need to be performed at any particular time. I make it clear to the patients that my primary concern is that they are comfortable so that I can perform the procedure to the absolute best of my ability. If at any time they feel that they are too nervous or uncomfortable, we can stop. Empowering the patient with this knowledge often gives them the confidence and strength needed to move forward.

This patient also illustrates the difficulty in dealing with an eccentric ablation. Although the authors presented a successful technique which involves using an astigmatic ablation with arcuate cuts, this technique is difficult. While not available at the time of this case presentation, topography-assisted LASIK would be the best potential option for this problem.

CASE D, LASER MALFUNCTION

Charlotte Burns, OD, MS, and Louis E. Probst, MD

Main Concern: Partial Ablation
Patient Age: 26

INITIAL PREOPERATIVE INFORMATION

	OD	OS	COMMENTS
Preoperative refraction	-4.50 – 1.00 X 075	-4.50 – 1.00 X 075	
BCVA	20/20	20/20	
Topography Details	normal	normal	
SimK Values	42.12/42.87 X 028	41.62/42.12 X 070	
Pachymetry	573 μm	563 μm	

PROCEDURES PERFORMED

	OD	OS	COMMENTS
1. Date/type	3/6/98 LASIK	3/6/98 LASIK	laser malfunction OU
Laser/keratome/plate	VISX Star/ACS/200	VISX Star/ACS/200	
2. Date/type		3/20/98 LASIK enhancement	
Laser/keratome/plate		VISX Star/lifted flap	
3. Date/type	6/5/98 LASIK enhancement		
Laser/keratome/plate	VISX Star/lifted flap		

CURRENT POSTOPERATIVE INFORMATION

	OD	OS	COMMENTS
Time Postoperative	1 year	1 year	excellent outcome
Postoperative Refraction	plano	-0.25 DS	
BCVA	20/20	20/20	
Topography Details	central flattening	central flattening	
Refractive Correction	none	none	

A 26-year-old male presented for LASIK on March 6, 1998. His twin brother also had surgery the same day. His presenting prescription was -4.50 – 1.00 X 075 OD and OS, with BCVA of 20/20 OD and OS. Topography was normal (Figure 5D-1), and pachymetry readings were 573 μm OD and 563 μm OS. The LASIK surgery was uneventful until the laser was applied for each eye. The laser was applied to the OD, but did not sound as if it was operating normally, and then shut down with 4 seconds left. The procedure was aborted after about half of the laser application OS. The VISX Star laser displayed a fluence error on the screen. We were unable to complete the procedure.

Three weeks later, the patient's refraction was -0.75 – 2.25 X 076 OD, and -2.25 – 1.50 X 085 OS with 20/20 BCVA OU. Topography indicated reasonably well-centered ablations (Figure 5D-2). An enhancement was performed on the OS only, with the full cycloplegic prescription programmed. Since the full laser treatment had been applied to the OD (except for the last 4 seconds), we wanted to wait 3 months to enhance. We also wanted to review the results OS before proceeding with the OD.

At 3 months postoperative the OS refraction was plano with an UCVA of 20/20. An enhancement was performed on the OD at this time. The result at one month was plano OD with 20/20 acuity. The topography found a well-centered regular ablation. At 1 year postoperative, the OD is still plano, 20/20, and the OS is -0.25 DS, 20/20.

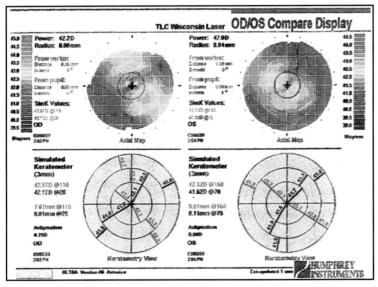

Figure 5D-1. Preoperative topography indicates a reasonably regular pattern OU.

Figure 5D-2. Topography prior to enhance OD demonstrating well-centered ablation after enhancement OS and slightly irregular decentered pattern OD.

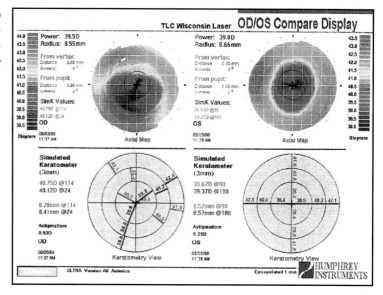

Editor's Notes

This case illustrates the rather unusual situation of laser failure during the excimer ablation. Following this case, the VISX technician was called and the laser was fully evaluated. A wire had come loose within the machine during the ablation, which had resulted in a sudden reduction of the fluence. Out of the 18,000 excimer laser procedures that I have performed, this is the only time that the laser has actually shut down in the middle of a procedure.

Prior to this case, the fluence was tested and found to be in normal range. An EXACT test plate was also used to test the beam homogeneity and this was found to be even and symmetrical. Approximately 20 procedures had been performed on this day prior to this case in which the laser had worked perfectly normally. On the following day, all these patients had achieved the normal predicted results. Therefore, this problem was unpredictable and unavoidable.

When the VISX laser is working properly and there is an inadvertent shut down from a power failure, the laser can be restarted and will restart the ablation where it prematurely ended. Unfortunately in this case, the laser was malfunctioning so this was not possible.

Despite this rather disconcerting problem, the patient's final visual result was excellent. We cautiously retreated each eye separately, waiting for refractive stability to ensure that we would achieve the optimum result on the second enhancement procedure.

CASE E, CENTRAL ISLAND

James D. Ferguson, OD, and Louis E. Probst, MD

Main Concern: Central Island
Patient Age: 47

INITIAL PREOPERATIVE INFORMATION

	OD	OS	COMMENTS
Preoperative Refraction	-3.00 – 1.25 X 005	-1.50 – 1.25 X 010	
BCVA	20/20	20/20	
Topography Details	normal astigmatic bow-tie formations OU		

PROCEDURES PERFORMED

	OD	OS	COMMENTS
1. Date/type	1/30/98 bilateral LASIK		persistent central
Laser/keratome/plate	VISX Star/ACS/180		island
2. Date/type		5/18/98 LASIK	
Laser/keratome/plate		central island/217/flap lifted	
3. Date/type		8/14/98 LASIK	
		central island formation	
Laser/keratome/plate		VISX Star/flap lifted	
4. Date/type		11/13/98 island correction,	
Laser/keratome/plate		VISX Star/flap lifted	

CURRENT POSTOPERATIVE INFORMATION

	OD	OS	COMMENTS
Time Postoperative		17 months	persistent island
Postoperative Refraction	-0.75 – 0.50 X 080	+1.25 – 1.00 X 032	
BCVA	20/20	20/20	
Topography Details	central flattening	island	
SimK Values	42.04/41.71	43.36/41.27	
Pachymetry	608 µm	513 µm	
Visual Complaints	none	blur	
Medications	none	none	
Refractive Correction	spectacles	spectacles	

This 47-year-old male underwent an uncomplicated bilateral LASIK procedure in January of 1998. Preoperatively, the corneal topography indicated mild irregular astigmatism OU (Figure 5E-1). Postoperatively he presented with complaints of ghosting and blur in the left eye (UCVA 20/30, BCVA 20/20 +1.50 −1.50 x 050). The right eye was essentially unremarkable and the patient was quite pleased with the result in the right eye. Refraction of the left eye showed a hyperopic astigmatic correction. Topographical analysis revealed a central island of 3 mm diameter (Figure 5E-2).

Four months postoperative, the patient was complaining of blur and ghosting in the left eye. The central island was persistent (which is not unusual in LASIK islands) (Figure 5E-3). The refractive error OS was +1.50 −1.50 X 050 20/20. The patient was quite anxious and his patience was running short.

A central island (-2.50 D, diameter 3 mm, VISX PRK program) treatment was done under the flap at 4 months postoperatively in the left eye without complications.

One day post-island treatment, the patient showed a residual island of approximately 2.00 D. UCVA declined once again (20/60). The patient was again educated as to the possibility of loss of BCVA and he was monitored closely.

Eight days post-island treatment, the central island increased to 4.00 D in height since the last treatment. The ghosting and blur was still pervasive subjectively. UCVA was 20/60 again but improved with a spectacle correction of OS +1.00 − 1.00 X 180 20/20. The patient was educated again, as we needed to wait for stabilization.

Eleven weeks post-island treatment, UCVA was measured at OS 20/70. BCVA was measured at OS +1.00 − 1.00 X 180 20/20. The topography indicated a decentered central island (Figure 5E-4). A hyperopic/astigmatic treatment was performed and reduced the SRX to +0.25 − 1.50 X 070 20/20. However, the central island persisted.

Nine months postoperatively (from the initial procedure) the patient demonstrated a persistent central island with complaints of ghosting and decreased acuity (-0.25 − 1.75 X 032 20/30). Since the island had increased to 5.00 D in height (Fig 5E-5), another island treatment was instituted. Again, -1.50 D to the central 3 mm zone.

One day post-central island treatment 3, the patient showed a decrease in the island to 3.00D (Fig 5E-6) with only a slight improvement in UCVA 20/60 and a decrease in BCVA (+1.00 − 1.75 X 035 20/25). An Orbscan was also performed to confirm that a central divot had not been formed by the repeated island treatment (Fig 5E-7). Since the last treatment, the island has yet again increased in magnitude to 5.00 D and the patient's symptoms remain the same. Another central island treatment will be attempted.

Persistent central island formations are common in LASIK patients. Unlike PRK central islands, LASIK islands do not tend to decrease in magnitude without treatment. This patient has quite an uncommon presentation of persistent islands. Fortunately, his cornea was thick enough to accommodate the multiple treatments. These patients need education and reassurance during stabilization. Both the comanaging doctor and the surgeon need to communicate the need for time and stabilization to the patient.

Central island formation is the most common topographical postoperative complication in LASIK. Many of the new excimer laser software packages include pretreatment programming to prevent such an episode. With improved surgical technique and proper pretreatment they can be prevented. Patients with central islands tend to complain of blur, distortions and ghosting out of proportion to clinical findings. They will present with reasonable acuities that can be corrected with a disproportionate amount of myopic and/or astigmatic correction (atypically hyperopic astigmatic corrections can be found). Topographical analysis is the gold standard for diagnosing central islands. Topographically they will appear as a central steepening of approximately 2 to 3 mm in diameter with a flattened surrounding area. The topographical printout will demonstrate a red 2 to 3 mm zone surrounded by a lake of blue or green.

Treatment of central island formations is focused on flattening the 2 to 3mm central cornea. Use the Munnerlyn formula: (depth of ablation = diameter^2 X diopter correction <height of the island>)/3.

However, a rule of thumb is to double pretreat in the 3 mm ablation zone and then perform one-half of the refractive error.

Figure 5E-1. Mild irregular astigmatism OU was seen preoperatively.

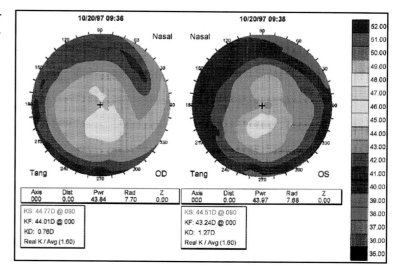

Figure 5E-2. A central island was evident on topography OS.

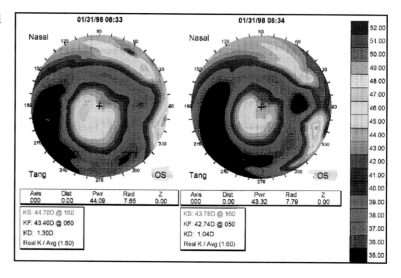

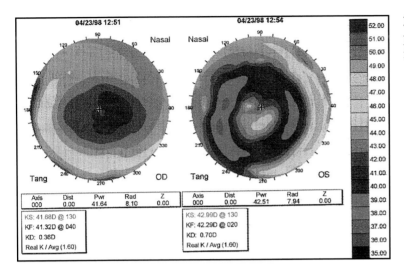

Figure 5E-3. Four months postoperatively the central island is persistent OS.

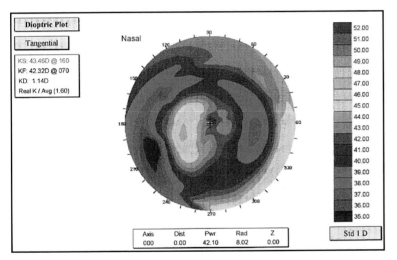

Figure 5E-4. Three months after the treatment of the central island with little improvement.

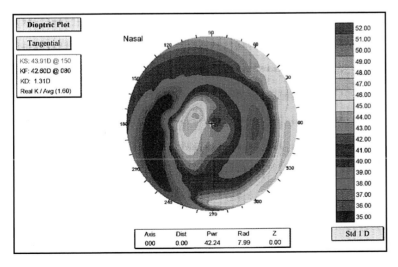

Figure 5E-5. Nine months after initial LASIK, the central island is still persistent despite treatment of the island and astigmatism with hyperopia.

Figure 5E-6. Third treatment of central island is not successful.

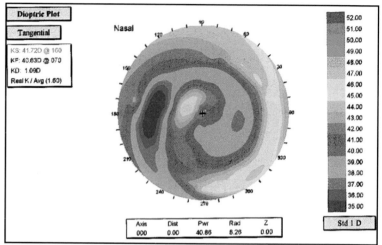

Figure 5E-7. Orbscan confirms persistent central steepening OD.

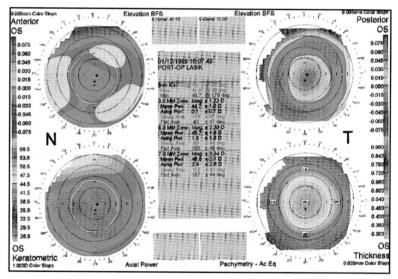

Editor's Notes

This patient illustrates some of the difficulties that can be encountered when trying to treat central islands. The patient had a small central island in the visual axis of the right eye, which had occurred after the primary procedure by the referring surgeon. This island had three retreatments with excimer laser applied in the central area, however, the island continues to persist. Because a central corneal divot can occasionally be mistaken for a central island on topography, the existence of the central island was confirmed with an Orbscan image of the right cornea.

When treating central islands, the height of the island in microns can be calculated by the Munnerlyn formula. The depth and diameter of the ablation can be set with a PTK card in the VISX laser. It is important not to overtreat central islands, as a large corneal divot could be created that would be difficult to correct and would induce significant hyperopia. Therefore, a conservative approach is appropriate. In this case, however the conservative approach resulted in unsuccessful result after three treatments of the central island. At this point we are waiting for the refraction to stabilize so that additional central island treatment can be performed.

6

EPITHELIAL INGROWTH

EPITHELIAL INGROWTH - SUMMARY NOTES

Clinical

Significant epithelial ingrowth requiring removal has been reported in 1.7% of LASIK eyes, however, refinements in LASIK with delicate preservation of the corneal epithelium have reduced this incidence to less than 0.5%. Epithelial ingrowth can occur in a number of patterns including lines, speckles, nest of pearls, strands, or sheets. Epithelial ingrowth that is significant and persistent will often result in a peripheral flap edge melt.

Identification of Epithelial Ingrowth

TEST	FINDING
tangential slit lamp illumination	white to gray material under flap
fluorescein staining	pooling at the flap edge
corneal topography	surface irregularities
retroillumination	margins of sheets of ingrowth

Risk Factors for Epithelial Ingrowth

- preoperative risk factors
- ABMD
- a history of recurrent corneal erosions
- advanced age
- a history of ingrowth in the other eye
- postoperative risk factors
- epithelial defects
- flap edema
- inflammation
- repeat LASIK
- flap slippage

Management

Jeffery J. Machat, MD, has devised a practical grading system for epithelial ingrowth that guides the management. Indications for treatment of epithelial ingrowth following LASIK include greater than 2 mm of ingrowth from the flap edge, documented progression, associated flap melting, or a disturbance of BCVA which can be attributed to the ingrowth.

Machat Epithelial Ingrowth Classification

GRADE 1: thin ingrowth, 1 to 2 cells thick, limited to within 2 mm of flap edge, transparent, difficult to detect, well delineated white line along advancing edge, no associated flap changes, non-progressive
  No retreatment required.

GRADE 2: thicker ingrowth, discreet cells evident within nest, at least 2 mm from the flap edge, individual cells are translucent, easily seen on slit-lamp, no demarcation line along nest, corneal flap edge rolled or gray, no flap edge melting or erosion, usually progressive

Requires nonurgent treatment within 2 to 3 weeks.

GRADE 3: pronounced ingrowth, several cells thick, greater than 2 mm from flap edge, ingrowth areas opaque, obvious on slit lamp, white geographic areas of necrotic epithelial cells with no demarcation line, corneal flap margins rolled with thickened whitish-gray appearance. Progression results in large areas of flap melting from collagenase release from the necrotic epithelium. Confluent haze develops peripheral to the flap edge as the flap pulls away leaving exposed stromal bed in contact with surface epithelium

Urgent treatment required with close follow-up, as recurrences are more common due to the altered flap edges.

Operative Technique for Removing Epithelial Ingrowth
- the edge of the corneal flap is marked at the slit lamp
- peripheral cornea alignment markings are placed
- the flap is then slowly dissected free at its temporal margin
- the flap is gently folded over its nasal hinge
- epithelium removed from underneath the flap
- peeling
- scraping
- irrigating
- epithelium is removed from the stromal side of the cap
- any epithelium hanging in the peripheral stromal bed is gently pushed back
- the flap is then replaced (as in primary LASIK)
- thorough irrigation is done underneath the cap to eliminate residual epithelial cells

Prevention
Epithelial ingrowth is avoided by eliminating epithelial defects with LASIK. Patients who will loose epithelium, such as those with ABMD, are best treated with PRK. Topical anesthesia should be used sparingly to avoid any epithelial toxicity. All surgical maneuvers should be performed with great delicacy in order to avoid any epithelial trauma.

CASE A, EPITHELIAL INGROWTH TREATED WITH ALCOHOL

Eric J. Linebarger, MD, David R. Hardten, MD, and Richard L. Lindstrom, MD

Main Concern: Epithelial Ingrowth
Patient Age: 51

INITIAL PREOPERATIVE INFORMATION

	OD	OS	COMMENTS
Preoperative Refraction	n/a		
UCVA	20/40		
Topography Details	peninsula		
SimK Values	n/a		
Pachymetry	n/a		

PROCEDURES PERFORMED

	OD	OS	COMMENTS
1. Date/type	removal of ingrowth		
Laser/keratome/plate			

CURRENT POSTOPERATIVE INFORMATION

	OD	OS	COMMENTS
Time Postoperative	1 week		
Postoperative Refraction	plano		
UCVA	20/20		
Topography Details	symmetrical		
SimK Values	n/a		
Visual Complaints	haloes		
Medications	none		

A 51-year-old male who underwent bilateral LASIK 2 months previous, presented for second opinion regarding ongoing halos and blurred vision in his right eye. The patient reported that his initial surgery was complicated by an epithelial defect at the time of treatment.

UCVA was 20/40- in the right eye with ghosting images, and no significant improvement on manifest refraction. UCVA in the left eye was 20/20.

Slit lamp examination of the right eye revealed a nasally hinged LASIK flap, with a whirled, putty-like membrane at the superior flap junction near the 1 o'clock position extending toward the visual axis approximately 3 mm (Figure 6A-1). An additional finger-like projection was noted at the 10 o'clock position. Careful inspection revealed this membrane to be in the lamellar interface. Slit lamp examination of the left eye revealed a well-positioned LASIK flap free of interface cells or debris. There were occasional maps and microcysts present in the surface epithelium.

Corneal topography of the right eye revealed a central peninsula encroaching on the visual axis with irregular astigmatism (Figure 6A-2).

This case illustrates a classic presentation of epithelial ingrowth, an infrequent but vision compromising complication of LASIK surgery.[1] Patients with epithelial defects at the time of surgery, particularly those associated with ABMD, are at increased risk of this complication. Findings of ABMD can be exceedingly subtle, and often missed on preoperative slit lamp examination. A loose, baggy epithelium, often accentuated by preoperative topical anesthetic, can be easily torn as the microkeratome makes its pass across the corneal surface. While the defect will frequently heal spontaneously, the irregular epithelial edge serves as a stimulus for abnormal cell growth into the lamellar interface.

The patient often has good visual acuity early in the postoperative course. As the cells migrate centrally into the flap interface, the patient will begin to notice worsening acuity and ghosting images. This usually occurs between 4 and 8 weeks postoperatively, although it may occur even later. Careful slit lamp examination with attention to the flap edges, as well as topography, can aide in making the diagnosis and instituting prompt intervention. While the majority of eyes will do well if identified and treated early, peripheral corneal melting has been reported in cases of extensive epithelial ingrowth resulting in compromised visual outcome.[2]

Several treatment strategies have been proposed to effectively deal with lamellar epithelial ingrowth, each with similar rates of success.[3,4] In general, treatment should consist of relifting the flap and removing the epithelium. This will frequently come off in a sheet, although paying meticulous attention to removing all cellular remnants on the flap bed, undersurface of the cap, and interface gutters is crucial to prevent recurrence. The authors have found that applying a solution of absolute alcohol (100% ethanol) can be used as an adjunct to prevent cellular regrowth and recurrence in particularly problematic cases.[3]

The patient underwent lifting of the LASIK flap, with manual scraping of the epithelial ingrowth with a bladed PRK spatula. Both the bed and undersurface of the cap were completely denuded of all epithelial remnants. The area was then treated with a solution of absolute alcohol soaked in a merocel sponge for approximately 30 seconds. The flap was then replaced and floated in to position with BSS. It was then allowed to dry for several minutes prior to removing the lid speculum. Postoperatively, the patient was placed on a regimen of ocuflox (Allergan Pharmaceuticals, Irvine, Calif) and FML (Allergan Pharmaceuticals, Irvine, Calif), which was tapered over 2 months.

At the 1 week postoperative visit, the patient's UCVA had improved to 20/20- in the right eye. At the 3 month visit, he had retained his 20/20- visual acuity, but noticed some occasional haloes in dim light conditions. Slit lamp examination revealed scant lamellar haze superiorly, but no recurrence of epithelial ingrowth (Figure 6A-3). His topography had normalized considerably (Figure 6A-4).

References

1. Helena MC, Meisler D, Wilson SE. Epithelial growth within the lamellar interface after laser in-situ keratomileusis (LASIK). *Cornea.* 1997;16:300-305.

2. Castillo A, Dias-Valle D, Gutierrez AR, Toledano N, Romero F. Peripheral melt of flap after laser in situ keratomileusis. *J Refract Surg.* 1998;14:61-63.

3. Hardten DR, Lindstrom RL. Management of LASIK complications. *Oper Tech in Cataract and Refract Surg.* 1998;1:32-39.

4. Lim JS, Kim EK, Lee JB, Lee JH. A simple method for the removal of epithelium grown beneath the hinge after LASIK. *Yonsei Medical Journal.* 1998;39:236-239.

Figure 6A-1. Epithelial ingrowth 2 months post-LASIK.

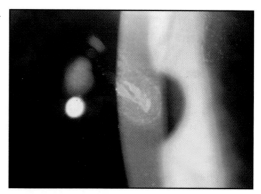

Figure 6A-2. Topography showing irregular astigmatism.

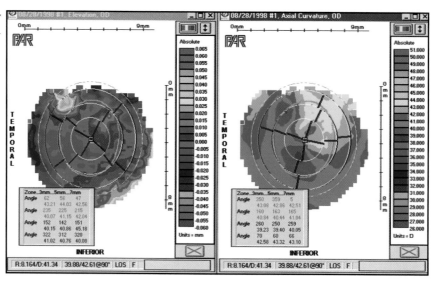

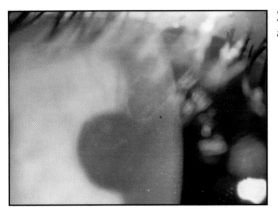

Figure 6A-3. Appearance 3 months after lifting and debriding flap.

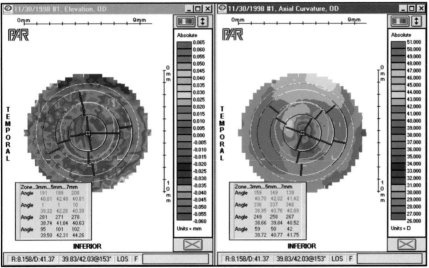

Figure 6A-4. Topography 3 months after lifting and debridement.

Editor's Notes

Epithelial ingrowth used to be a relatively common complication of LASIK, occurring in up to 2% of cases. Over the last several years, the incidence of epithelial ingrowth has declined significantly. This is in part due to the improvement in the technique of LASIK with the goal to preserve the integrity and health of the corneal epithelium. The absolute minimum topical anaesthetic is used to avoid corneal toxicity. Lubrication is used during the microkeratome cut and careful attention is paid to the epithelium during the procedure. Patients are instructed to keep their eyes closed and given lubricants to use post-LASIK, all in order to preserve the epithelium and minimize any epithelial defects that can occur. Any epithelial defects that do occur will result in epithelial healing that will increase the risk of epithelial ingrowth.

Preoperatively, any patients with a history of recurrent corneal erosions should be carefully evaluated for any signs of anterior basement membrane dystrophy. Older patients tend to have a greater incidence of epithelial ingrowth. Patients who have had previous radial keratotomy or other corneal surgical procedures also have a greater risk.

Another reason for the decrease in the incidence of epithelial ingrowth may be related to the quality of the LASIK flap. The older suction units used on the ACS machine provided less powerful suction with readings in the range of 24 mmHg. This would result in an elevation in the IOP sufficient to achieve a corneal flap, however insufficient to achieve a sharp flap edge that could serve as a barrier to epithelial ingrowth. My personal experience with this situation illustrates this problem. When using the Technolas 217 Laser, which comes equipped with its own new suction unit, we have had a very low incidence of epithelial ingrowth. We have had a similar experience with the Hansatome that comes with a new suction unit designed for this machine. When we recently obtained another excimer laser, we used our older suction base unit that was approximately 2 years old. Suddenly we noticed an increase in the incidence of epithelial ingrowth for the LASIK cases performed with the older suction base unit. Therefore any suction unit suspected to have low levels of suction should be serviced to ensure that the suction levels are appropriate.

CASE B, GRADE 3 EPITHELIAL INGROWTH

Ted Smith, OD, and Jeffery J. Machat, MD

Main Concern: Grade 3 Ingrowth
Patient Age: 41

INITIAL PREOPERATIVE INFORMATION

	OD	OS	COMMENTS
Preoperative Refraction	-6.00 – 2.50 X 27		
UCVA	20/cf@1ft		
BCVA	20/20-		
Topography Details	44.37/42.25 X 28		
SimK Values	0.51		
Pachymetry	632 μm		

PROCEDURES PERFORMED

	OD	OS	COMMENTS
1. Date/type	03/02/99 LASIK		uncomplicated
Laser/keratome/plate	LaserSight LSX/ACS/180		
2. Date/type	04/08/99		
Laser/keratome/plate	lift/ingrowth		

CURRENT POSTOPERATIVE INFORMATION

	OD	OS	COMMENTS
Time Postoperative	2 weeks		post lift/ingrowth
Postoperative Refraction	+0.25 – 0.75 X 120		
UCVA	20/25+		
BCVA	20/20-		
Topography Details	39.37/38.37 X 034		on lift/ingrowth day
SimK Values	2.98		
Pachymetry	580 μm		
Visual Complaints	none		
Medications	none		
Refractive Correction	none		

This patient was a 41-year-old white female with an unremarkable medical history. Her surgical history consisted of bilateral LASIK performed on March 4, 1999, in attempt for full correction of OD -6.00 – 2.50 X 27, and monocorrection OS -6.75 – 2.00 X 165. Preoperative BCVAs were 20/20 OU. Topography showed smooth, regular corneas with cylinder corresponding to the spectacle refraction (Figure 6B-1). The procedure was performed using a Chiron ACS keratome and the Lasersight LSX LaserSight Technologies, Inc., Orlando, Fla) for ablation. Both procedures were uncomplicated. At 1 week postoperative, this patient showed a manifesting *Rx* of OD -0.50 – 0.50 X 120, with unaided and corrected acuities of 20/40 and 20/20- respectively. The left eye showed an *Rx* of -0.50 – 1.00 X 125 with UCVA 20/40- and BCVA 20/25. The inferior of the right cornea showed a 1.5 mm invasion of epithelial ingrowth from 4 o'clock to 8 o'clock along the flap edge. It was left untreated to monitor progression.

At 4 weeks postoperatively, the patient was referred to our center because the ingrowth OD had progressed 2.5 mm inward from the inferior flap edge (Figure 6B-2). Topography showed K values of 39.37/38.37 X 34 with a CIM value of 2.98 (Figure 6B-3). Pachymetry showed a central corneal thickness of 580 µm. The flap was subsequently lifted and the ingrowth scraped. A small 2.5 mm epithelial defect was left in the region of the previous ingrowth. A bandage contact lens was not indicated. A regimen of Inflamase Forte Q1h and Ocuflox q.i.d. was prescribed as per standard LASIK postoperative care.

At 2 weeks post-lift and ingrowth removal, no reoccurrence of ingrowth was noted. The epithelial defect was essentially healed with only slight roughening visible. Unaided acuity was 20/25- with a manifest *Rx* of +0.25 – 0.75 X 20 giving 20/20-. The patient was given artificial tears prn for comfort and to encourage epithelial healing.

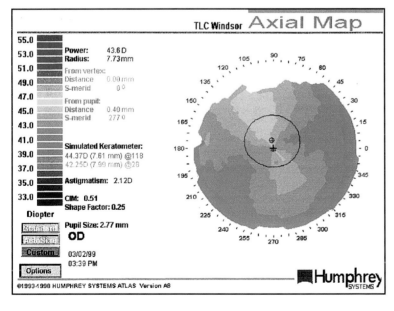

Figure 6B-1. Preoperative topography OD demonstrates a regular pattern.

Figure 6B-2. Grade 3 epithelial ingrowth.

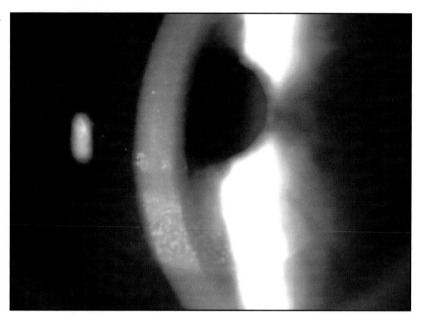

Figure 6B-3. Postoperative topography OD shows a well-centered slightly irregular ablation.

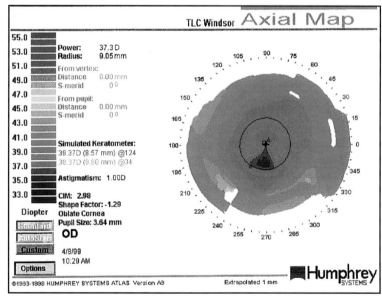

Editor's Notes

Epithelial ingrowth is generally a fairly innocuous condition that can be effectively treated without altering compromising the outcome. A typical case of epithelial ingrowth generally occurs 1 week to 3 months following the original procedure. Patients should be followed closely after the removal of the epithelial ingrowth to ensure that it does not reoccur.

This case illustrates a typical temporal sequence for epithelial ingrowth with the first appearance at 1 week, with progression over 4 weeks postoperatively.

CASE C, EPITHELIAL INGROWTH THROUGH BOWMAN'S LAYER RENT
John Doane, MD

Main Concerns: Corneal Stromal Melt, Irregular Astigmatism, and Lost Lines of BCVA
Patient Age: 43

INITIAL PREOPERATIVE INFORMATION

	OD	OS	COMMENTS
Preoperative Refraction		-5.50 + 1.25 x 003	
BCVA		20/20	
Topography Details		normal	
SimK Values		45.5@180/45.37@090	
Other			tight fissure squeezer

PROCEDURES PERFORMED

	OD	OS	COMMENTS
1. Date/type		2/11/97 LASIK	referring center
Laser/keratome/plate		VISX Star/ACS/160	
2. Date/type		5/9/97 removal of epithelial ingrowth	referring center
3. Date/type		7/24/97 removal of epithelial ingrowth	referring center
4. Date/type		11/5/97 removal of epithelial ingrowth	referring center
5. Date/type		Doane sees 1/19/98	
6. Date/type		1/28/98 removal of epithelial ingrowth	
7. Date/type		2/12/98 removal of epithelial ingrowth	
8. Date/type		3/4/98 flap removed	
9. Date/type		1/18/99 LASIK	
Laser/keratome/plate		VISX S2/Hansatome/160	

CURRENT POSTOPERATIVE INFORMATION

	OD	OS	COMMENTS
Time Postoperative		2 months	excellent final outcome
Postoperative Refraction		+0.50 + 0.50 X 123	
BCVA		20/30+1	
Topography Details		regular	
SimK Values		42.75@120/41.37@030	
Visual Complaints or Medications		none	
Refractive Correction		none	

This 43-year-old Caucasian female presented with a complicated history OS after bilateral LASIK. She was referred after the initial surgeon was unable to cure recurrent episodes of epithelial ingrowth in the left eye despite valiant efforts. In February 1997, she underwent bilateral LASIK with the Bausch and Lomb ACS and VISX Star excimer laser targeting plano OD and -1.5 OS. Her preoperative refractive error of the left eye was -5.5 + 1.25 X 003 for 20/20 visual acuity. Her simulated keratometry values on topography of OS were 45.5@180/45.37@090 (Figure 6C-1). Anatomically she did have relatively tight eyelid fissures and was prone to eyelid squeezing. Approximately 3 months after her original surgery her flap was lifted for inferior epithelial ingrowth. Epithelial ingrowth recurred in the same location after two more attempts to lift the flap and actively remove the epithelial ingrowth process.

The patient presented to me on January 19, 1998. Her UCVA was 20/200, which improved to 20/50+ with -1.5 + 3.25 X 167. Frank epithelial ingrowth was seen (Figure 6C-2a and b). Topography revealed inferior flattening and irregularity on photokeratoscope view was suggestive of corneal flap stromal loss from melting (Figure 6C-3 and 6C-4). The flap was lifted on January 28, 1998, and the epithelial cells were removed. At the conclusion of the case no epithelial cells were evident in the interface. Careful attention to the stromal bed, gutter edge, and back surface of flap were maintained to make certain no cells were present. No alcohol was used.

On January 29, 1998, 24 hours later, her UCVA in the left eye was 20/400, which improved to 20/40 with a refraction of -5 D. Small retroillumination Bowman's folds were noted. On February 9, 1998, the patient's UCVA was 20/100, which improved to 20/60+ with -4.0 + 3.75 X 165. An island of epithelial cells was noted in same location as on presentation. No epithelial demarcation line was present that would suggest the gutter as the source of ingrowth.

On February 12, 1998, a second lift and scrape was attempted by myself. On lifting the flap the area of ingrowth was firmly adherent in almost a "tendinous fashion" to the stromal bed. There was no peripheral connection of epithelial cells to the gutter. At this point I was fairly certain that the ingrowth had come from a rent in the anterior stroma and Bowman's layer, allowing basal epithelial cells to track through this rent into the interface. A history of difficulty lifting from the primary surgeon and having seen a similar case prior led me to this assumption. On the first and fifth postoperative days no epithelial cells were present at the original location. On the 13th day after my second attempt at epithelial removal, the patient's UCVA was 20/50 and then improved to 20/25 with a refraction of -1.25 + 3.75 X 002. Slit lamp examination again revealed epithelial cyst formation in the original location.

On March 4, 1998, approximately 3 weeks after my second lift for epithelial removal, her UCVA was 20/50- which improved to 20/30 with a refraction of -1.25 + 3.5 X 180. Pachymetry was 505 μm. The cysts were increasing in size. At this point I recommended flap removal since it was obvious that this situation would progress and five previous attempts had failed to cure the problem. A second reason for removal was the irregular astigmatism induced by inferior flap stromal melting. At this point, removal of flap and lamellar graft could have been a consideration.

On March 11, 1998, the flap was removed with a 64-blade and the patient was placed on topical Polytrim, FML, and Ketorlac. A soft bandage contact lens was placed. Nine days after removal the UCVA was 20/60. FML was continued until August 24, 1998. At that time the UCVA was 20/100 and then improved to 20/25+ with a refraction of -5.0 + 4.5 X 090. Trace haze was noted on slit lamp examination. Pachymetry was 429 μm. The FML was stopped.

On January 18, 1999, UCVA was 20/100. Refraction revealed -5.50 + 5.50 x 090 for 20/25 acuity. Corneal topography revealed regular with-the-rule astigmatism (Figure 6C-5). Since there was sufficient stroma left, a repeat LASIK was completed on February 10, 1999, with the Bausch and Lomb Hansatome, 9.5 mm ring and 160 µm head. In my hands the Hansatome creates, on average, a flap thickness 75% of what was predicted. Therefore, I was certain I would leave more than 200 µm of posterior stroma after ablation. Corneal topography at 1 day and 1 month (Figures 6C-6 and 6C-7) revealed a regular surface and no distortion on photokeratoscopy. Two months postoperatively her UCVA is 20/30 and she refracts to 20/30+ with +0.5 + 0.5 X 123. Her uncorrected near vision is J2. She is not wearing glasses and is on no topical medications. She is extremely happy with her current visual status of the left eye and her binocular function overall.

Figure 6C-1. Topography of left eye revealing normal preoperative examination.

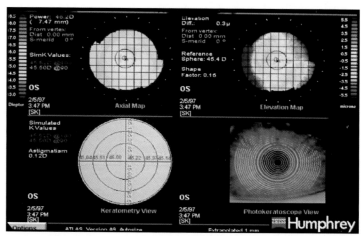

Figure 6C-2a. Direct slit lamp view. Note prominent islands of epithelial cells.

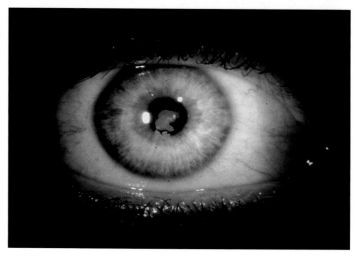

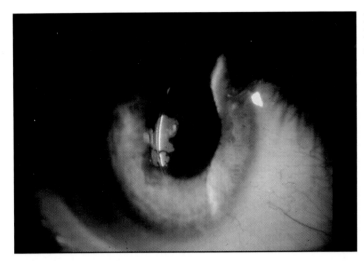

Figure 6C-2b. Oblique slit lamp view. Note prominent islands of epithelial cells.

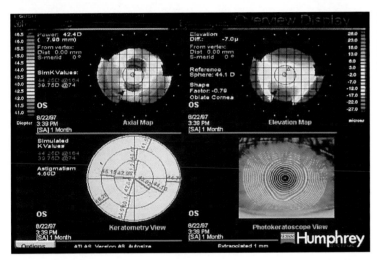

Figure 6C-3. Topography from prior visit revealing inferior flattening suggesting corneal flap stromal loss from melting.

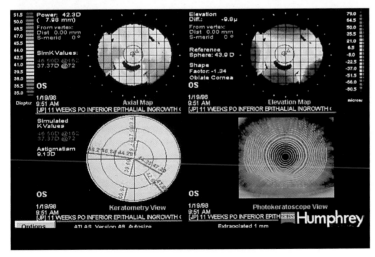

Figure 6C-4. Topography on initial visit of consulting physician revealed a similar picture to Figure 6C-3.

Figure 6C-5. Topography 10 months after flap removal revealing regular with-the-rule astigmatism.

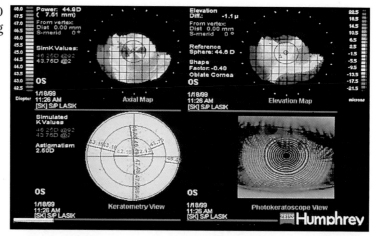

Figures 6C-6. Corneal topographies of the left eye 1 day after repeat LASIK (after flap removal 10 months prior). Note regular pattern and no distortion on photokeratoscopy.

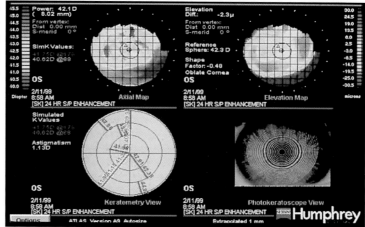

Figures 6C-7. Corneal topographies of the left eye 1 month after repeat LASIK (after flap removal 10 months prior). Note regular pattern and no distortion on photokeratoscopy.

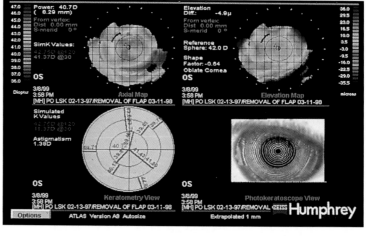

Editor's Notes

While there was no mention of ABMD, there is certainly a possible explanation for the recurrence of the ingrowth. The rent in Bowman's layer that allowed the epithelial cells to extend underneath the flap may have been caused by an unrecognized buttonhole flap. Perhaps this buttonhole flap was not complete and only extended to the epithelial layer. This allowed the epithelial layer to extend underneath the flap once altered by the enhancement procedures.

In this case, Dr. Doane achieved excellent results by removing the flap and then performing a LASIK enhancement. Another technique of removing central epithelial cells when the flap is weak, as with a buttonhole flap, is to make an incision in the primary flap and milk the epithelial cells out through the small incision.

It is fortunate that this patient had a regular astigmatism pattern that could be corrected with LASIK following flap removal. Unfortunately, many cases of irregular flaps have an irregular stromal bed. Once the flap is removed the patient develops an irregular astigmatism that cannot be effectively corrected with further LASIK procedures. Often there is associated loss of BCVA, along with distortion of the images, that requires a hard contact lens to correct.

CASE D, EPITHELIAL INGROWTH WITH LOSS OF TISSUE

Ioannis G. Pallikaris, MD, Theokliti Papadaki, MD, and Dimitrios S. Siganos, MD

Main Concern: Epithelial Ingrowth
Patient Age: 45

INITIAL PREOPERATIVE INFORMATION

	OD	OS	COMMENTS
Preoperative Refraction		-16.5 – 0.75 X 075	high myopia
BCVA		20/20	

PROCEDURES PERFORMED

	OD	OS	COMMENTS
1. Date/type		1995 M-LASIK	uncomplicated
Laser/keratome/plate		ACS/161	
2. Date/type		6 month postoperative ingrowth removal	

CURRENT POSTOPERATIVE INFORMATION

	OD	OS	COMMENTS
Time Postoperative		1 month	
Postoperative Refraction		+2.75 – 4.0 X 110	irregular astigmatism
BCVA		20/25	
Topography Details		20/25	
SimK Values		irregular	

A 45-year-old woman underwent LASIK in OS for the correction of -16.5 – 0.75 X 75. The BCVA was 20/20.

The ACS microkeratome was used to create a flap 8 mm wide and 161 μm thick. Apart from a small irregularity at the borders of the temporal edges of the flap, no other intraoperative complications were recorded.

The preoperative and 1 month postoperative topographic patterns are compared in Figure 6D-1. The wide, dark blue area corresponding to the ablation zone is inferotemporally decentered, while no irregularities within the ablation zone can be detected on this scale. On slit lamp examination (Figure 6D-2), interface accumulation of dense exogenic material was detected in two sites in the central and paracentral zones of the cornea. The patient experienced a loss of two lines in BCVA, which was 20/32 with a correction of +2.0 – 4.0 X 90.

At the third postoperative month, refraction remained stable, although on slit lamp examination, the central material seemed to be growing in size and density, while in the paracentral material, the cells tended to coalesce and melt (Figures 6D-3 and 6D-4).

Further deterioration in vision was detected at the sixth postoperative month interval. BCVA had reduced to 20/40 with a correction of +3.75 – 4.75 X 130. Slit lamp view of the cornea at 6 months is presented in Figure 6D-5. The change in corneal topography from 1 to 6 postoperative months is presented in Figure 6D-6. A steepening at the temporal half of the cornea was detected corresponding to the areas of material accumulation. Steepening was more prominent at the upper temporal quadrant, indicating the location of the growing focus.

In order to prevent further vision loss, we decided to remove the material. The flap was partially detached from the bed until the areas of accumulation were exposed. The exogenic material was then scraped away from the bed and the stromal side of the flap using the aspiration/irrigation cannula. Both surfaces were thoroughly irrigated with BSS, the flap was sealed back using dry air, and a bandage soft contact lens was applied. Microscopic examination of a smear taken from the material removed showed that the latter consisted mainly of dead epithelial cells.

The appearance of the cornea 4 days after retreatment is presented in Figure 6D-7. A mild opacification indicates the areas where the epithelial accumulations were located. The differential topographic map revealed a marked flattening of the area corresponding to the removed material and a simultaneous steepening of the opposite inferotemporal half of the cornea (Figure 6D-8).

For the first postoperative month after retreatment, the cornea retained normal clarity (Figure 6D-9), while BCVA was restored to 20/25 with a correction of +2.75 – 4.0 X 110.

Epithelial ingrowth at the outer edge of a hinged flap can be left undisturbed unless it induces irregular astigmatism, causes a flap melt, or extends centrally and affects visual acuity (at which time it should be removed).

Figure 6D-1. The differential map comparing preoperative to 1 month postoperative topographic patterns reveals an inferotemporal decentration of the ablation zone.

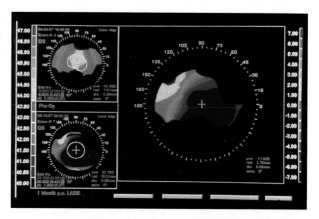

Figure 6D-2. On slit lamp examination, interface accumulation of dense exogenic material is detected in two sites in the central and paracentral zone of the cornea.

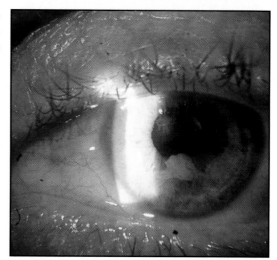

Figure 6D-3. In the third postoperative month, the central focus seems to be growing in size and density, while in the paracentral focus the cells tend to coalesce and melt.

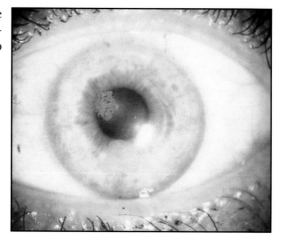

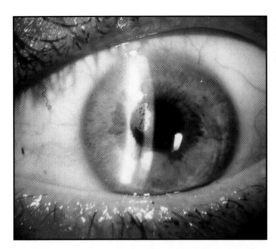

Figure 6D-4. Third postoperative month: narrow beam view reveals that the epithelial accumulation is located within the interface.

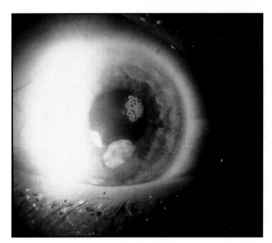

Figure 6D-5. Six months postoperatively: slit lamp view shows no further growth of the accumulation. On the contrary, the cells within the ingrowth seem to coalesce, forming a liquid mass demarcated by a surrounding groove.

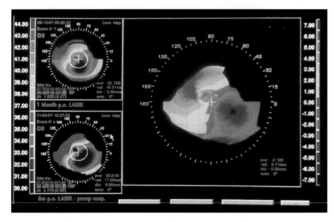

Figure 6D-6. On the difference map a steepening at the temporal half of the cornea is detected from 1 to 6 months postoperatively, corresponding to the areas of material accumulation.

Figure 6D-7. Four days after epithelial removal: a mild opacification just indicates the areas where the epithelial accumulations have been located.

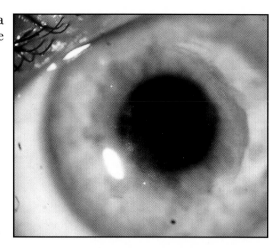

Figure 6D-8. The differential topographic map reveals a marked flattening of the area corresponding to the removed material and a simultaneous steepening of the opposite inferotemporal half of the cornea.

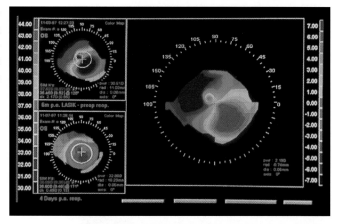

Figure 6D-9. In the first postoperative month after retreatment, the cornea appears clear at slit lamp examination.

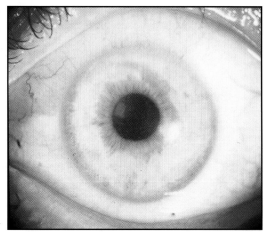

Editor's Notes

With the improved techniques of LASIK, epithelial ingrowth has become a much less common problem. Nevertheless, any case of epithelial ingrowth identified to be a progressive, or extending greater than 2 mm beyond the flap edge, should be treated immediately. Epithelial ingrowth that extends underneath the flap and is not treated will result in collagenase production from the hypoxic epithelial cells, which can result in stromal melting.

This case demonstrates the sequelae of epithelial ingrowth when it is not treated immediately. The epithelial ingrowth was removed after 6 months. This resulted in a loss of tissue in the area of the ingrowth and an irregular astigmatic pattern. If treated earlier, this irregularity of the cornea may have been avoided.

It is important to note that recurrence of epithelial ingrowth occurs in approximately 10% of cases, so patients should be followed weekly for a least 1 month after the removal of epithelial ingrowth to ensure that this problem does not reoccur.

CASE E, RECURRENT EPITHELIAL INGROWTH

Michael Lawless, MBBS, FRACO, FRACS, FRCOphth, Sue Webber, BSc(Hons), FRCOphth, and Gerard Sutton FRACO, FRACS

Main Concern: Epithelial Ingrowth
Patient Age: 33

INITIAL PREOPERATIVE INFORMATION

	OD	OS	COMMENTS
Preoperative Refraction	+2.5/-0.25 X 70	+3.25/-0.5 X 100	flat corneas, deep
BCVA	6/6	6/6	set eyes
Topography Details	regular spherical	small regular astigmatism	
SimK Values	40.76/41.05@94	41.10/41.56@54	
Pachymetry	n/a	n/a	

PROCEDURES PERFORMED

	OD	OS	COMMENTS
1. Date/type	12/16/97 M-LASIK		epithelial defect
Laser/keratome/plate	Summit Apex Plus/ACS/200		
2. Date/type	1/8/98 lifted LASIK flap and removed epithelial ingrowth		
3. Date/type	9/15/98 lifted LASIK flap and removed epithelial ingrowth		

CURRENT POSTOPERATIVE INFORMATION

	OD	OS	COMMENTS
Time Postoperative	6 weeks after last epithelial ingrowth removal		
Postoperative Refraction	+1.25/-1.75 X 100		
BCVA	6/7.5		
Topography Details	irregular astigmatism		
SimK Values	39.10/42.08@147		
Pachymetry	613 μm		
Visual Complaints	none		
Medications	none		
Refractive Correction	none		

This patient attended for correction of his hypermetropia. At initial assessment it was recognized that this patient had K readings lower than average (Figure 6E-1) and deep set eyes. In view of these findings, a 200 μm plate for the microkeratome was selected to reduce the chance of a buttonhole flap.

Immediately after the flap was cut, an epithelial defect was noted. It is our clinical impression that patients who sustain a perioperative epithelial defect are at higher risk of epithelial implantation. Therefore, one should take the opportunity to be particularly assiduous when cleaning and irrigating the flap interface. On the first postoperative day the epithelial defect persisted, however, by the third day it had healed, except for a small length at the flap edge. Clinical observation has suggested that delayed closure at the wound edge may portend the onset of epithelial ingrowth problems.

On the sixth day, early epithelial ingrowth was noted at the temporal edge of the flap. At this stage the topography shows a central regular astigmatism. However, 2 weeks later the area of ingrowth had increased, so the flap was lifted and the epithelium removed. Immediately postoperatively the cells appeared to regress. However, 6 weeks after the first epithelial ingrowth removal the cellular ingrowth appeared viable. Over the ensuing 3 months, the ingrowth seemed to stabilize and then improve. Despite some progression on topography (Figures 6E-2 and 6E-3) the patient's acuity corrected to 6/7.5, so we elected not to intervene.

However, at 29 weeks after ingrowth removal there was no longer any clinical improvement and the patient's spectacle acuity had dropped to 6/12. Two weeks later this had fallen to 6/15. Over the same period, the area of ingrowth appeared to be thickening (Figure 6E-4), as seen through localized steepening on the topography. At this stage, we elected to lift the flap again and remove the epithelial material (Figure 6E-5). Postoperatively the patient has regained a BCVA of 6/7.5, the topography has minor aberrations and the corneal appearance is much improved (Figure 6E-6).

This case highlights two points in the management of epithelial ingrowth; when to intervene, and how the epithelial cells might most effectively be removed. The answer to the first is perhaps the most difficult as we do not yet fully understand the mechanism of cell replication and survival. Clinically one can observe areas of epithelial implantation behaving quite differently to each other. On the one hand, there are some epithelial cell deposits in the flap interface that are isolated and do not change or grow. Yet, there are also other areas that spread and cause increasing irregular astigmatism. These differences in behavior may be explained by differences in cell type. Transient amplifying cells from deep in the epithelium may become dislodged at the time of the lamellar cut and these cells may have the potential for continued replication. Alternatively, surface epithelial cells may not have the genetic ability for continued cell multiplication and therefore will cause no clinical problem.

The key to deciding when to intervene is by careful observation of the ingrowth. When an increase in size can be demonstrated and it threatens the visual axis or it is causing an increase in irregular astigmatism, then its removal would be considered. Conversely, if the cells are forming a quiet, isolated, translucent, stable area away from the visual axis then perhaps it would be preferable not to intervene.

The procedure is performed at the operating microscope, preferably in sterile operating room conditions. The eye is anaesthetized with topical anaesthetic and the existing flap is lifted. We have found it useful to mark and weaken the flap edge beforehand at the slit lamp. This may be done by performing a series of epithelial perforations using an instrument such as a dialing hook. The patient is then taken to the operating room for the remainder of the procedure. The flap edge is lifted by insinuating a blunt pointed instrument. Once it has been achieved, a flat spatula may be used to elevate the remainder of the flap. The mechanism of ingrowth removal depends on the consistency of the material. Usually the epithelial cells form a sheet, which may be scraped or peeled off using a blunt hockey blade. However, the second time this procedure was performed on this patient the ingrowth material was like a viscous fluid. The ingrowth should be removed from both sides of the flap interface. The cap should be supported on a moist merocel sponge (Solan Ophthalmic Products, Jacksonville, Fla) when the underside of the flap is cleared. There is always a risk of residual cells regrowing, as occurred here. In an attempt to prevent this, adjunctive treatments have been used. Some surgeons apply a very light PTK to the areas involved and others apply alcohol in an attempt to lyse and kill any few remaining cells.

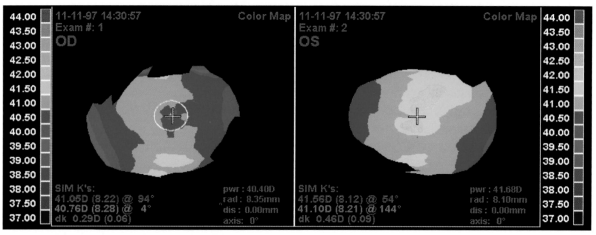

Figure 6E-1. Preoperative topography OU.

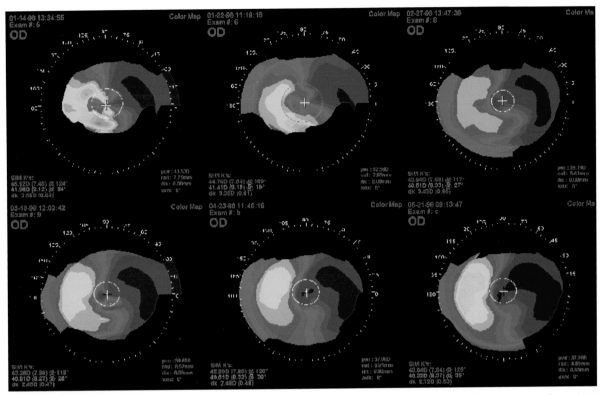

Figure 6E-2. Postoperative topography. All maps on an absolute scale of 1 D steps from 37 to 51 D. Mid-range = 44 D, green. (Top row a through c, bottom row d through f.)

a) One week after first epithelial ingrowth removal. The area of high power overlies the affected area.

b) Two weeks after epithelial ingrowth removal. Clinically the residual cells appeared to be clearing. Note the slight decrease in power of the temporal area compared to the previous week.

c) Seven weeks after epithelial ingrowth removal. Clinically the involved area appeared to have increased in size.

d) Nine weeks after epithelial ingrowth removal. Clinically the involved area appeared to be decreasing in size. The corrected acuity was 6/7.5.

e) Fifteen weeks after epithelial ingrowth removal. Area still decreasing in size clinically.

f) Nineteen weeks after epithelial ingrowth removal. Area becoming less opaque.

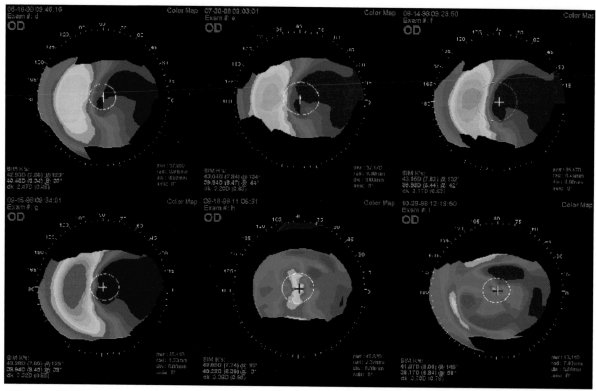

Figure 6E-3. Postoperative topography. All maps on an absolute scale of 1 D steps from 37 to 51 D. Mid-range = 44 D, green. (Top row a through c, bottom row d through f)

a) Twenty-three weeks after epithelial ingrowth removal. Clinically there appears to be no change between this and the previous examination but topographic progression is seen.

b) Twenty-nine weeks after epithelial ingrowth removal. The patient's BCVA has dropped to 6/12. Clinically the area of ingrowth appears stable, but the area of astigmatism on topography has increased.

c) Thirty-one weeks after epithelial ingrowth removal. Clinically the involved area appeared to have increased the BCVA decreased to 6/15.

d) Thirty-six weeks after first epithelial ingrowth removal. (Immediately prior to second procedure.)

e) Three days after second epithelial ingrowth removal.

f) Six weeks after second epithelial ingrowth removal.

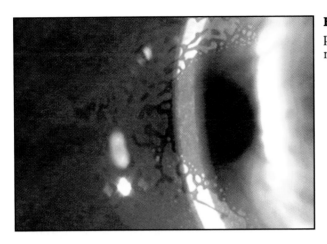

Figure 6E-4. The appearance of the eye just prior to the second epithelial ingrowth removal.

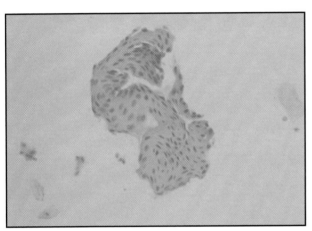

Figure 6E-5. The histological appearance (haematoxylin and eosin stain) of the tissue removed from the flap interface. The histology reports reads 'tiny fragments of squamous epithelium'.

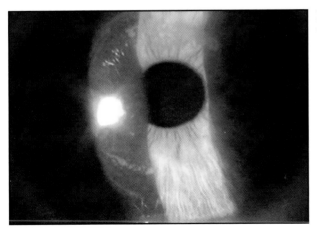

Figure 6E-6. The appearance 6 weeks after the second epithelial ingrowth removal.

Editor's Notes

It is interesting that this case of epithelial ingrowth was reported in a case of hyperopic LASIK. Epithelial ingrowth is definitely more common with hyperopic LASIK. This may be because there is a greater edge gape along the keratectomy, allowing cells to grow underneath the flap. Epithelial defects also seem to occur more commonly in hyperopic individuals. This may be because the hyperopic population that undergoes LASIK tends to be older, with a less adherent epithelium.

For the treatment of epithelial ingrowth, the key concept is meticulous removal of all epithelial cells. The stromal bed should be thoroughly scraped and then cleaned to ensure that no residual epithelial cells persist. The stromal side of the flap should also be cleaned to ensure that there are no epithelial cells present. Finally, epithelial defects should not be induced during the epithelial removal procedure so that epithelial healing is not required to a large extent following this procedure. This will help reduce the chance of the healing epithelium from growing underneath the flap again.

CASE F, EPITHELIAL INGROWTH AFTER LASIK ENHANCEMENT

Roberto Zaldivar, MD, Susana Oscherow, MD, and Giselle Ricur, MD

Main Concern: Referral Due to Loss of BCVA at 1 Year Post-LASIK
Patient Age: 36

INITIAL PREOPERATIVE INFORMATION

	OD	OS	COMMENTS
Preoperative Refraction		-2.50 – 0.50 X 165	
UCVA		20/40	
BCVA		20/30	
Topography Details:		(Figure 6F-1)	decentered ablation
SimK		38.79 D/37.16 D@105	
Pachymetry		534 μm	
Other		epithelial ingrowth peripheral melt, central microstriae (Figure 6F-2)	

PROCEDURES PERFORMED

	OD	OS	COMMENTS
1. Date/type		1998 M-LASIK	referring center
Laser/keratome/plate		NIDEK EC5000/ACS/160	
2. Date/type		1998 LASIK enhancement	referring center
3. Date/type		1998 LASIK enhancement	referring center
4. Date/type:		9/28/98 interface cleaning and hydration	

CURRENT POSTOPERATIVE INFORMATION

	OD	OS	COMMENTS
Time Postoperative		3 months	excellent outcome
Postoperative Refraction		n/a	
UCVA		20/30	
Medications		artificial tears	
Refractive Corrections		none	
Other		slit lamp exam: flap aligned no epithelial ingrowth, melts, or striae	

Adequate treatment of epithelial ingrowth can successfully restore lost visual acuity. The presence of epithelial cells in the corneal interface post LASIK constitutes the entity known as epithelial ingrowth. This event can be produced by true seeding of the interface or by cell growth from the periphery of the flap.

Risk factors have been described in the literature both pre- and intraoperatively, as well as its different patterns and grades of clinical presentation.

Undetected or left untreated, isolated cells or cysts of epithelial cells may coalesce, growing progressively and form pearls, strands, or sheets of epithelial ingrowth with subsequent loss of corneal transparency. Irregular astigmatism and disturbance of the visual axis can lead to dramatic decrease of BCVA. Corneal surface irregularities may also lead to disruption of the precorneal tear film. This may lead to scarring and haze, and the final outcome is the patient's complaints regarding night halos and glare. If persistent in time, this condition increases the incidence of stromal melting with potential ulceration and corneal infection.

In this case, the incidence of epithelial ingrowth was directly related to excessive flap manipulation; common in retreatments. Inadequate or repeated manipulation of the borders of the flap induces epithelial cell migration towards the interface with consequent trapping of the cells, once the flap is repositioned. Trapped epithelial cells in the interface presumably release collagenase, the main cause of melting.

The patient mentioned having being retreated twice before being referred for evaluation. Retroilluminated images captured with the Nidek EAS 100 camera clearly showed the epithelial ingrowth and stromal melts the patient's cornea presented on her first visit (Figure 6F-2).

This event requires prompt diagnosis and treatment is mandatory. Flaps must be raised and everted carefully. In my experience, scraping of the interface with a Beaver blade aided by a merocel sponge has been very useful. Once free of all epithelial cells, both surfaces are irrigated and the flap is repositioned. Excessive fluid must be carefully squeezed out with gentle stroking of the flap from the center to the periphery. Rapid adhesion is favored with the application of air along the edges of the flap.

Postoperative treatment should include topical antibiotics, steroids, as well as frequent instillation of ocular lubricants, and close follow-up examinations should be arranged.

Follow-up controls revealed marked improvement (Figure 6F-3) and gain of BCVA was the final outcome.

Experience as well as excimer laser and microkeratome proficiency are essential for minimizing the incidence of retreatments. One must put extra care in manipulating the flap in order to avoid epithelial cell dispersion and migration. If epithelial ingrowth is the case, fulfillment of proposed treatment and close patient follow-up ensures low rates of its recurrence.

Suggested Reading

Buratto L, Brint S. *LASIK Principles and Techniques.* Thorofare, NJ: SLACK Incorporated; 1998.

Machat JJ, Slade SG, Probst LE. *The Art of LASIK.* 2nd ed. Thorofare, NJ: SLACK Incorporated; 1999.

Zaldivar R, Davidorf J, Oscherow S, et al. Results and complications of laser in situ keratomileusis by experienced surgeons. *J Refract Surg.* March/April 1998;14(2).

Figure 6F-1. Topographic image 1 year after the original LASIK procedure.

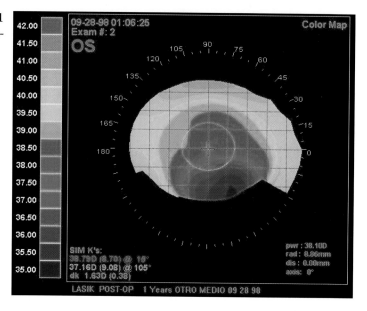

Figure 6F-2. Infrared image showing the epithelial ingrowth in the inferior part of the flap.

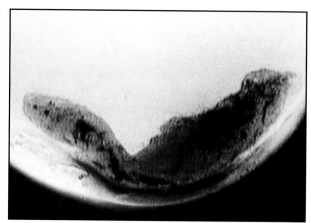

Figure 6F-3. Infrared image of the same cornea 1 day after the flap was lifted and the interface was scraped clean.

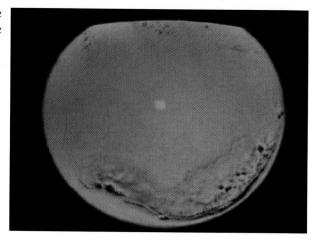

Editor's Notes

This case represents a typical case of epithelial ingrowth, except that it presented over 1 year after the primary procedure. Epithelial ingrowth usually occurs within 1 week to 3 months following the primary LASIK. While it is certainly possible this ingrowth did occur at a later date, it is more likely that the epithelial ingrowth occurred much earlier and has been present underneath the flap for an extended period of time. Epithelial ingrowth of this severity should definitely be removed, as it will induce flap melting. The topography does show some elevation inferiorly, which is a result of the elevation of the flap from epithelial ingrowth.

Case G, Grade 3 Ingrowth with Loose Epithelium

Ted Smith, OD, and Jeffrey J. Machat, MD

Main Concern: Epithelial Ingrowth
Patient Age: 51

INITIAL PREOPERATIVE INFORMATION

	OD	OS	COMMENTS
Preoperative Refraction	-1.25 – 2.50 X 97		no ABMD identified
UCVA	20/150		
BCVA	20/20		
Topography Details	46.37/45.87 X 096		
SimK Values	0.83		
Pachymetry	580 µm		

PROCEDURES PERFORMED

	OD	OS	COMMENTS
1. Date/type	3/25/99 LASIK		loose epithelium
Laser/keratome/plate	Technolas 217/ACS/180		defects
2. Date/type	5/08/99 Lift		
Laser/keratome/plate	lift/scrape ingrowth		

CURRENT POSTOPERATIVE INFORMATION

	OD	OS	COMMENTS
Time Postoperative	7 weeks		on day of lift for
Postoperative Refraction	n/a		ingrowth
UCVA	20/70		5/13/99
BCVA	20/20		
Topography Details	43.50/42.37 X 100		
SimK Values	1.82		
Visual Complaints	blur		
Medications	none		
Refractive Correction	none		

This patient was a 51-year-old white male. His surgical history consisted of bilateral LASIK performed on March 25, 1999, in an attempt to correct refractions of OD -1.25 – 2.50 X 097 and OS -1.75 – 1.75 X 087. Topography showed symmetrical, smooth corneas with minimal astigmatism, indicating that there was a significant lenticular component (Figure 6G-1). The procedure was uncomplicated OU, other than weak epithelial adhesion that resulted in bilateral epithelial defects requiring bandage contact lens insertion OU.

On the second postoperative day, the comanaging doctor reported grade 1 NSDIK in both eyes. Unaided acuities were 20/150 but no refraction was performed. Maxidex was prescribed Q1h OU. The following day unaided acuities improved to 20/80 OU and the bandage contact lens was removed. The regimen of Maxidex was reduced to Q2h and tapered to q.i.d. over the next week and was then discontinued.

At 7 weeks postoperative, the patient presented for an assessment at TLC on referral from his comanaging doctor for a consultation in regard to epithelial ingrowth OD. Unaided acuities were OD 20/70 and OS 20/30+ with refractions of +1.75 – 1.25 X 120 and +0.75 – 0.50 X 105 respectively. Biomicroscopy showed grade 3 ingrowth advancing in the superior cornea OD, with grade 2 ingrowth presenting inferiorly (Figure 6G-2 and 6G-3). The left cornea showed minimal grade 1 ingrowth. The right and left pachymetry readings were 530 µm and 526 µm respectively. Topography OD showed areas of peripheral flattening that corresponded to the areas of the observed ingrowth. The corneal astigmatism also corresponded to the observed topography, with K values 43.50/42.37 X 100 and CIM 1.82 (Figure 6G-4). It was felt that the ingrowth was likely to be responsible for the observed residual *Rx*.

The right flap was subsequently lifted and the epithelial ingrowth scraped. The resulting epithelial defects in the flap indicated insertion of a bandage contact lens in the right eye (Figure 6G-5). The patient was prescribed Inflamase Forte Q1h and Ciloxan q.i.d. as per standard LASIK postoperative regimen. The patient is currently being followed for stabilization.

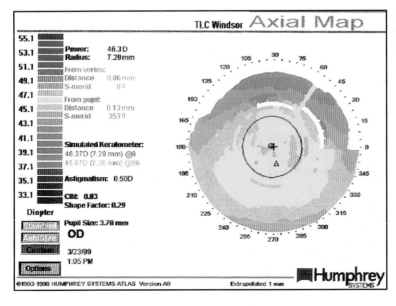

Figure 6G-1. Minimal astigmatism was noted on preoperative topography.

Figure 6G-2. Grade 3 ingrowth can be seen advancing in the cornea superiorly.

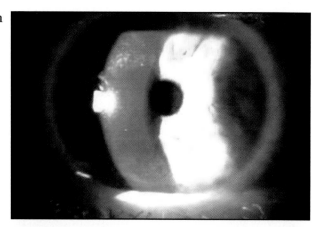

Figure 6G-3. Higher magnification view of superior ingrowth.

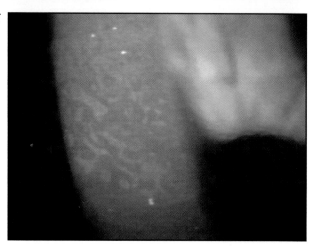

Figure 6G-4. Peripheral corneal flattening in areas of ingrowth.

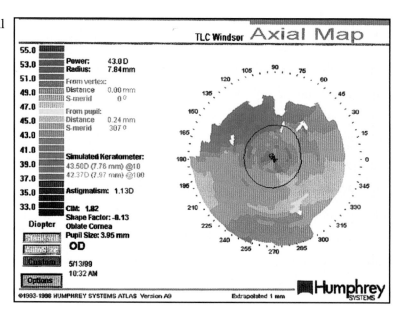

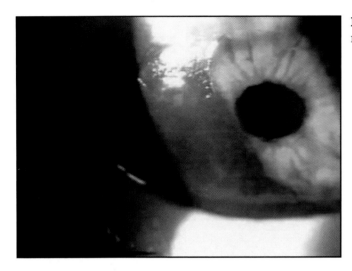

Figure 6G-5. Epithelial defects after removal of ingrowth.

Editor's Notes

This case demonstrates how epithelial defects occurring because of loose epithelium during LASIK often lead to epithelial ingrowth following the procedure. Preventative treatment is best in these situations. Minimal topical anesthesia, a lot of intraoperative lubrication, and very delicate manipulation of the flap are all important to preserve the epithelium during the procedure so epithelial ingrowth does not occur.

An effective technique that I have found useful to prevent epithelial defects in cases suspected to have loose epithelium is to use extra lubrication on the cornea prior to the keratectomy. In these situations, I will place one drop of Celluvisc on the cornea followed by one drop of proparicaine. This slightly viscous solution seems to allow the keratectomy to be performed in a very smooth manner with minimal trauma to the epithelium. If I am surprised by an epithelial defect in the right eye then I will use this mixture for the left eye and often have no epithelial defects there whatsoever.

7

LASIK Flap Striae

Summary Notes

LASIK FLAP STRIAE - SUMMARY NOTES

Clinical

Flap striae become more difficult to remove as the length of the postoperative course increases. Therefore, identification of the striae on the first postoperative day is imperative. Retroillumination of the fixation light and aiming the beam through the dilated pupil provides accurate localization of the flap striae and will help identify microstriae in cases of unexplained reduction of BCVA. Normally the striae are oriented horizontally with a nasal hinge and vertically with a superior hinge.

Etiology of Flap Striae

- misalignment of the corneal flap after flap replacement
- movement of the corneal flap during the first postoperative day
- the "tenting effect" of the corneal flap over the ablated stromal bed

Management

Most flap striae occur within the first hour after LASIK. Flap striae become more difficult to remove as the length of the postoperative course increases. Therefore identification of the striae on the first postoperative day is imperative. Even 1 week postoperatively, flap striae are becoming imbedded in the corneal flap tissue.

Indications for Treatment of Flap Striae

- flap striae extend through the visual axis
- causes a decrease in BCVA
- induce irregular astigmatism

Removal of Flap Striae

- phenylephrine 2.5% to allow intraoperative retroillumination
- the flap edge is marked at the slit lamp
- no flap alignment markings are made
- the flap is reflected back
- stromal surface of the flap is hydrated with BSS solution for 30 seconds
- the flap is replaced in the stromal bed and floated into position
- the flap is left for 5 minutes to attach to the stromal bed and dry the epithelial surface
- the side of the blunt forceps is used to stretch the flap perpendicular to the striae

Prevention

Intraoperative attention to the repositioning of the flap with minimal manipulation once it has been replaced into the correct position will help reduce the occurrence of flap striae. Postoperatively, patients are instructed to avoid rubbing or squeezing the eye. Patients wear eye protection 24 hours a day for the first week to prevent any trauma while the flaps are healing.

CASE A, MACROSTRIAE

Eric J. Linebarger, MD, David R. Hardten, MD, and Richard L. Lindstrom, MD

Main Concern: Striae/Blurred Vision
Patient Age: 18

INITIAL PREOPERATIVE INFORMATION

	OD	OS	COMMENTS
Preoperative Refraction	n/a		post-LASIK
UCVA	20/20		
Topography Details	n/a		
SimK Values	n/a		
Pachymetry	n/a		
Other	ghosting/distortion		

PROCEDURES PERFORMED

	OD	OS	COMMENTS
1. Date/type	1998 M-LASIK		striae
Laser/keratome/plate	VISX Star/ ACS/160		
2. Date/type	stretch/refloat		

CURRENT POSTOPERATIVE INFORMATION

	OD	OS	COMMENTS
Time Postoperative	4 weeks		no striae
UCVA	20/20		
Topography Details	n/a		
SimK Values	n/a		
Visual Complaints	none		

An 18-year-old male who underwent bilateral LASIK for correction of low myopia complained of ongoing ghost images and distortion in his right eye several weeks after surgery. His surgery was performed by creating a nasal-hinged lamellar flap using the Chiron ACS with a 7.5 mm diameter and 160 μm cutting plate in both eyes. No intraoperative complications were reported.

UCVA in the right eye was 20/20, although he noted distortion of visual images. Slit lamp examination of the right eye revealed a nasal hinged lamellar LASIK flap with significant obliquely oriented flap striae over the visual axis (Figure 7A-1). Examination of the left eye was unremarkable.

Visually significant flap striae are a rare, but often frustrating, complication for both physician and patient. The affected eye will often have excellent acuity by Snellen testing, although the patient will complain vociferously about the quality of the image.

Eliminating striae is best accomplished at the time of the original surgery. Meticulous attention to alignment after refloating the flap, and limiting the amount of irrigation used during the floating procedure will help reduce striae formation. In addition, gently stroking the flap with a lightly moistened merocel sponge along the long axis of orientation (nasal to temporal for nasal hinged flaps, top to bottom for superior hinged flaps) can also be of benefit. Milking of the flap edge by gently stretching the flap from center to edge with a dry merocel has also been advocated.

However, in spite of all efforts to reduce their formation, striae will occasionally occur. Mild microstriae are often seen on high magnification with oblique illumination and are rarely visually significant. More severe macrostriae are usually easily visible on slit lamp inspection (Figure 7A-2).

The earlier striae are dealt with, the easier they are to treat, as collagen memory becomes more permanent over time. Several techniques have been described, ranging from relifting the flap and then stretching the flap with a dry merocel or the blunt end of a spatula, irrigating canula, or other instrument. Several flap roller instruments (similar to a paint roller in design) are currently in prototype development stages and may prove useful in future striae management.

Striae that are particularly prominent and have been left untreated for several months may require flap relifting and suturing. A series of interrupted 10-0 nylon with radial orientation are placed through the flap edge to place it on "stretch". These sutures are left in place for several weeks.

The patient underwent flap relifting and refloating with massage and milking to restretch the flap approximately 4 weeks after the initial LASIK procedure (Figure 7A-3). The eye was then taped closed overnight. Post-lift day 1 examination revealed an UCVA of 20/25- with significant resolution of striae. By post-lift week 4, the vision had returned to 20/20 uncorrected with no complaints of ghosting or distortion. The striae had been entirely resolved.

Suggested Reading

Pannu JS. Incidence and treatment of wrinkled corneal flap following LASIK. *J Cataract Refract Surg.* 1997;23:695-696.

Probst LE, Machat J. Removal of flap striae following laser in situ keratomileusis. *J Cataract Refract Surg.* 1998;24:153-155.

Figure 7A-1. Striae in LASIK flap with distortion of mire.

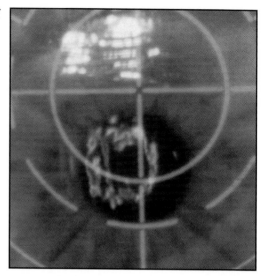

Figure 7A-2. Macrostriae in LASIK flap.

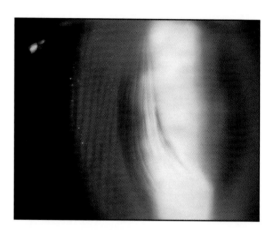

Figure 7A-3. Clearing of striae after relifting and stretching of flap with noticeable improvement in mire quality.

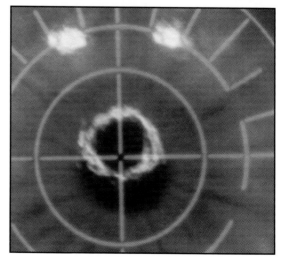

Editor's Notes

While epithelial ingrowth has declined in incidence with LASIK because of improved technique, LASIK flap striae do still continue to occur. Striae can occur because of misalignment of the flap during the original procedure, but more commonly they occur due to some trauma to the flap after the original LASIK procedure. The most critical time is the first 24 hours as the flap is sealing into the stromal bed and the epithelium is healing along the keratectomy edge.

Out of a total of 16,000 LASIK cases, I have had approximately 8 dislodged flaps, giving an incidence of approximately 1 in 2,000. It would appear that it is the postoperative management of the patient that is most crucial in avoiding dislodged flaps. I personally instruct each patient to try to keep their eyes closed on the first postoperative day as much as possible. I tell the patient that this will help their eye heal and keep their eye protected. We also instruct the patients not to rub or squeeze the eyes and give them protective sunglasses to wear during the day and eyeshields to wear at night. We always examine the patients 20 minutes after the procedure and they are also examined the following day to ensure that no striae are present. Any flap striae are treated immediately, as early treatment gives the best results. When treated effectively, most flap striae can be eliminated. This often results in a full restoration of the BCVA.

CASE B, SEVERE STRIAE WITH FLAP DISPLACEMENT

Ted Smith, OD, and Jeffery J. Machat, MD

Main Concern: Severe Macrostriae
Patient Age: 47

INITIAL PREOPERATIVE INFORMATION

	OD	OS	COMMENTS
Preoperative Refraction		-6.50 DS	
UCVA		20/cf@1ft	
BCVA		20/16	
Topography Details		43.12/43.12	
SimK Values		0.73	
Pachymetry		537 μm	

PROCEDURES PERFORMED

	OD	OS	COMMENTS
1. Date/type		12/22/98	uncomplicated
Laser/keratome/plate		LaserSight LSX/ACS/180	
2. Date/type		12/23/98	
Laser/keratome/plate		lift/striae	

CURRENT POSTOPERATIVE INFORMATION

	OD	OS	COMMENTS
Time Postoperative		2 weeks	post-lift
Postoperative Refraction		+1.00 DS	
UCVA		20/40-	
BCVA		20/25-	
Topography Details		38.75/38.50 X 90	
SimK Values		1.50	
Pachymetry		not performed	
Visual Complaints		none	
Medications		none	
Refractive Correction		none	

This patient was a 47-year-old white male with an unremarkable medical history. LASIK was performed on his right and left eyes on December 22, 1999. We attempted for full correction of OD -5.75 DS and OS -6.50 DS using a Chiron ACS keratome with a 160 μm flap and the LaserSight LSX for ablation. Topography showed smooth spherical corneas (Figure 7B-1). The procedure was uncomplicated OU. At 1 day postoperatively, severe central striae were noted OS, indicating that his left flap had torqued overnight (Figures 7B-2 and 7B-3). Unaided acuity was 20/80 and could be improved only to 20/60 with an *Rx* OS -0.25 + 1.25 X 055. The right flap was well-positioned with BCVA 20/20 and a manifesting *Rx* OD +1.00 DS.

The left flap was lifted and the striae were stretched and smoothed. At 2 weeks post-flap lift the striae were minimal. A manifest *Rx* of OS +100 sphere gave unaided and aided acuities of 20/40- and 20/25- respectively. Topography and biomicroscopy showed slight central corneal irregularity with K values of 38.75/38.50 X 90 and CIM value 1.50 (Figure 7B-4). The patient claimed to be experiencing ghost imaging even with correction.

At 3 months postoperatively, the information from the comanaging doctor indicated that he had an improvement in unaided acuity to 20/30+. The manifest *Rx* had decreased to a stable endpoint of OS +0.75 + 0.75 X 170, which gave an acuity of 20/15-. No ghosting of images was reported. Biomicroscopy showed a smooth corneal surface. The patient reported difficulty with near work, attributable to the residual hyperopia. The hyperopia may be enhanced if it stabilizes and produces persistent asthenopia with near work.

Figure 7B-1. Preoperative topography OS demonstrates a regular pattern.

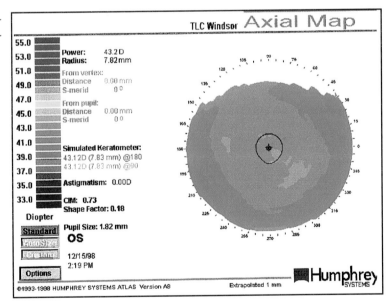

Figure 7B-2. Flap displacement with oblique flap striae through the visual axis.

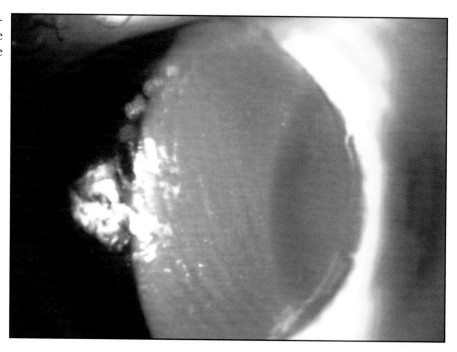

Figure 7B-3. Retroillumination view of the same flap striae.

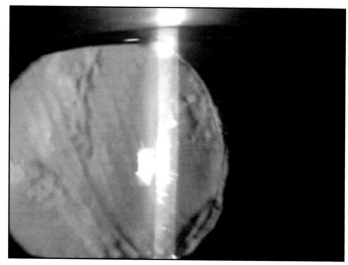

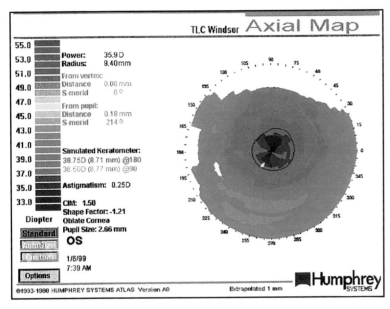

Figure 7B-4. Postoperative topography OS shows a well-centered small zone ablation.

Editor's Notes

The striae in this case are likely a result of excessive eyelid squeezing or rubbing that resulted in movement of the flap. This caused a significant loss of BCVA. The flap striae were treated the first postoperative day, which allowed the most effective management of striae.

In this case, the overcorrection can be treated with hyperopic LASIK. Since the patient was 47 years old, he will likely find this degree of hyperopia quite disturbing. As the original procedure was performed with the ACS system (which generally produces a 8.5 mm flap), the transition zone for the hyperopic LASIK can be adjusted to extend from 5.5 to 8.5 mm.

CASE C, STRIAE AND HAZE

Ted Smith, OD, and Jeffery J. Machat, MD

Main Concern: Striae and Haze
Patient Age: 48

INITIAL PREOPERATIVE INFORMATION

	OD	OS	COMMENTS
Preoperative Refraction	-0.50 – 2.00 X 148		post-irregular flap and
BCVA	20/80-		LASIK enhancement
UCVA	20/150		referring center
Topography Details	39.50/38.37 X 162		
SimK Values	2.08		
Pachymetry	430 µm		

PROCEDURES PERFORMED

	OD	OS	COMMENTS
1. Date/type	7/24/97 LASIK		referring center
Laser/keratome/plate	Classic/ n/a		
2. Date/type	8/26/97 LASIK		referring center
Laser/keratome/plate	lift/enhance		
3. Date/type	10/21/97		
Laser/keratome/plate	epithelial scrape		referring center
4. Date/type	11/5/98 PRK/PTK(6 and 7 mmOZ)		
Laser/keratome/plate	Technolas 217		

CURRENT POSTOPERATIVE INFORMATION

	OD	OS	COMMENTS
Time Postoperative	1 month (12/3/98)		post PTK/PRK
Postoperative Refraction	+0.50 – 1.00 X 165		
UCVA	20/60		
BCVA	20/30-		
Topography Details	37.00/36.50X112		
SimK Values	2.30		
Pachymetry	387 µm (intraoperative)		
Visual Complaints	diplopia/blur		
Medications	levobunolol 0.5% b.i.d.		
	fluoromethalone 0.1% q.i.d.		
Refractive Correction	none		

This patient was a 48-year-old white male with an unremarkable medical history. He was referred from another center as a complex case. His surgical history consisted of bilateral LASIK performed on July 24, 1997, in an attempt to correct refractions of OD -9.00 + 0.75 X 112 and OS -9.00 + 0.50 X 70. The right LASIK flap had been thin and irregular. We have little more information other than to know that the surgeon proceeded to ablate, despite poor flap quality. Furthermore, a subsequent enhancement was apparently performed OD on August 26, 1997, and a further epithelial debridement procedure occurred on October 21, 1997.

The left surgical procedure was uncomplicated. However, striae occurred postoperative and were left untreated. The unaided acuity was 20/50 OS, *Rx* OS of +2.00 – 2.00 X 129 with BCVA of 20/30+. His topography shows K values 39.12/38.50 X 026 and CIM 2.84 (Figure 7C-1). Biomicroscopy shows central basket-weave striae that are fibrosed with 2 years of no treatment. It is felt that a rigid gas permeable contact lens or lamellar graft surgery may be the only alternatives to providing clearer vision.

The patient presented to our center for treatment on his right eye on November 5, 1998, with a manifesting *Rx* OD of -0.50 – 2.00 X 148 that corresponded to a BCVA of 20/80-. There was dense central confluent corneal haze visible by biomicroscopy (Figure 7C-2). The flap appeared thin and irregular. The central cornea was thinned to a pachymetry reading of 419 µm. Topography showed K values of 39.87/38.87 X 158 with a corresponding CIM value of 1.76 (Figure 7C-3). The patient had been taking Pred Forte q.i.d.

To attempt to reduce the corneal haze, 50 µm of PTK was applied with an optic zone of 6 mm. Secondly, an ablation of PRK for a correction of -0.25 – 1.50 X 160 was performed. Lastly, 30 µm of PTK at OZ. 7 mm was applied as well as 300 shots of PTK with a 2 mm spot over the corneal periphery. Intraoperative pachymetry indicated a central corneal thickness of 387. The patient was managed as an atypical PRK with a regimen of dexamethosone 1% Q2h and ofloxacin 0.3% until the bandage contact lens was removed at day 4 postoperative, at which time the medications were changed to Flarex q.i.d. and tapered over 4 months.

At 4 weeks postoperative, the patient presented with an unaided acuity OD of 20/60. A manifest *Rx* of OD +0.50 – 1.00 X 165 improved the acuity to 20/30-. There was mild central diffuse corneal haze which was markedly reduced from preoperative measurements. Topography showed a relatively spherical cornea centrally with temporal flattening, with slight central irregularity, K values 37.00/36.50 X 112, CIM value 2.3 (Figure 7C-4). A slight steroid induced ocular hypertension (IOP 24 mmHg) indicated prescribing levobunolol b.i.d. until the steriod was tapered off.

At 6 months postoperative, the patient presented with an unaided acuity OD of 20/60-. A refraction of +0.75 – 1.25 X 163 improved visual acuity to 20/25-. Pachymetry showed a central corneal thickness of 439 µm. Topography indicated K values of 36.62/36.37 X 090, CIM 2.56. The cornea was essentially clear, with only trace reticular haze. All medications had been discontinued. With the minimal equivalent sphere *Rx* that is residual OD, combined with the considerably flat K values, it was decided that the most appropriate course would be to be fit him with a right rigid gas permeable contact lens.

Figure 7C-1. Preoperative topography indicating a normal cornea.

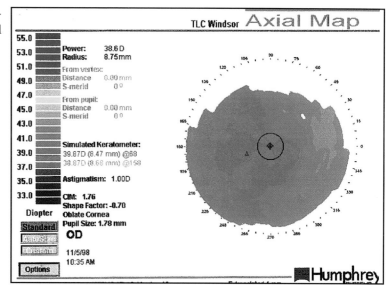

Figure 7C-2. Confluent corneal haze OD.

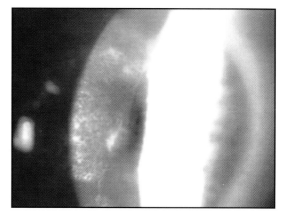

Figure 7C-3. Topography 3 months post-LASIK shows irregularity and temporal flattening.

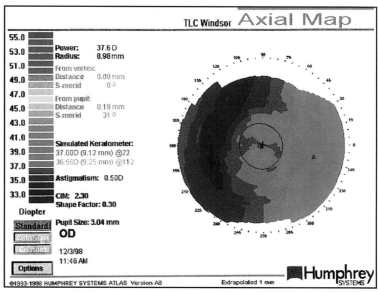

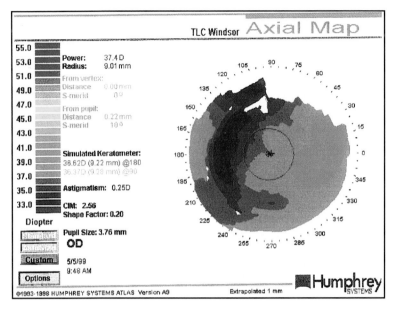

Figure 7C-4. One month post-PTK. The cornea is flattened temporally with slight central irregularity.

Editor's Notes

This patient developed central confluent haze that decreased the BCVA to 20/80. This necessitated a PTK procedure with an epithelial ablation of 50 μm of PTK. PRK correction was done to remove some of the astigmatism indicated on the topography. Finally, an additional PTK procedure was done to remove the residual haze that was still present on the cornea. The patient was kept on topical steroids following the procedure in order to reduce the final amount of haze that occurred.

At the 6 month follow-up, the patient's BCVA had improved to 20/25. There was minimal central stromal haze. There was some increased corneal thickening, likely as a result of stromal and epithelial remodeling. The corneal topography indicates significant corneal flattening, temporally in the right eye with irregularity in the visual axis. Although a hard contact lens would provide a temporary solution for this patient, topography-assisted LASIK would be the ideal procedure to restore the UCVA.

CASE D, DENSE FIBROSED STRIAE

Ted Smith, OD, Jeffery J. Machat, MD, Stephen G. Slade, MD, and Louis E. Probst, MD

Main Concern: Striae
Patient Age: 51

INITIAL PREOPERATIVE INFORMATION

	OD	OS	COMMENTS
Preoperative Refraction	+4.50 – 1.50 X 45		post-LASIK/PTK
BCVA	20/30		referring center
Topography Details	38.37/37.87 X 40		
SimK Values	2.46		
Pachymetry	531 µm		

PROCEDURES PERFORMED

	OD	OS	COMMENTS
1. Date/type	1/97 LASIK		referring center
Laser/keratome/plate	n/a		
2. Date/type	4/30/97 PTK		referring center
Laser/keratome/plate	n/a		
3. Date/type	12/22/97 LASIK/PTK (6 mm OZ)		
Laser/keratome/plate	Technolas 217/lift		
4. Date/type	5/7/98 PRK/PTK (6 mm OZ)		
Laser/keratome/plate	Technolas 217/flap removed		
5. Date/type	6/11/98 PRK		
Laser/keratome/plate	Technolas 217		
6. Date/type	9/8/98 PK		

CURRENT POSTOPERATIVE INFORMATION

	OD	OS	COMMENTS
Time Postoperative	6 months		post-PK
Postoperative Refraction	-5.25 – 6.50 X 104		
UCVA	20/200		
BCVA	20/40		
Topography Details	46.26/42.22 X 120		
Pachymetry	562 µm		
Visual Complaints	blur/haloes		
Medications	levobunolol/steriod q.i.d.		
Refractive Correction	none		

This patient was a 51-year-old white male with an unremarkable medical history. His surgical history consisted of bilateral LASIK performed in January, 1997. Unfortunately we do not have the information for the initial preoperative data, however, we do know that the surgical procedure for the right eye was complicated by a thin and irregular flap. The left eye was apparently successful with a UCVA of 20/25 at 2 years postoperative. Due to subsequent complications involving untreated dense fibrosed striae in the right eye, PTK was attempted 4 months later to remove the associated haze. At that time, the preoperative Rx OD was apparently -4.25 – 0.50 X 170, with a BCVA of 20/20. With minimal success in reducing the central haze, the patient was referred to our center for treatment on December 22, 1997.

Preoperative assessment at our center showed a manifest Rx of OD +4.50 – 1.50 X 45 that provided a BCVA of 20/30. Topography showed central irregular astigmatism with a suspect central island with K values 38.37/37.87 X 40, CIM value 2.46 (Figure 7D-1). Biomicroscopy showed dense fibrosed striae with surrounding haze and an irregular flap contour (Figure 7D-2). The flap was lifted to perform a hyperopic ablation and PTK using the Technolas 217. An ablation correction of +2.25 – 0.75 X 120 was performed, as well as 35 µm of PTK to the stromal bed at an optic zone of 6 mm. Since the flap was thin, it split across the visual axis intraoperatively. Despite a high likelihood of the flap being unviable, it was replaced and followed for healing potential.

Over the next few months, there was no significant improvement in corneal clarity/striae and BCVA. On May 7, 1998, the right eye showed an Rx of OD +3.00 – 0.50 X 100 that provided an acuity of 20/30. Topography indicated K values of 39.12/39.00 X 180 and CIM 2.12 (Figure 7D-3). Dense fibrosed striae and haze were still present. The flap was lifted and removed because it became unviable, as well as a primary source of haze. PRK was subsequently performed with an attempted correction of +2.50 sphere and 20 µm of PTK was applied to the stromal bed at an optic zone of 6 mm. A bandage contact lens was inserted and the patient was managed as a PRK postoperative with Ocuflox and Flarex q.i.d.

One month later, the patient had developed a stromal nodule with overlying epithelial irregularity and severe confluent haze central to his visual axis. Unaided acuity was cf@2 feet, which could only be slightly improved to 20/200 with pinhole. No reasonable topography could be obtained due to poor tear stability. A 3 mm area of epithelium was debrided, the underlying stroma scraped and dissected and a correction of -0.50 D of PRK was ablated. A bandage contact lens was inserted and dexamethasone 1%, and antiscore drop q.i.d. was prescribed.

Over the next 3 months the patient was followed. Examination at that time showed that there remained to be persistent severe confluent corneal haze and surface irregularity. Visual acuity had dropped further to a BCVA of 20/400. It was decided that penetrating keratoplasty was the only solution to try to improve visual function. Corneal transplant surgery was consequently performed on September 8, 1999. The surgery was uncomplicated and the patient achieved an unaided acuity of 20/70 that pinholed to 20/30 by 2 weeks postoperative. Unfortunately, the patient developed steroid induced ocular hypertension (IOP 38 mmHg) by 2 to 3 months postoperatively. By 6 months post PK, the IOP was stabilized at 20 mmHg and the BCVA was 20/40 with a manifest Rx of OD -5.25 – 6.50 X 104. The patient was continued on medications of levobunolol b.i.d. and Eflone q.i.d. and will be monitored monthly.

Figure 7D-1. Topography after LASIK at referral center demonstrates a small ablation zone and mild island pattern.

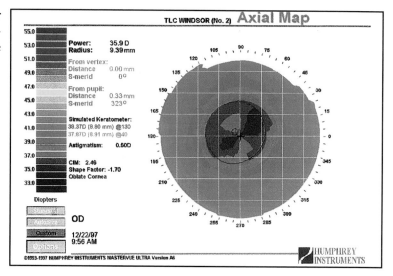

Figure 7D-2. Fibrosed striae in visual axis.

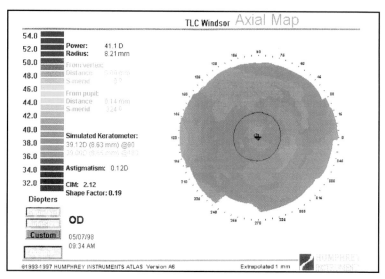

Figure 7D-3. Irregular topography after initial corrective LASIK.

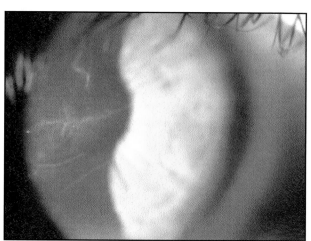

Editor's Notes

This case represents one of the worst potential outcomes from a LASIK procedure. This patient eventually had over six procedures in the right eye that culminated with a PK. The ongoing anxiety and concerns with the right eye have proven to be devastating for this patient's personal life. The patient has stopped working and is completely preoccupied with his vision in his right eye. The psychological component of this LASIK complication has been terrible.

The initial corrective procedure performed by lifting the flap illustrates the problems with lifting thin buttonhole flaps. The flap tore in the middle. This ripping of the flap made it extremely difficult for the flap to heal afterwards, so the flap was eventually removed. PTK procedures were done in an attempt to smooth the stromal bed, unfortunately this was not successful. With the multiple PTK procedures, the cornea became excessively flattened and distorted, which resulted in a reduction in the patient's UCVA. The patient was then referred to my center for follow-up care.

When I first evaluated this patient, I was most concerned about his mental status. He picked at his arms and body more and more frequently the more we discussed his eye. His conversation was broken and repetitive. He would always return to the question, "When will I be able to see 20/20?" From our discussions with the family, we learned that this previously healthy productive man was now out of work and separated from his wife. We contacted the patient's family doctor and family to discussed the need for further care and support.

With a hard contact lens the patient had a BCVA of 20/20, unfortunately prolonged hard contact lens use was not acceptable to the patient. The patient was evaluated for a potential homograft, but the irregularity of the corneal surface and the inadequate corneal thickness made this option less attractive. The patient did eventually have a PK, however the residual myopia and astigmatism further upset him. The situation was further complicated on another follow-up visit, when the BCVA began to diminish to the 20/50 level. It became evident that the patient had started to develop posterior subcapsular cataracts in both eyes, likely due to the prolonged use of topical steroids.

This patient is currently under evaluation for cataract surgery in the right eye. The IOL will be carefully selected so that myopic sphere and astigmatism are preserved, as this can be treated with LASIK and the VISX S2 laser. Full correction using the average K values would result in a mixed astigmatism pattern that would require that the patient travel to a scanning excimer laser to have the astigmatism corrected.

In the 16,000 LASIK cases that I have performed and examined, this is the absolute worst result. The multiple procedures and reduction in the vision in the right eye have been psychologically devastating for the patient. Although severe complications in LASIK are rare, this outcome must always be considered when the preoperative risks are discussed with each patient.

CASE E, FLAP STRIAE WITH LOSS OF BCVA

Ioannis G. Pallikaris, MD, Theokliti Papadaki, MD, and Dimitrios S. Siganos, MD

Main Concern: Flap Striae
Patient Age: 51

INITIAL PREOPERATIVE INFORMATION

	OD	OS	COMMENTS
Preoperative Refraction	-9.75 – 1.50 X 90	-0.75 –1.5 X 085	high myopia
BCVA	20/20	20/25	

PROCEDURES PERFORMED

	OD	OS	COMMENTS
1. Date/type	1995 M-LASIK	1995 PRK	flap striae OD
Laser/keratome/plate	ACS/160		
2. Date/type	3 months postoperative realign flap		

CURRENT POSTOPERATIVE INFORMATION

	OD	OS	COMMENTS
Time Postoperative	1 month after lift	3 months	smooth anterior
Postoperative Refraction	+1.50 – 1.50 X 80	n/a	cornea, BCVA
UCVA	n/a	20/25	restored
BCVA	20/25	20/25	

A 25-year-old woman underwent LASIK OD for the correction of -9.75 – 1.50 X 90. OS was simultaneously operated with astigmatic PRK for the correction of -7.5 – 1.5 X 85. Preoperative BCVA was the same in both eyes (20/25).

The procedure was completed successfully. The ACS microkeratome was used to cut a 8.5 mm wide and 160 μm thick flap. This was repositioned using the dry technique. Reattachment was enhanced by exposing the cornea to dry air for a few seconds. The eye was left unpatched.

The corneal topography at the same interval reveals a well-centered flattening of the central cornea of approximately 7 D (Figure 7E-1 and 7E-2).

In the early postoperative period, the patient complained of blurred vision in the LASIK eye, which did not improve with time. At the third postoperative month's examination, achieved correction was within emmetropia (+1.5 – 1.5 X 90), yet one line loss in BCVA was detected (20/32). The Ast-PRK eye, although presenting the expected hyperopic shift (+4.0 – 0.75 X 90), had reached a UCVA equal to the BCVA (20/25). The difference map between 2 days and 3 months postoperatively in OD revealed nothing but a satisfactorily centered, round 5 mm ablation zone and confirmed a progressive steepening of the central cornea due to a normal healing response (Figure 7E-3). On retroillumination, flap striae were prominent and created an uneven corneal surface of poor optical quality (Figure 7E-4), when compared to the smooth surface of the fellow PRK eye (Figure 7E-5).

The loss in BCVA was attributed to the anterior corneal surface undulations. The decision was made to raise and realign the flap.

The Holladay Diagnostic Summary prior to flap retreatment (Figure 7E-6) indicated that the optical quality of the corneal surface within the 3 mm pupil zone was adequate with minimal distortion (distortion map). A CU index of 60%, however, indicated a nonuniform cornea throughout the 3 mm pupil zone, while PC acuity was evaluated as 20/40, which corresponded well to the patient's actual BCVA in this eye.

On the first postoperative day after flap repositioning, the Holladay map confirmed that uniformity of the corneal surface had reached normal levels (CU index = 80%), while potential visual acuity had increased to 20/25 (Figure 7E-7). One month after reoperation, a BCVA of 20/25 had been achieved with a correction of +1.5 – 1.50 X 80. A smoother anterior corneal surface was detectable with slit lamp examination (Figure 7E-8).

Flap striae are more common when using the dry technique. The patient should be reevaluated under the operating microscope 30 to 60 minutes after the operation to ensure proper alignment of the flap. A misaligned or striated flap should be lifted back and repositioned immediately as it may cause a loss in BCVA and induce irregular astigmatism.

Postponing repositioning is pointless because flap striation is not a self-limiting condition. On the other hand, delayed intervention may involve permanent damage to Bowman's membrane with subsequent failure of any attempt to realign the flap and eliminate the striae.

Figure 7E-1. On the second postoperative day fine vertical striae can be detected within the flap area.

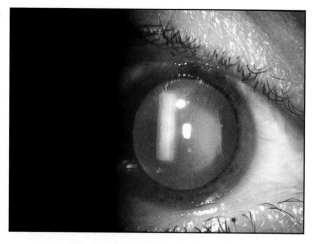

Figure 7E-2. Difference map comparing the preoperative corneal topographic pattern to that obtained immediately postoperatively.

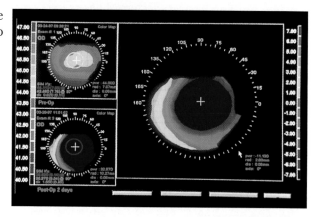

Figure 7E-3. Difference map showing the topographic changes throughout the first 3 postoperative months.

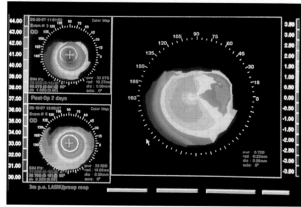

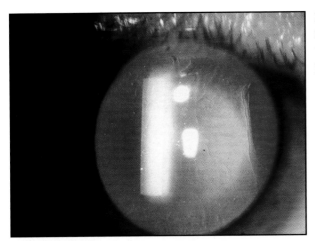

Figure 7E-4. Three months postoperatively: flap striae are prominent on retroillumination creating an uneven corneal surface of poor optical quality.

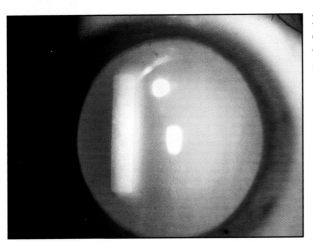

Figure 7E-5. Three months postoperatively: compare the previous picture to this one, which presents the smooth, even surface of the PRK fellow eye.

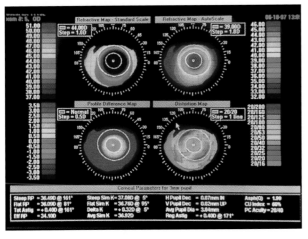

Figure 7E-6. The Holladay Diagnostic Map prior to repositioning.

Figure 7E-7. The Holladay Diagnostic map 1 month after repositioning.

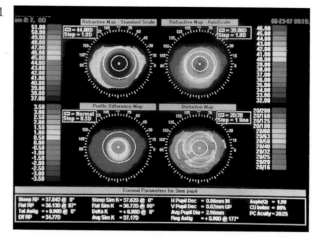

Figure 7E-8. Slit lamp view of the corneal surface 1 month after repositioning.

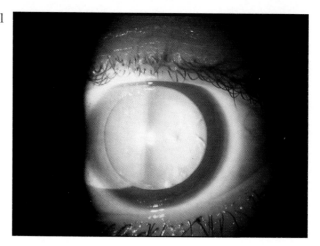

Editor's Notes

Significant flap striae continue to occur after LASIK with an incidence of approximately 1 in 300 cases. This can be due to misalignment of the flap during the original procedure or movement of the flap in the first postoperative day. The dry technique is more prone to develop striae as the interface irrigation allows precise alignment and hence reduces the incidence of flap striae.

When striae cause a reduction of BCVA or induce astigmatism, they should be treated. Ideally, striae are treated within the first week, as this is when the flap is most malleable. We have successfully treated striae up to 7 months after the original LASIK procedure with success. Retroillumination is an important way of identifying small striae that could be the reason for an unexplained loss of BCVA.

It is important to note that the PRK eye in this case achieved an excellent result, demonstrating that PRK is still an excellent procedure despite the overwhelming popularity of LASIK.

CASE F, IMMEDIATE SEVERE POSTOPERATIVE STRIAE

Ted Smith, OD, and Jeffery J. Machat, MD

Main Concern: Severe Striae
Patient Age: 56

INITIAL PREOPERATIVE INFORMATION

	OD	OS	COMMENTS
Preoperative Refraction		+4.25 − 0.50 X 010	
UCVA		20/cf	
BCVA		20/20	
Topography Details		42.12/41.50 X 180	
SimK Values		0.68	
Pachymetry		556 μm	

PROCEDURES PERFORMED

	OD	OS	COMMENTS
1. Date/type		5/6/99	
Laser/keratome/plate		Technolas217/	
		Hansatome/180	
2. Date/type		5/6/99	
Laser/keratome/plate		lift 20 minutes	
		postoperative	

CURRENT POSTOPERATIVE INFORMATION

	OD	OS	COMMENTS
Time Postoperative		1 week	no striae
Postoperative Refraction		+1.00 DS	
UCVA		20/30−	
BCVA		20/25−	
Topography Details		42.62/41.50 X 090	
SimK Values		3.50	
Pachymetry		n/a	
Visual Complaints		none	
Medications		none	
Refractive Correction		none	

This patient was a 56-year-old white male. Both his blood pressure and glucose levels were well-controlled and stable. His surgical history consisted of bilateral LASIK on May 6, 1999, for attempted correction of OD +4.00 – 0.50 X 075 and OS +4.25 – 0.50 X 010. His preoperative topography showed smooth, symmetrical corneas with minimal astigmatism, which corresponded to the spectacle Rx (Figure 7F-1). The procedure was uncomplicated OU.

At the 20 minute postoperative flap assessment, the patient showed significant debris under the left flap. He was subsequently returned to the surgical suite to refloat the flap. Ironically, upon the second 20 minute postoperative check following the debris removal, the patient showed severe striae OS (Figure 7F-2 and 7F-3). The right flap was well-positioned. The patient was once again returned to the surgical suite for the flap to be relifted and replaced. The subsequent flap assessment at 30 minutes postoperative showed the flap to be well-positioned.

At 1 week postoperative, the patient presented for an assessment to determine whether there were any residual striae OS. Unaided acuities were 20/30 OU with manifest Rx of OD pl + 0.50 X 075 and OS +1.00 DS, providing BCVAs of 20/25 OU. There was no observable striae OS. Topography OS showed slight central corneal irregularity with K values of 42.62/41.50 X 090 and CIM 3.50. However, the CIM value was likely inflated due to poor corneal wetting despite lubrication (Figure 7F-4). The patient is currently being monitored by his comanaging doctor for stabilization. As healing progresses, it is expected that improved corneal wetting should improve the left corneal topography.

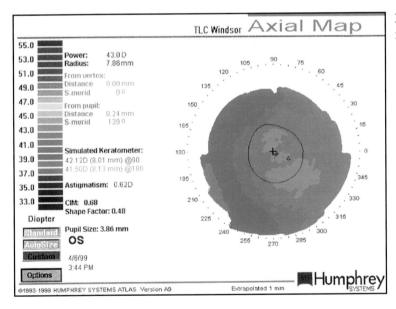

Figure 7F-1. Preoperative topography OS.

Figure 7F-2. Severe striae noted on 20 minute postoperative check.

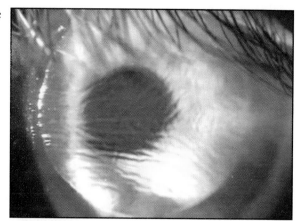

Figure 7F-3. Severe striae noted on 20 minute postoperative check.

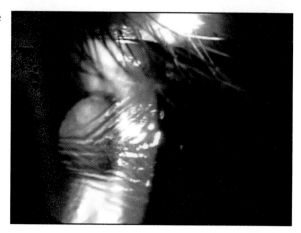

Figure 7F-4. Postoperative topography 1 week after treating striae.

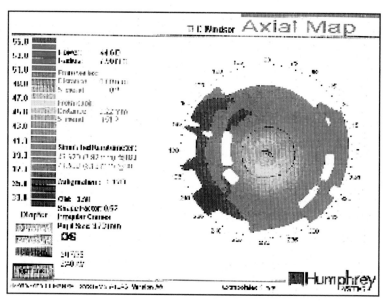

Editor's Notes

This case demonstrates the importance of checking the flap following the LASIK procedure. This patient originally had his flap checked 20 minutes after LASIK and debris was found under the left flap. The patient returned to the surgical suite to have the interface cleaned and the debris removed. When his flap was checked again 20 minutes following the procedure, significant striae were noted. It is much easier to correct flap striae immediately following LASIK rather than waiting until the next postoperative day to discover the striae and then fix the problem. It should also be noted that when the flap is refloated, the flap will become more edematous and this will decrease flap adhesion. Therefore if a large amount of interface irrigation is performed or the flap needs to be refloated for any reason it would be wise to let the flap adhere for a longer period of time in order to reduce the risk of flap displacement.

LASIK Interface Keratitis

8

LASIK INTERFACE KERATITIS - SUMMARY NOTES

Names for LASIK Interface Keratitis (LIK)
- Sands of the Sahara
- sands
- non-specific diffuse interface keratitis (NSDIK)
- diffuse lamellar keratitis (DLK)

Clinical
LIK presents as postoperative interface inflammation in the 24 to 72 hour postoperative period. The interface inflammation has a "sifted sand" appearance with a dusting of a powder-like material in the interface which is generally more dense centrally. The rest of the eye is usually unaffected with no conjunctival injection, anterior chamber inflammation, epithelial defects, or corneal infection. It is unilateral in 70% of cases. Clusters of cases have been reported from various surgeons and centers. LIK can occur in a limited localized form under epithelial defects after LASIK.

Hatsis Classification of LIK

	INTERFACE	TOPOGRAPHY	VISION
Grade I	partial	no change	excellent
Grade II	complete	changes	excellent
Grade III	complete	changes	foggy
Grade IV	complete	changes	foggy

+ injection, lid edema, a/c cells

Proposed Causes of LIK
- betadine
- BSS
- contaminants on instruments
- environmental agents
- lubricant
- metallic debris
- topical medications
- benzene
- contaminants from eyelids
- corneal abrasions
- laser thermal effect
- meibomian gland secretions
- talc
- bacterial cell wall hypersensitivity

Bacterial Cell Wall Hypothesis
It has been proposed that LIK represents a hypersensitivity reaction to bacterial cell proteins that have accumulated on the autoclaved instruments. The bacteria multiply on the wet instruments or the autoclave overnight. While the sterilization kills the bacteria, the cell walls persist on the instruments, and this material is transferred to the corneal interface.

Management

Early identification of LIK allows the prompt initiation of topical steroid treatment, which can cause rapid resolution. More severe cases can take 4 to 8 weeks to resolve. Topical steroids are started every hour and then slowly taper over several weeks. Severe cases of interface inflammation can be treated with interface irrigation, which has been reported as successful by some surgeons. LIK associated with epithelial defects should be treated with topical steroids to suppress the inflammation and lubrication and prophylactic antibiotics for the defect.

Management of LIK

- ensure sterility (no epithelial defects)
- topical steroids
- start quickly
- frequent application of topical steriods (Q1H initially)
- antibiotics have no obvious role
- irrigation of flap interface
- avoid scraping or laser to interface

Prevention

The bacterial cell wall hypothesis has led to some precautions that should reduce the potential for bacterial accumulation. At the end of each surgical day, the instruments are autoclaved and then dried to prevent bacterial replication on the surface. The tray of the autoclave is removed and dried as well. The water collection container for the autoclave is also drained to prevent bacterial accumulation. The microkeratome head is autoclaved and dried. The microkeratome motor end is rotated in a bath of ethanol and dried. Finally, disposable instruments are used when possible. Postoperatively, all patients are instructed to use topical steroid drops every hour on the second postoperative day in an effort to suppress any potential cases of LIK. While we have followed all these precautions since January 1999, we have continued to have LIK occur in 1 in 500 cases, suggesting that further measures may be necessary.

CASE A, DIFFUSE LAMELLAR KERATITIS WITH A LOSS OF BCVA

Eric J. Linebarger, MD, David R. Hardten, MD, and Y. Ralph Chu, MD

Main Concern: LASIK Interface Inflammation
Patient Age: 28

INITIAL PREOPERATIVE INFORMATION

	OD	OS	COMMENTS
Preoperative Refraction	-2.25 – 0.50 X 90		
BCVA	n/a		
Topography Details	n/a		
SimK Values	n/a		
Pachymetry	n/a		

PROCEDURES PERFORMED

	OD	OS	COMMENTS
1. Date/type	1998 M-LASIK		interface
Laser/keratome/plate	VISX Star/ACS/160		inflammation
2. Date/type	flap lifted		
Laser/keratome/plate	interface scraped		

CURRENT POSTOPERATIVE INFORMATION

	OD	OS	COMMENTS
Time Postoperative	1 month		residual hyperopia
Postoperative Refraction	+1.75 DS		and irregular
BCVA	20/60		astigmatism
Topography Details	inferior flattening		
SimK Values	n/a		
Pachymetry	n/a		
Visual Complaints	distortion		
Medications	none		

A 28-year-old white female with a history of keloid scarring underwent bilateral LASIK for treatment of low myopia with no reported intraoperative complications (preoperative Rx: OD -2.25 + 0.50 X 090, OS -1.25 + 0.25 X 090). Her 1 day postoperative exam revealed well-positioned LASIK flaps OU with a few scattered cells in the lamellar interface, more pronounced in the right eye. She was started on a normal postoperative course of FML 1% and Ocuflox drops q.i.d. OU. She was seen at her 1 week postoperative visit complaining of decreased vision in the right eye.

UCVA in the right eye was 20/100 with double images and halos, and no improvement with pinhole. UCVA in the left eye was 20/20.

Slit lamp examination of the right eye revealed a dense, white, corrugated plaque in the lamellar interface (Figure 8A-1). It measured approximately 3 x 3 mm and was located in the inferior visual axis (Figure 8A-2). The remaining peripheral cornea was clear, and there were a few rare cells present in the anterior chamber. Examination of the left eye revealed a few scant cells in the peripheral lamellar interface, and a clear visual axis.

This case describes a severe form of DLK. Interestingly, it occurred in a patient with a history of keloid formation, which, while associated with severe haze formation after PRK, has not previously been a known contraindication to LASIK.

The etiology of DLK is currently unknown, although anecdotal reports have implicated a host of possible sources. Attention has focused on possible contaminants of the microkeratome/blade system, such as oil, rust, silicates, metallic fragments, bacterial cell wall fragments (endotoxin), and poor autoclave cleaning. These antigenic stimuli are hypothesized to be inoculated into the lamellar interface, a normally immune privileged site, where they incite migration of a mixed leukocyte response.

The cellular infiltrate is granular in appearance, and initially located in the peripheral cornea, near the flap border. It is often present in the first 24 hours after treatment, although visual acuity may be unaffected (Figure 8A-3). Meticulous slit lamp examination on the first postoperative day is crucial in identifying eyes with DLK, as prompt intervention can prevent irreversible visual morbidity later on.

The majority of eyes with DLK will respond to intensive topical steroid treatment if identified early. However, a minority of eyes will progress even after several days of topical steroid, and it is these eyes which must be followed closely. Movement of the cellular infiltrate centrally (the so-called "shifting sands" or "sands of the Sahara" syndrome) with clumping, aggregation, and a hyperopic shift is an ominous sign (Figure 8A-4). If left untreated, these eyes will go on to lose several lines of BCVA that can be irreversible.

The visual morbidity in these cases results from both scarring and necrosis of the central flap. The cells appear to collect centrally in the deepest part of the ablation zone, and settle slightly inferiorly with gravity. The cells coalesce to form a focal area of hypertonic and enzymatic fluid collection which causes overlying flap edema, necrosis, and eventually melt. Topography will frequently show a focal area of intense flattening do to stromal melting, with a resultant hyperopic shift.

The authors have found that prompt relifting of the LASIK flap at the first sign of central cellular migration, with cleaning and irrigation of the flap bed, can successfully manage this condition with near 100% success rate. While speculation will continue on the etiology of this uncommon, but frustrating complication, prompt identification on the first postoperative day along with daily follow up visits and flap lifting and irrigation if necessary can prevent unwanted visual outcomes.

The patient received topical Pred Forte 1% drops every hour along with FML ointment at bedtime to the affected eye for 48 hours. The visual acuity and appearance of the infiltrate remained unchanged. The flap was eventually lifted on postoperative day 8 and the bed was cultured, gently scraped, and irrigated. A collection of soggy cellular debris was removed from the inner surface of the cap, and a bullae formation was noted overlying the affected area. The flap was then floated back in place and allowed to dry.

The patient was maintained on intensive topical steroid medication. Culture results were negative, and the area of infiltrate slowly decreased in both size and intensity over the next few weeks. The patients BCVA remained in the 20/60 range with a +1.75 sph refraction. Topography revealed an inferior zone of intense flattening with associated superior steepening, and irregular astigmatism (Figure 8A-5).

Suggested Reading

Wilson SE. LASIK: Management of common complications. *Cornea.* 1998;17:459-467.

Maloney RK. *Interface keratitis after LASIK.* Presented at the American Academy of Ophthalmology annual meeting. San Francisco, Calif; November 1997.

Figure 8A-1. Slit lamp exam 1 week after LASIK.

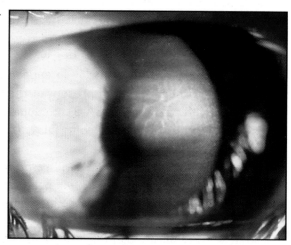

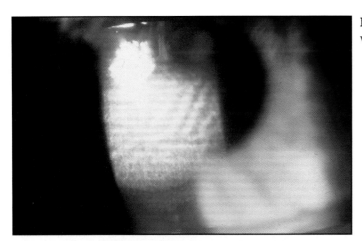

Figure 8A-2. High power magnified view of corrugated infiltrate.

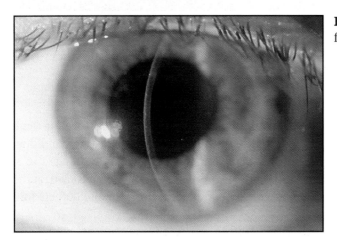

Figure 8A-3. Granular cells in flap interface.

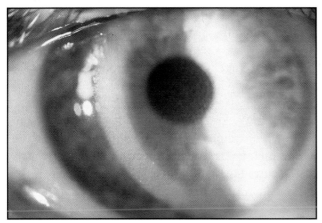

Figure 8A-4. Central involvement of cells in flap interface.

Figure 8A-5. Topography showing flattening and irregular astigmatism associated with area of flap necrosis.

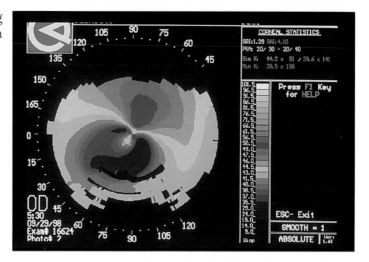

Editor's Notes

This case illustrates a severe form of LASIK interface keratitis which occurs to a less severe extent in approximately 1 in 300 LASIK cases. While the etiological factor associated with this condition remains to be clearly identified, it is currently hypothesized that in many cases it may be related to a hypersensitivity reaction to bacterial cell wall proteins left on the instruments following the sterilization process. Localized areas of interface keratitis are also known to occur underneath epithelial defects following LASIK.

Since LASIK interface keratitis tends to occur 1 to 3 days following LASIK, any patients complaining of decreased vision or demonstrating inflammatory material at the interface at this time should be reviewed on an urgent basis in order to determine whether frequent topical steroids would be useful. A mild case of LASIK interface keratitis can be controlled with a frequent use of topical steroid preparation. If epithelial defect is associated with a localized interface keratitis, frequent lubrication is also helpful to heal the epithelial defect along with antibiotic coverage to prevent infection. In severe cases of LASIK interface keratitis, irrigation of the interface may also be helpful to remove the inflammatory stimuli.

Further laser application to the stromal bed or scraping of the stromal bed should be avoided if at all possible. Since the inflamed tissue is edematous, there will be removal of significant amounts of tissue that will alter the refractive outcome significantly. The final topography of this case demonstrates the inferior area of flattening following the scraping that occurred in the inferior part of the cornea.

Case B, Diffuse Lamellar Keratitis with a Central Island

Richard Duffey, MD

Main Concern: Interface Inflammation
Patient Age: 28

Initial Preoperative Information

	OD	OS	Comments
Preoperative Refraction	-7.25		
BCVA	20/20		
Topography Details	normal		
SimK Values	46.0 X 69/45.4 X 159		
Pachymetry	575 μm		

Procedures Performed

	OD	OS	Comments
1. Date/type	10/31/96 LASIK		
Laser/keratome/plate	VISX Star/ACS/160		
2. Date/type	2/6/97 flap lifted and PTK		central island
Laser/keratome/plate	VISX Star		

Current Postoperative Information

	OD	OS	Comments
Time Postoperative	12 months		persistent small
Postoperative Refraction	pl + 1.50 X 30		central island
BCVA	20/30		
Topography Details	central island		
SimK Values	39.7/39.2		
Pachymetry	n/a		
Visual Complaints	less glare		
Medications	none		
Refractive Correction	none		

On October 31, 1996, a 28-year-old male underwent uneventful LASIK with a VISX Star laser on his right eye. His preoperative refraction was -7.00 DS. On the first postoperative day, UCVA was 20/20 with a refraction of +0.25 also yielding 20/20 visual acuity. There was +1 interface debris and no striae with a fully epithelialized flap gutter.

The patient returned 1 week later complaining of decreased visual acuity OD and irritation. UCVA was 20/80 improving to 20/40 with a refraction of -0.75 + 1.00 X 140. There was a small epithelial break centrally on the flap with anterior stromal edema diffusely throughout the center of the flap and anterior stromal bed and a 2+ cellular reaction diffusely in the flap interface (Figure 8B-1).

The decision was made not to lift the flap and the patient was placed on hourly ofloxacin and fluorometholone drops. The following day visual acuity had improved to 20/40 without correction with less flap edema and fewer white cells and haze throughout the flap interface and bed. The drops were decreased to every three hours and he was asked to return in one week.

On November 18, 1996, UCVA was 20/50 improving to 20/40+ with a +0.25 refraction. A small amount of anterior stromal haze remained primarily at the interface and the epithelium was intact. Fluorometholone was continued at 4 times a day and the ofloxacin was discontinued.

On December 2, 1996, visual acuity without correction was 20/60 improving to 20/30 with refraction of +0.75 with only minimal anterior stromal haze at the flap interface and he was placed on a tapering dose of fluorometholone over the next 2 months.

He was next examined on February 3, 1997, at which time UCVA was 20/50, improving to 20/30 with a refraction of +0.50 + 1.50 X 175. A corneal map was done (Figure 8B-2) that noted a paracentral island/peninsula extending to the edge of the visual axis. The patient had complaints of ghosting and halos, as well as glare and light sensitivity. The paracentral island was treated by lifting the original flap and applying the excimer laser in a PTK mode on February 6, 1997. One day following PTK treatment of the island, UCVA was 20/30 with no further improvement and a refraction of -0.50 + 0.75 X 075. He was treated with a tapering dose of fluorometholone over a 2 week period and topical ofloxacin for 1 week.

At 2 weeks, visual acuity remained 20/30 with a normal flap. He was again seen on April 11, 1997, with visual acuity of 20/30 both UCVA and BCVA. He was then last seen on October 13, 1997, with visual acuity of 20/30 improving to 20/25 with a refraction of pl + 150 X 30 and minimal complaint of light sensitivity or glare. The topography showed a persistent central island (Figure 8B-3).

At the time of this patient's development of DLK in 1996, LASIK was still relatively new in the US and DLK had not been formally described. The less aggressive treatment of this entity (frequent use of topical steroids and topical antibiotics) as opposed to a more aggressive approach (lifting and irrigating beneath the flap to remove the inflammatory nidus) probably contributed to the prolonged inflammation and ultimate minimal scar formation on this patient's cornea. A paracentral island formation was probably a direct consequence of this DLK suggested by the fact that the patient's UCVA was 20/20 on day 1.

In the future, I would recommend treating this type of patient's complication with a much more aggressive approach of lifting and irrigating beneath the flap to remove any inflammatory debris or nidus that may contribute to the DLK. Whether or not the island formation is a direct consequence of the DLK is not provable in this case; however, certainly a less prolonged course of inflammation would have been advantageous to this patient by lessening the corneal scarring that was a consequence of this inflammation.

Figure 8B-1. Nine days post-LASIK with consolidating white blood cells in the region of the DLK.

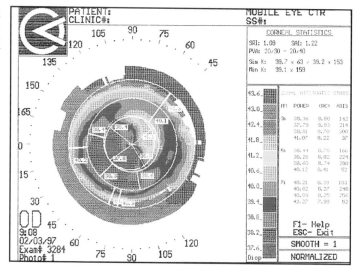

Figure 8B-2. Paracentral island topography map 3 months post-LASIK and immediately before PTK and treatment under the flap.

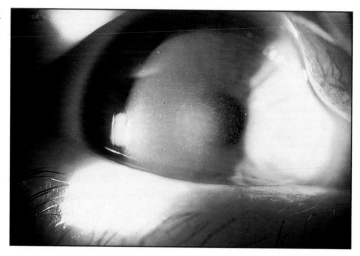

Figure 8B-3. One year post-LASIK and 9 months post-PTK treatment under the flap. Small central island remains.

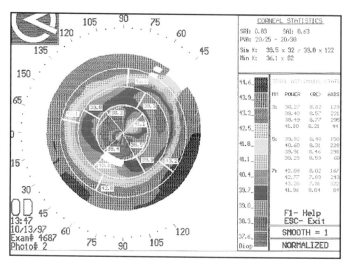

Editor's Notes

This is an unusual presentation of LIK for several reasons. The onset of the condition occurred at approximately 9 days postoperatively. Generally LIK occurs 1 to 3 days following the LASIK procedure. This case also occurred in 1996, prior to the identification of this condition, so little was known about its diagnosis or treatment. The interface inflammation was associated with an epithelial defect and the eye was uncomfortable, which are also uncommon findings with LIK.

While LIK is a very possible diagnosis in this situation, other considerations would be an early form of infectious keratitis that gained access to the cornea through the epithelial defect. In this situation, the treatment with topical antibiotics was very appropriate. Infection could also be an explanation for the central corneal scar that resulted in the paracentral corneal island.

Case C, Grade 3 Sands with Striae

Ted Smith, OD, Jeffery J. Machat, MD, and Louis E. Probst, MD

Main Concern: Sands with Hyperopia
Patient Age: 20

Initial Preoperative Information

	OD	OS	Comments
Preoperative Refraction	+5.75 − 8.00 X 003		pre-AK
UCVA	20/40-		
BCVA	20/25		
Topography Details	47.75/41.37 X 180		
SimK Values	0.56		
Pachymetry	548 µm		

Procedures Performed

	OD	OS	Comments
1. Date/type	11/20/98 AK		
Laser/keratome/plate	2 x 4 mm incisions		
2. Date/type	2/12/99 LASIK		
Laser/keratome/plate	Technolas 217/ACS/180		
3. Date/type	2/24/99 PTK (OZ 6 mm)		
Laser/keratome/plate	Technolas 217/lift		
4. Date/type	2/25/99 PTK (OZ 6 mm)		
Laser/keratome/plate	Technolas 217/lift		

Current Postoperative Information

	OD	OS	Comments
Time Postoperative	6 weeks		from last PTK/lift
Postoperative Refraction	+525 DS		iatrogenic hyperopia
UCVA	20/50-		irregular topography,
BCVA	20/30		loss of BCVA
Topography Details	44.75/34.12 X 28		
SimK Values	6.17		
Pachymetry	352 µm		
Visual Complaints	blur		
Medications	none		
Refractive Correction	none		

This patient was a 20-year-old white male with an unremarkable medical history. To reduce his severe corneal cylinder, AK surgery was performed on both his right and left eye on November 20/98 on a preoperative *Rx* of +5.75 – 8.00 X 003 OD and +6.25 – 7.50 X 180 OS (Figures 8C-1 and 8C-2). Two 4 mm incisions were made at 12 and 6 o'clock. At 4 months postoperative the stabilized *Rx* was OD +4.50 – 5.00 X 006 with BCVA of 20/25 and OS +5.25 – 6.50 X 002 with BCVA 20/20. Topography showed K values OD of 47.50/42.00 X 008 CIM 0.62 and OS 47.00/41.62 X 004 CIM 0.66 (Figures 8C-3 and 8C-4). At that time, LASIK was performed with the aim for full correction OU with an ACS keratome and 180 µm flap. Remarkably, this patient had unaided acuities of 20/20- OU, with a minor *Rx* OD +0.50 + 0.25 X 090 and OS -050 – 0.75 X 0.70 OS at 1 day postoperative.

By day 4 postoperative, the left eye was stable at 20/20-, however the right eye developed grade 3 NSDIK and BCVA had reduced to 20/200. Unfortunately this was treated as stromal edema by the comanaging doctor, Pred Forte and Muro 128 (Bausch and Lomb Pharmaceuticals, Inc. Tampa, Fla) were prescribed q.i.d. Upon examination at our center at day 12 postoperative, the patient. had an *Rx* of +2.25 – 1.00 X 180 and a BCVA of 20/400, pinholing to 20/60. Biomicroscopy confirmed grade 3 NSDIK, with dense central haze and striae (Figure 8C-5). At this time the corneal flap was lifted and 25 µm of PTK was applied to the stromal bed and 5 µm of PTK to the undersurface of the flap, both at optic zones of 6 mm. In addition, the hyperopia was treated with a desired correction of +1.75 – 0.50 X 180. The dense striae, which had developed from the corneal edema, were stretched and smoothed. Ocuflox q.i.d. and Maxidex q30min, tapered to qhr, q2hr and q.i.d. each day were prescribed. A bandage contact lens was inserted to cover epithelial defects from flap manipulation.

On examination the next day, biomicroscopy showed absence of the central striae, however, the central haze and edema were reduced only slightly (Figure 8C-6). An *Rx* of OD +6.75 + 1.25 X 150 was exhibited, which corresponded to unaided and aided acuities of 20/400 and 20/40 respectively. The corneal flap was relifted and 10 µm of PTK was applied to the stromal bed and 10 µm of PTK was applied to the undersurface of the flap, again at optic zone 6 mm. A refractive correction of +4.50 D was ablated. The patient was instructed to continue with the medications listed above. At the 1 week postoperative assessment, the patient exhibited an *Rx* of OD +7.75 + 1.00 X 150 with unaided and BCVAs of 20/400 and 20/40- respectively. the patient. claimed to be experiencing multiplopia. All medications were discontinued other than ocular lubrication prn.

At 5 weeks postoperative, the patient showed improved unaided acuity OD of 20/50-. There was still a manifest *Rx* of OD +5.25 DS that provided a BCVA of 20/30. Central corneal clouding had reduced markedly, showing only mild reticular haze (Figure 8C-7). Topography was not reliable due to persistent tear instability despite lubrication, however it indicated high paracentral corneal irregular astigmatism and substantial central flattening, with K values of 41.00/34.50 and CIM value 9.48 (Figure 8C-8). Pachymetry showed a substantially thinned cornea with central thickness of 352 µm.

Despite the remarkable improvement in corneal clarity, it appears that lamellar or full thickness corneal graft surgery may be the only alternative to restore functional vision in the right eye, due to the residual multiplopia, high hyperopia and minimal central corneal thickness.

Figure 8C-1. Preoperative topography OD demonstrates a regular with-the-rule astigmatism.

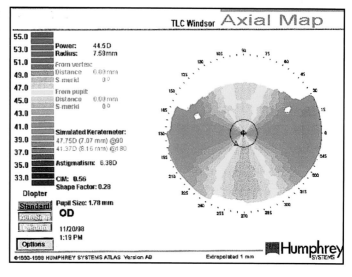

Figure 8C-2. Preoperative topography OS demonstrates a regular with-the-rule astigmatism.

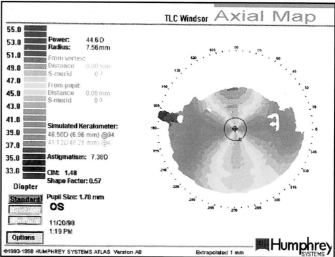

Figure 8C-3. Post-AK topography OD shows a reduction in the astigmatism by about 2 D.

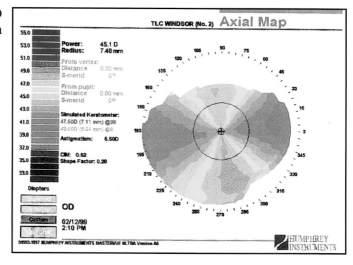

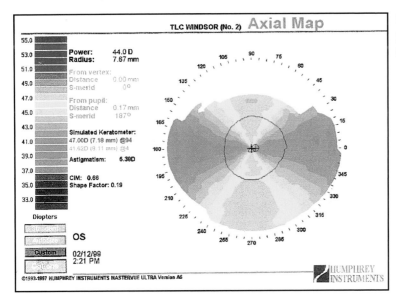

Figure 8C-4. Post-AK topography OS shows a reduction in the astigmatism by about 2 D.

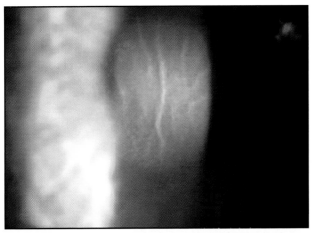

Figure 8C-5. Dense interface inflammation causing striae in the flap OD.

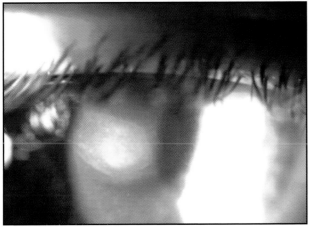

Figure 8C-6. Slight improvement in the interface inflammation OD.

Figure 8C-7. Marked improvement in the interface inflammation and the striae after 5 weeks.

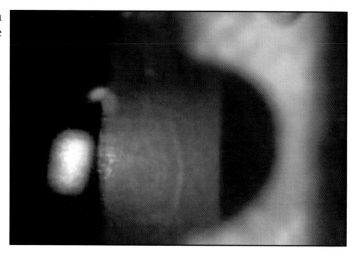

Figure 8C-8. Tremendous central flattening due to the interface keratitis and the multiple PTK applications.

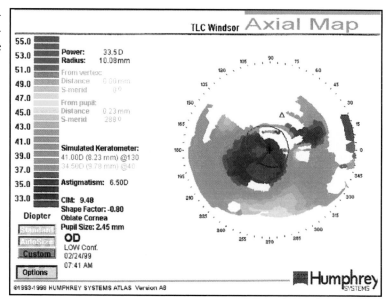

Editor's Notes

This case represents the most undesirable sequelae of LIK. This patient originally presented with an extreme amount of astigmatism which was treated with AK to reduce the astigmatism into the range that could effectively treated with the Technolas 217 excimer laser. On the initial follow-up topography after the initial AK procedure, the astigmatism had been reduced by approximately 2 D in both eyes. After the bilateral LASIK procedure, the result in the left eye was outstanding with an UCVA of 20/20-. The initial result in the right eye also yielded a UCVA of 20/20- on day 1 but unfortunately on the third postoperative day the UCVA had been reduced to 20/200 due to the LIK.

When the patient returned to our center, there was a dense central corneal interface haze that was evident with central flap striae in the interface. This was treated with multiple PTK applications to the interface, as well as a compensatory hyperopic correction because of the expected induced hyperopia from the PTK. Despite these measures, the patient has ended up significantly hyperopic with a prescription in the +4.50 D range. The BCVA has been substantially restored. However, the cornea is excessively thinned and therefore further corrective procedures will be difficult.

The most conservative surgical option would be holmium laser thermal keratoplasty (LTK) in an effort to correct the hyperopia. Since the cornea is thin, LTK will have an enhanced effect with one ring at 7.0 mm, reducing the hyperopia by about 3.0 D. A homograft may be required in order to restore the corneal thickness, and the refractive error could be corrected in a second procedure. PK may become the only adequate solution.

This case illustrates two important points with LASIK. Any patient with a sudden loss of visual acuity on the first few postoperative days should be evaluated immediately in order to ensure that any correctable situation is rectified. In this situation, early interface irrigation or early topical steroids may have had some beneficial effect on the cornea. Secondly, any tissue removal type of procedure such as scraping of the interface or applying PTK pulses to an inflamed interface should be done with great caution. Removal of this inflamed tissue will result in an alteration of the refractive error. This could result in an irregular astigmatism or an extreme hyperopic shift that can significantly alter the final outcome.

CASE D, BILATERAL SANDS

Ted Smith, OD, and Jeffery J. Machat, MD

Main Concern: Interface Inflammation
Patient Age: 53

INITIAL PREOPERATIVE INFORMATION

	OD	OS	COMMENTS
Preoperative Refraction	-14.50 – 0.25 X 60		high myope
UCVA	hm@1ft		
BCVA	20/20-		
Topography Details	46.12/44.87 X 012		
SimK Values	0.99		
Pachymetry	580 µm		

PROCEDURES PERFORMED

	OD	OS	COMMENTS
1. Date/type	7/29/98 LASIK		
Laser/keratome/plate	Technolas 217/ACS/160		

CURRENT POSTOPERATIVE INFORMATION

	OD	OS	COMMENTS
Time Postoperative	9 weeks		interface inflammation
Postoperative Refraction	-1.25 – 0.75 X 070		resolved
UCVA	20/40-		
BCVA	20/20-		
Topography Details	40.37/38.87 X 176		
SimK Values	1.70		
Pachymetry	469 µm		
Visual Complaints	none		
Medications	none		
Refractive Correction	none		

This patient was a 53-year-old white female. Her surgical history consisted of bilateral LASIK done on July 29, 1998 in attempt for full correction of OD -14.50 – 0.25 X 60 and OS -13.00 – 0.25 X 090 with BCVA OU of 20/25. An ACS keratome and a 160 µm flap was used with the Technolas 217 laser. Prior to the procedure, topography showed K values of OD 46.12/44.87 X 12 CIM 0.99 and OS 45.37/44.37 X 022 CIM 0.70 (Figure 8D-1). The surgery was uneventful other than a small epithelial defect OD, which was believed to have originated from minor undiagnosed anterior basement membrane dystrophy. A bandage contact lens was inserted to cover the defect. At 1 day postoperative, the corneas were clear OU and UCVA was 20/60 OD and 20/70 OS. There was still residual epithelial cell disruption inferiorly OD, hence the bandage contact lens was left in place.

At postoperative day 2, dense grade 2 NSDIK was observed OD, BCVA was 20/40 with a slight hyperopic *Rx* of +0.50 DS (Figure 8D-2). The left eye showed mild grade 1 NSDIK with BCVA 20/30. Treatment with Pred Forte q1h was initiated as well as Ocuflox q.i.d. maintained for antibiotic coverage OU. At one week postoperative the sands had cleared substantially OD, however persistent corneal inflammation was present. The left cornea was completely clear. There was no residual refraction OD and BCVA had improved to 20/30. The left eye showed an *Rx* of +0.50 – 2.25 X 025 and BCVA 20/30. The regimen of Pred Forte was reduced to q.i.d. OU and tapered over the next 2 weeks.

At 9 weeks postoperative the right cornea had cleared, and the UCVA of 20/40- was correctable to 20/20- with a manifest *Rx* of OD -1.25 – 0.75 X 070. Pachymetry showed central corneal thickness of 469 µm. Topography showed a smooth, regular central cornea with a CIM value of 1.70 and K values of 40.37/38.87 X 176 (Figure 8D-3). The patient has been content to remain at the above *Rx* OU without an enhancement, as she uses the unaided myopia OD to aid in reading at near.

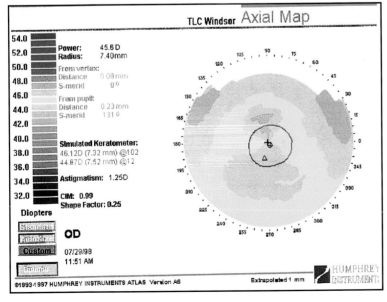

Figure 8D-1. Preoperative topography OD demonstrates a regular pattern.

Figure 8D-2. Grade 2 interface inflammation on day 2.

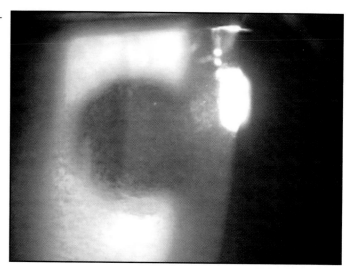

Figure 8D-3. Postoperative topography OD shows a smooth, regular central cornea.

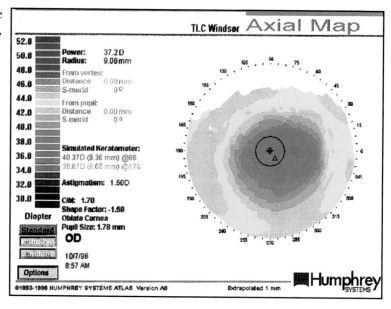

Editor's Notes

LIK is generally a mild condition that does not significantly affect BCVA and can be effectively treated with topical steroids. This case demonstrates a typical case of LIK. The original procedure was complicated by a small epithelial defect necessitating the placement of a bandage contact lens in order to improve patient comfort following the procedure. Epithelial defects can be one of the predisposing factors to LIK. The quick initiation of frequent topical steroids assists with the quick resolution of LIK. Although the refraction did take almost 2 months to stabilize, the final refractive outcome yielded a BCVA of 20/20-. Often LIK will cause an alteration of the refractive outcome with a more hyperopic prescription after myopic LASIK has been performed, however in this case the result was a small under-correction.

CASE E, FOCAL LASIK INTERFACE INFLAMMATION

Michael Lawless, MBBS, FRACO, FRACS, FRCOphth, and Sue Webber, BSc(Hons), FRCOphth

Main Concern: Interface Inflammation
Patient Age: 38

INITIAL PREOPERATIVE INFORMATION

	OD	OS	COMMENTS
Preoperative Refraction	-3.75	-3.75	
BCVA	6/6	6/6	
Topography Details	spherical cornea	small regular astigmatism	
SimK Values	47.0@51/46.48	47.07@105/46.42	
Pachymetry	not performed	not performed	

PROCEDURES PERFORMED

	OD	OS	COMMENTS
1. Date/type	1/5/97, LASIK	1/5/97, LASIK	
Laser/keratome/plate	OU: Summit Apex Plus/Chiron ACS/160 µm, standard anti-island pretreatment, then -3.8 D		

CURRENT POSTOPERATIVE INFORMATION

	OD	OS	COMMENTS
Time Postoperative	4 months	4 months	excellent results OU
Postoperative Refraction	0/-0.75 X 97	+2.25/-0.75 X 115	
BCVA	6/6	6/6	
Topography Details	some irregular astigmatism OU		
SimK Values	42.82@20/42.50	42.08@159/41.25	
Visual Complaints	none	none	
Medications	none	none	
Refractive Correction	reading correction OU		

This patient had routine LASIK correction of -3.75 D to both eyes with no preoperative abnormalities (Figure 8E-1). On the day after surgery ocular examination was unremarkable and he was prescribed Tobramycin 0.3% and Pred Forte t.i.d. to both eyes. He returned on the fifth postoperative day complaining of pain in the left eye. Examination at that stage demonstrated UCVAs of 6/12 OD and cf OS. There was a central epithelial defect in the left eye. Both corneas had a 3 mm circular area of stromal opacity at the interface of the flap and the stromal bed (Figures 8E-2 and 8E-3). There were folds in the corneal cap that were highlighted by the inflammatory material (Figure 8E-4). The anterior chambers were quiet. At this stage, the differential diagnosis included infective keratitis, medication toxicity and sterile reactive inflammation. The current treatment was ceased and g. ciprofloxacin (3 mg/ml) q.i.d. was commenced. Over the next 2 weeks the visual acuity and interface changes improved. A diagnosis of noninfective inflammation was made and the treatment was changed to FML b.i.d. Five weeks after surgery both eyes showed some hypermetropic shift, with residual interface changes. At 2 months after LASIK the FML was ceased, and 2 months later the visual acuity and refraction were as reported above (Figure 8E-5).

This case raises several interesting questions. First, what is the source of the inflammation? The clinical course in both this case and others we have observed, would suggest that the lesion is not infective.[1] In this case, the opacity decreased with only ciprofloxacin q.i.d.. If this were infective, it is unlikely that this medication would represent adequate treatment. Alternatively, this could represent a tissue reaction to foreign material introduced at the time of surgery or an extreme reaction to epithelial cells or meibomian secretions deposited at the time of surgery. At no time was any foreign material or ectopic ocular matter seen in the flap interface.

Smith and Maloney[2] described a series of patients with a condition they named DLK. While the case here is in a different order of severity than those reported by Smith and Maloney, it is possible that they both represent manifestations in a spectrum of the same disease etiology. In at least some of the Maloney cases, fibrous foreign bodies were identified in the interface. It is possible that all these patients are exhibiting a reaction to foreign or ectopic material.

Clinical differentiation is at the heart of the management of these cases. Clearly, if the inflammation seen is sterile, the treatment would pivot around the use of anti-inflammatory medication. Yet, if infective, microbiological sampling should be undertaken before the use of fortified antibiotics. How to tell the difference is difficult, especially if there is a spectrum of sterile inflammatory disease. The sterile and infective conditions may present in a similar fashion with pain, photophobia, epiphora, decreased acuity and redness. There are a few key points in the differentiation of the two conditions. First, sterile inflammatory disease is more likely to be confined to the flap interface with little or no extension into the anterior or posterior stroma. Second, in sterile inflammatory disease there is little or no anterior chamber inflammation, whereas with infection intense cellular reaction, KPs and hypopyon might occur. Third, in sterile conditions the infiltrate is more likely to be diffuse and bilateral, whereas in infective conditions the disease may be focal and unilateral. Time will also help, infection usually rapidly progresses unless appropriate treatment is given.

This inflammatory response has resulted in a hypermetropic refraction in this and other patients we have seen.[1] We postulate that this is because tissue necrosis has occurred and caused extreme flattening in the central corneal area. However, it is also reassuring to note that these patients can achieve a normal final BCVA.

References

1. Fraenkel GF, Cohen PR, Sutton GS, Lawless MA, Rogers CM. Central focal interface opacity after laser in situ keratomileusis. *J Refract Surg.* 1998;14:571-576.
2. Smith RJ, Maloney RK. Diffuse lamellar keratitis. *Ophthalmology.* 1998; 105(9):1721-1726.

Figure 8E-1. Preoperative topography.

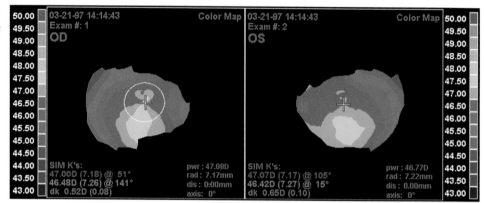

Figure 8E-2. Corneal appearance 1 week after surgery.

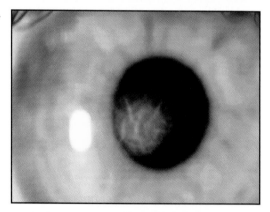

Figure 8E-3. Slit beam showing interface inflammation restricted to flap interface.

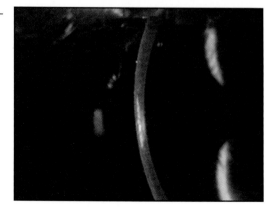

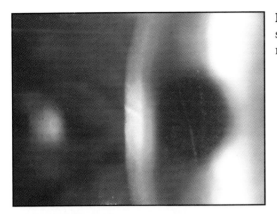

Figure 8E-4. Photograph 1 week after surgery showing corneal flattening due to probable stromal necrosis.

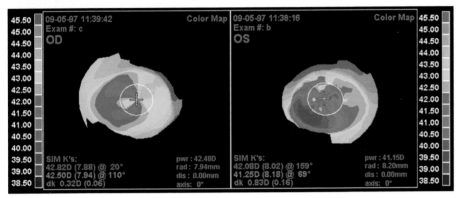

Figure 8E-5. Topography 4 months after surgery. Note considerable flattening of left cornea.

Editor's Notes

Prevention of LIK involve sterilizing the instruments at the end of each surgical day followed by a complete drying so no moisture would build up. The autoclave should be cleaned as well, with all fluid being removed. All autoclave trays should be left open in order to dry. The motor tip should be wiped down with alcohol and the microkeratome head should be sterilized and left open to dry as well. While the bacterial cell wall hypothesis remains to be definitely proven, this seems to be the most plausible explanation for LIK at the present time.

9

BACTERIAL KERATITIS
AFTER LASIK

BACTERIAL KERATITIS AFTER LASIK - SUMMARY NOTES

Clinical

Infections or corneal ulcers are extremely uncommon after LASIK with an incidence of less than 1/5000 cases. Since the corneal epithelium protects against infection, the risk of infection is minimal once the epithelium is completely healed. The short time of exposure of the stroma and the lack of epithelial disruption helps to minimize this risk. Infections begin as infiltrates in the area of an epithelial defect. If left untreated, they can progress into a typical corneal ulceration with infiltration, ocular inflammation, and pain.

Management

Any corneal infiltrate associated with an epithelial defect after LASIK should be assumed to be infective and treated immediately and aggressively. Corneal cultures can be performed, however, the utility of corneal cultures at this early stage of infection is controversial.

Treatment of Corneal Infection / Infiltrate
- stop nonsteroid medications
- stop topical steroid drops
- topical fluoroquinolone every hour
- lubrication
- daily follow-up
- switch to fortified topical antibiotics (if no resolution)

Prevention

Any patient with an epithelial defect after LASIK needs to be followed daily to ensure that no infection occurs until the defect has healed.

Prevention of Infection
- prophylactic antibiotics
- sterilization of the microkeratome
- lid hygiene
- preoperative antiseptic eyewash
- talc-free gloves

CASE A, BACTERIAL KERATITIS AFTER LASIK

Stephen Slade, MD, Ted Smith, OD, and Jeffery J. Machat, MD

Main Concern: Corneal Ulcer and Subsequent Confluent Haze
Patient Age: 38

INITIAL PREOPERATIVE INFORMATION

	OD	OS	COMMENTS
Preoperative Refraction	-13.75 – 1.75 X 180		high myopia
UCVA	cf@1ft		
BCVA	20/20		
Topography Details	45.00/43.00 X 178		
SimK Values	n/a		
Pachymetry	n/a		

PROCEDURES PERFORMED

	OD	OS	COMMENTS
1. Date/type	4/17/95 LASIK		
Laser/keratome/plate	Technolas 117/ACS/180		
2. Date/type	10/9/95 PRK/PTK		corneal haze
Laser/keratome/plate	6 mmOZ		
3. Date/type	1/9/97 lamellar keratoplasty		irregular cornea
4. Date/type	8/29/97		cataract
Laser/keratome/plate	phaco and IOL		
5. Date/type	12/12/97 Ptosis surgery		ptosis
6. Date/type	3/23/98 Yag capsulotomy		opacified capsule

CURRENT POSTOPERATIVE INFORMATION

	OD	OS	COMMENTS
Time Postoperative	9/4/98 (6 months post Yag)		considering clear
Postoperative Refraction	+0.75 – 3.00 X 106		lens extraction OS
UCVA	20/100		
BCVA	20/30-		
Topography Details	n/a		
SimK Values	n/a		
Visual Complaints	blur		
Refractive Correction	none		

This patient was a 38-year-old white female with an unremarkable medical history. Her surgical history consisted of LASIK performed on her right eye on April 17, 1995, for attempted correction of OD -13.75 – 1.75 X 180. Her left Rx was -10.75 – 2.00 X 178, however, due to her severe myopia, only her right eye was attempted. At that time, topography OD showed a smooth cornea with the expected astigmatism corresponding with the spectacle Rx, with K values 45.00/43.00 X 178 (Figure 9A-1). The procedure was uncomplicated.

On the second day postoperative, the patient presented to her comanaging doctor complaining of a foreign body sensation with UCVA 20/40. Biomicroscopy showed two epithelial infiltrates 2 mm in from the flap edge. The patient was prescribed a regimen of Ocuflox q1h and Tobradex q.i.d. The following morning the patient presented with a 2 x 3 mm corneal ulcer in the bottom third area of the flap. She was treated aggressively with fortified broad spectrum antibiotics until the ulcer was cultured, which showed the presence of Serratia marcescens. The patient was subsequently placed on Tobramycin fortified drops Q1h and subconjunctival injection. The corneal flap was debrided.

At 6 months postoperatively, the patient presented for evaluation for stabilization. During the past months the ulcer had healed with substantial corneal thinning and scarring despite aggressive intervention with steroids over several months. (Figure 9A-2). Refraction showed O.D. -9.50 – 1.50 X 005, providing a BCVA of 20/40 from the UCVA of cf at 2 feet. Pachymetry showed a cornea thinned to 394 µm. Topography showed severe, but reasonably symmetrical corneal astigmatism, with K values of 3.37/37.37 X 002 (Figure 9A-3). In attempt to address the corneal haze and residual Rx, PTK and PRK were applied with OZ 6 mm with an ablation correction target of -2.60 – 1.50 X 003 and depth 47 µm.

Over the next 6 months, management consisted of standard post PRK therapeutic treatment with Flarex q.i.d. tapered over 4 months. During that time, it was difficult to determine the residual refraction due to severe persistent corneal irregularity that also rendered topographical analysis futile due to tear instability. A series of attempts were made to provide decent functional vision with rigid gas permeable contact lens designs over the next 8 months. However, reasonable comfort with a contact lens could not be achieved and visual acuity tended to fluctuate frequently between BCVA 20/25 and 20/60.

It was decided that lamellar corneal homograft surgical intervention was the only alternative, since the corneal irregularity and limited thickness of 372 µm could not allow further ablations. The lamellar keratoplasty was performed on January 8, 1997, by Dr. Steve Slade. At 2 months postoperatively, the cornea was clear centrally and showed only the inferior peripheral scarring left over from the corneal ulcer. Unaided acuity was still reduced, at cf@2ft and refraction could not be determined accurately. It was believed that there was at least 9 D of myopia, however, this Rx only improved acuity to BCVA 20/400. Pinhole acuity achieved 20/70. Topography showed severe asymmetrical astigmatism with paracentral nasal flattening. K values were 46.25/40.87 X 020 with a CIM value 3.90 (Figure 9A-4).

Over the next 6 months, while the patient was being monitored for corneal stabilization following the lamellar homograft, the patient developed a substantial right posterior subcapsular cataract, undoubtedly as consequence to the repeated topical corticosteroid use over the previous 2 years. BCVA became reduced to cf@3ft, however, PAM indicated an acuity potential of 20/50.

The right cataract was removed via phacoemulsification on Aug 29, 1997, and a posterior chamber lens inserted. Refraction at 2 weeks postoperatively showed an *Rx* OD of -2.00 − 1.00 X 025 with unaided and aided acuities of 20/100 and 20/30 respectively. Topography still showed substantial corneal astigmatism that did not manifest in the above refraction, but the previously seen nasal flattening 6 months previously had reduced markedly. K values were 45.00/41.87 X 180 (Figure 9A-5).

As Murphy's Law dictates, the patient developed right ptosis and lid surgery was performed December 12, 1997. Incredibly, secondary posterior capsule opacification also developed over the next few months and a YAG capsulotomy was performed on March 23, 1998.

At last assessment on September 4, 1998, patient showed an UCVA OD of 20/100. The refraction had stabilized at +0.75 − 3.00 X 106 giving BCVA 20/30+. Topography indicated improved corneal regularity with reasonable symmetry about the visual axis (Figure 9A-6). There was an arcuate ridge of corneal steepening temporocentrally. Keratometry values were 45.12/42.25 X 012 with CIM 3.16. The central cornea was clear and there was still inferior haze from the corneal ulcer. The patient is currently using a contact lens OU. Due to the severe myopia OS, and resulting poor contact lens tolerance in that eye, the patient is currently investigating clear lens extraction. This will relieve the myopia and the anisometropia so that spectacle wear will be an option.

Figure 9A-1. Preoperative topography OU.

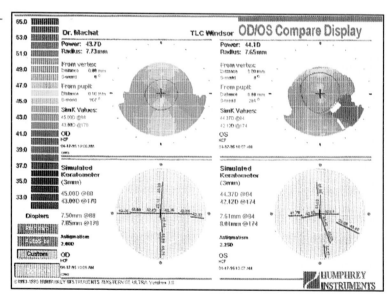

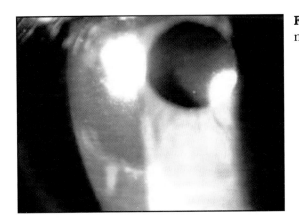

Figure 9A-2. Corneal scarring and thinning six months after corneal ulcer following LASIK.

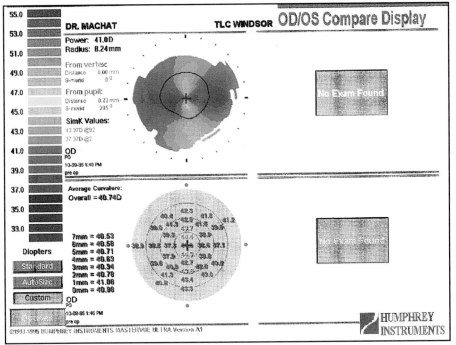

Figure 9A-3. Topography 6 months after corneal ulcer following LASIK showing severe regular astigmatism.

Figure 9A-4. Topography 2 months following lamellar keratoplasty OD.

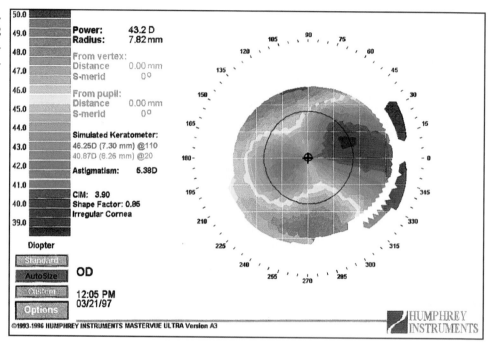

Figure 9A-5. Topography 7 months after lamellar keratoplasty shows some decrease in corneal irregularity.

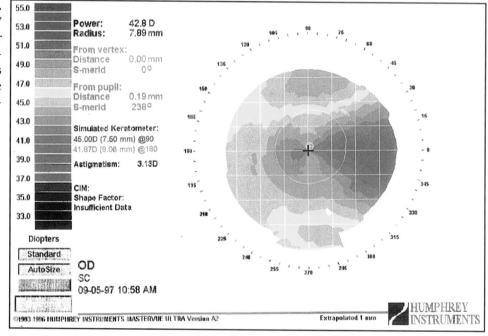

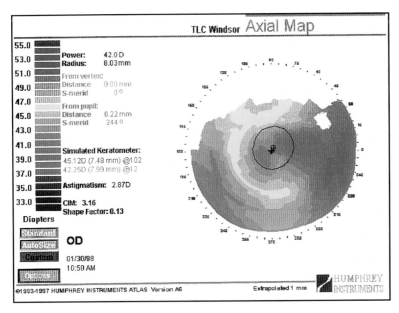

Figure 9A-6. One year and a half after lamellar keratoplasty OD, the cornea is more regular around the visual axis.

Editor's Notes

This case is the only severe LASIK infection that has occurred at our center since we began performing LASIK 5 years ago. Although the infection was treated successfully, the corneal scarring resulted in a reduction of BCVA. This eventually necessitated a homoplastic lamellar keratoplasty which did restore the BCVA. Unfortunately, the long term topical steroid use resulted in a posterior subcapsular cataract requiring cataract surgery. The patient still has residual astigmatism in the right eye. Since a YAG capsulotomy was performed in the right eye as well, the patient needs to be followed closely for a potential retinal detachment in that eye.

Due to the patient's problems with contact lens intolerance, and the significant anisometropia present between the two eyes, the patient is now exploring her options for refractive surgery in the left eye. The other two options currently available are insertion of a phakic IOL or clear lens extraction. Clear lens extraction certainly may offer her a simpler option, however the main risk with clear lens extraction is retinal detachment. She is now at the same risk for retinal detachment in the right eye. While retinal detachment is not an uncommon problem following cataract surgery in high myopia, this patient's experience with the right eye has demonstrated that LASIK can also have significant complications.

CASE B, INTERFACE INFECTION

Michael Lawless, MBBS, FRACO, FRACS, FRCOphth, and Sue Webber, BSc(Hons), FRCOphth

Main Concern: Interface Infection
Patient Age: 30

INITIAL PREOPERATIVE INFORMATION

	OD	OS	COMMENTS
Preoperative Refraction	-7.0D	-6.5D	
BCVA	normal	normal	
Topography Details	n/a		
SimK Values	n/a		
Pachymetry	n/a		
Other	surgery performed elsewhere		

PROCEDURES PERFORMED

	OD	OS	COMMENTS
1. Date/type	5/26/98 M-LASIK	5/26/98 M-LASIK	referral center
2. Date/type		6/7/98 corneal abscess	referral center
		left anterior chamber tap	
3. Date/type		6/8/98, left flap lifted	
		and corneal scrape	
4. Date/type		6/18/98, left flap lifted	
		and corneal scrape	

CURRENT POSTOPERATIVE INFORMATION

	OD	OS	COMMENTS
Time Postoperative	14 weeks	14 weeks	loss of BCVA OS
Postoperative Refraction	-0.5/-0.5 X 157	0/-1.25 X 167	
BCVA	6/6	9/6	
SimK Values	41.00@86, 39.75	42.37@62, 40.62	
Pachymetry		421 µm	
Visual Complaints	none	slight photophobia	
Medications	none	none	
Refractive Correction	none	none	

This patient received bilateral LASIK at another center for moderate myopia. She presented for her 1 week postoperative appointment complaining that the left eye was sore and had poorer vision than the right eye. She was advised to reduce her postoperative steroids (FML) from q.i.d. to b.i.d. in the right eye, but to continue them as before in the left eye. Five days later she was awakened by severe pain in the left eye and she presented to an ophthalmologist who performed an anterior chamber tap.

She was referred to us the next day. On presentation she had visual acuities of 6/5OD and HM OS. The left eye was intensely injected, painful and watering. The corneal epithelium was edematous with a large epithelial defect and there were multifocal stromal abscesses. The anterior chamber had a fibrin clot and a one-quarter hypopyon. The patient was taken to the operating room where the LASIK flap was lifted and samples taken for microbiological investigation. The flap bed was irrigated with chloramphenicol before the cap was replaced. She was commenced on alternate half-hourly fortified cephalothin 5% and gentamicin 0.9%. A gram stain revealed profuse gram-positive cocci confirmed later as staphylococcus aureus. The gentamicin was ceased and the cephalothin continued hourly. Over the next few days the epithelium healed, the anterior chamber reaction resolved and the stromal infiltrate diminished (Figures 9B-1a and 9B-1b). The cephalothin was reduced to Q2h. However, the clinical picture worsened 2 days later (Figure 9B-2) and despite increasing the treatment, continued to do so (Figure 9B-3). Ten days after her first corneal scrape the patient returned to the operating room for repeat flap lifting and corneal scrape. The stromal bed was again irrigated with chloramphenicol and the patient was commenced on gentamicin 0.9% and ciprofloxacin 0.3% alternate half-hourly, with the addition of systemic ciprofloxacin. Over the next few days the eye improved and the topical treatment was reduced. Two days later, after further improvement topical prednisolone phosphate 0.5% was introduced. The corneal appearance continued to settle (Figures 9B-4a, 9B-4b, and 9B-5) and the treatment reduced. She was finally taken off all treatment 9 weeks after her second corneal scrape.

This case raises many questions about infections after LASIK. Firstly, and perhaps most importantly, how should one recognize and diagnose an infection? The differential diagnosis would include epithelial ingrowth, diffuse lamellar keratitis[1] or the more severe focal interface opacities.[2] All these conditions may present with blurred vision and photophobia. However, other signs will lead the clinician towards a diagnosis of infection. Infections will tend to cause a red painful eye, whereas the noninfected eye will perhaps just be sore and gritty. The corneal opacity in an infection is more likely to be focal or multifocal than have a diffuse appearance. It may also extend into the anterior or posterior stroma, whereas in sterile conditions the opacity is generally confined to the flap interface. Finally, in sterile conditions there is usually mild or no anterior chamber reaction, whereas infective keratitis may be accompanied by hypopyon. When there is a strong index of suspicion for infection, we would advocate microbiological investigation. Lifting of the flap to obtain a direct sample of the suspect material would be our preferred method. An anterior chamber tap has the risk of introducing the infecting organism into what has hitherto been a sterile anterior chamber reaction. Simply performing a swab from the ocular surface is less likely to obtain a positive result and is more likely to give a picture confused by commensal organisms.

The treatment of LASIK flap infection may well prove to be more challenging than the usual corneal ulcer and abscess. The crucial difference with LASIK infections is that the infection is deep in the stroma, with no connection to the corneal surface. Thus, we are relying on the absorption and penetration of antibiotics into the corneal stroma, sometimes through an intact corneal epithelium. In view of this we would advocate the use of a flouroquinolone, as the corneal penetration is good (once past the epithelium) and the MIC90 for most common infecting organisms is very low. Once the infiltrate is sterilized, it would seem prudent to use topical steroids in an attempt to minimize inflammatory damage. It is recognized that even sterile inflammation can be severe enough to cause tissue loss and so alter the corneal shape.[2] For a more complete discussion of this case the reader is referred to the published case report.[3]

Despite this severe infection our patient has had a satisfactory outcome with a visual acuity that is compatible with a noncomplicated procedure.

References
1. Smith RJ, Maloney RK. Diffuse Lamellar Keratitis. *Ophthalmology.* 1998; 105(9):1721-1726.
2. Fraenkel GF, Cohen PR, Sutton GS, Lawless MA, Rogers CM. Central focal interface opacity after laser in situ keratomileusis. *J Refract Surg.* 1998;14:571-576.
3. Webber SK, Lawless MA, Sutton GL, Rogers CM. Staphylococcal infection under a LASIK flap. *Cornea.* 1999;18(3):361-365.

Figure 9B-1a. Appearance of left eye 2 days after presentation to our practice.

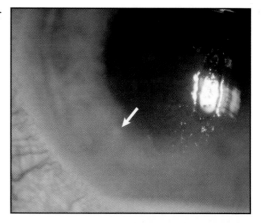

Figure 9B-1b. Appearance of left eye 2 days after presentation to our practice.

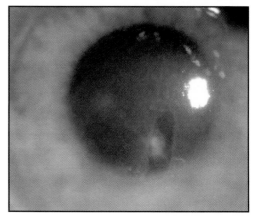

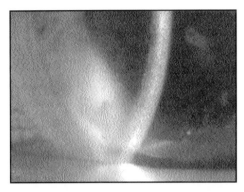

Figure 9B-2. The corneal appearance 8 days after the first corneal scrape, the inferonasal focus has worsened.

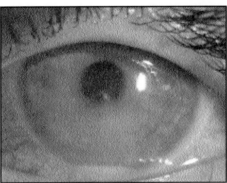

Figure 9B-3. The corneal appearance 10 days after the first scrape. Keratic precipitates and a hypopyon have reformed.

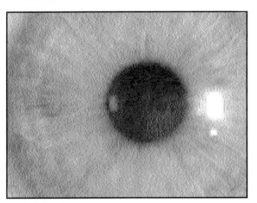

Figure 9B-4a. Appearance 8 weeks after presentation: stromal haze is visible within the visual axis.

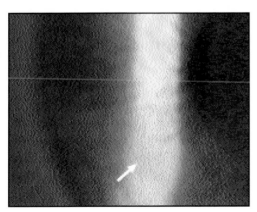

Figure 9B-4b. Appearance 8 weeks after presentation: flap microwrinkles are visible inferonasally.

Figure 9B-5. Corneal topography 2 months after presentation.

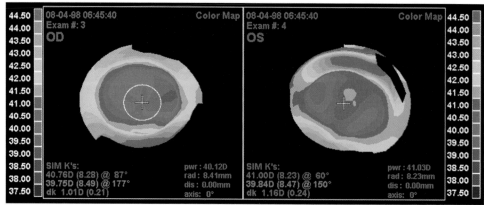

Editor's Notes

Any severe pain following LASIK requires immediate assessment. Epithelial defects often cause discomfort, however they do not cause severe pain. A dislodged flap will cause severe pain which often leaves the patient disabled. This case demonstrates another cause of severe pain. This infectious interface inflammation must be differentiated from the LIK as it is generally not associated with pain.

The source of the infection in this case is of considerable interest. Since the infection was present at interface, it may have occurred during the procedure itself. It is possible that contamination occurred from one of the instruments or the interface irrigating solution. While infections of this nature are extremely rare, this does demonstrate that it is important to autoclave all instruments prior to LASIK and suggests that all technicians and surgeons should be gloved while performing the procedure to ensure reasonable sterility during the procedure.

10

COMPLEX POSTOPERATIVE FLAP PROBLEMS

SUMMARY NOTES

COMPLEX POSTOPERATIVE FLAP PROBLEMS - SUMMARY NOTES

PAIN FOLLOWING LASIK

Clinical
Most patients do not experience pain following LASIK because of the minimal epithelial disruption and the regularity of the post-LASIK corneal surface. Therefore, any patients with significant pain should be evaluated, as this could indicate a complication.

Causes of Pain after LASIK
- epithelial defect
- dislodged flap
- toxic epithelial keratopathy
- residual pressure from suction ring/lid speculum
- infection (rare)

Management
Any complaint of significant pain following LASIK should be addressed with an eye examination to ensure that the flap is in place and the epithelium is intact. Generally, no major problems are identified, and reassurance and a mild narcotic to assist with sleeping is all that is required. Topical nonsteroid drops are helpful in controlling pain related to epithelial defects. The superficial punctate keratitis identified on the flap epithelium immediately after LASIK is best treated with generous lubrication.

Prevention
Pain is minimized after LASIK by ensuring that the procedure is as least traumatic as possible. Preoperative topical anesthesia is minimized to reduce the post-operative epithelial toxicity. One drop of a topical nonsteroid medication will reduce the immediate foreign body sensation experienced after LASIK. Patients are advised to avoid rubbing or squeezing their eye, which can disturb the flap position and cause significant pain. All surgical maneuvers should be performed with great delicacy to avoid any epithelial trauma.

DISLODGED FLAP

Clinical
Dislocation of the flap after LASIK is uncommon, occurring in 1/500 to 1/1000 cases. This is usually due to some type of eye trauma or vigorous eyelid squeeze immediately after LASIK in the first 12 hours. The patient is aware as soon as this occurs, as the vision becomes blurred and the eye becomes painful with an acute foreign body sensation similar to the pain of a corneal abrasion.

Management

The corneal flap must be replaced as soon as possible to avoid infection, reduce pain, and avoid permanent striae and damage to the flap. The incidence of epithelial ingrowth increases with both displacement and free caps.

Management until flap replacement involves lubrication every 30 minutes with sterile preservative-free artificial tears to check the flap hydration and improve the discomfort. Patients will usually keep their eye closed due to discomfort, or the eye can be taped shut until treated.

The technique by which the flap is replaced involves the same principles used for the treatment of flap striae.

Prevention

The stability of the flap is checked by ensuring it is secure at the conclusion of the procedure with the striae and blink tests. Waiting an adequate amount of time after the corneal flap has been properly realigned, usually in the range of 1 to 3 minutes, and avoiding excessive interface irrigation allows for a strong seal to form. Patients are advised not to rub or squeeze the eye. Eye protection for both day- and nighttime use is provided so that the eyes are always protected.

CASE A, LOST CAP WITH A LOSS OF BCVA

Ted Smith, OD, and Jeffery J. Machat, MD

Main Concern: Partial/Free/Lost Cap
Patient Age: 54

INITIAL PREOPERATIVE INFORMATION

	OD	OS	COMMENTS
Preoperative Refraction	-8.75 – 2.75 X 040		pre-free cap
UCVA	cf@1ft		referring center
BCVA	20/25-		
Topography Details	45.40/43.50 X 32		
SimK Values	0.35		
Pachymetry	584 µm		

PROCEDURES PERFORMED

	OD	OS	COMMENTS
1. Date/type	10/14/98 M-LASIK		free cap
Keratome/plate	Moria/130		referring center

CURRENT POSTOPERATIVE INFORMATION

	OD	OS	COMMENTS
Time Postoperative	4 months		irregular topography
Postoperative Refraction	-9.00 – 3.25 X 044		and loss of BCVA
UCVA	cf@1ft		
BCVA	20/100-		
Topography Details	46.75/43.37 X 56		
SimK Values	5.54		
Pachymetry	558 µm		
Visual Complaints	blur		
Medications	none		
Refractive Correction	none		

This patient was a 54-year-old white female. Her surgical history consisted of LASIK surgery attempted on October 14, 1997. At that time, suction was lost with the Moria keratome (130 μm flap) and a partial, free, and subsequently lost flap occurred on her right eye. Her left eye was consequently left untreated with *Rx* -7.25 − 2.75 X 168 and BCVA 20/25+.

At 4 months postoperatively, the patient was referred to our center for management. Over the previous month, there was development of central corneal scarring and haze (Figure 10A-1). The patient's topography showed irregular astigmatism, with K values of 46.75/43.37 X 056 and a corresponding CIM value of 5.54 (Figure 10A-2). There was a residual *Rx* OD of -9.00 − 3.25 X 044 which gave a BCVA of 20/100-. Pachymetry showed a central corneal thickness of 558 μm.

This was a very difficult case. The irregularity in the cornea reducing best-corrected vision will require some type of topography-controlled procedure, such as LASIK with TopoLink. However, to address the lack of clarity of the visual axis, transepithelial PRK may be required to remove the scar tissue, in combination with the TopoLink. A partial or full thickness corneal graft may be required if visual function cannot be recovered adequately.

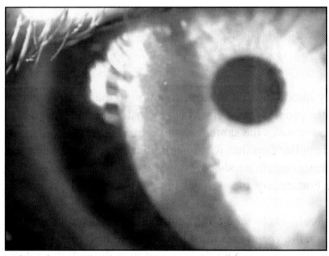

Figure 10A-1. Slit lamp photograph demonstrates peripheral corneal haze after lost cap OD.

Figure 10A-2. Severe corneal irregularity after lost cap.

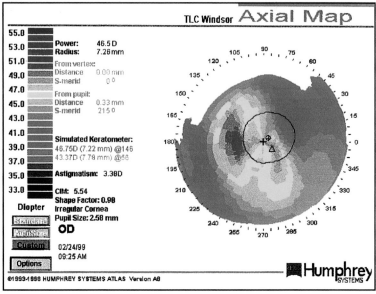

Editor's Notes

With a thin or incomplete flap, it is extremely important to pay close attention to the replacement of the flap so it is not lost. This case demonstrates the problems associated with a lost incomplete flap. The large keratectomy cut in the center of the cornea provokes the same response of a large PRK correction with a very high risk of haze. In this case, the lamellar flap that was lost did not significantly alter the refractive error, so the high level of myopia and astigmatism persisted. However the central corneal haze that developed reduced the BCVA to 20/100. Fortunately the corneal thickness was still preserved, allowing for further treatment.

We first need to wait for stabilization. This would likely take a minimum of 6 months after the primary procedure. Following refractive stabilization, the visual axis must be cleared to restore the BCVA. This could be done with a PTK procedure ablating through the epithelium and then through the anterior stromal haze. Unfortunately, this would be associated with a risk of recurrent corneal stromal haze. Therefore postoperative drops would be needed to reduce this haze risk which could include topical steroids or thiotepa. A second refractive procedure would then be performed once it was insured that the haze had not reoccurred. This would be most successfully done with LASIK. The total corneal thickness would need to be monitored to ensure that adequate thickness (400 μm) would remain after the LASIK procedure to maintain the long-term corneal integrity.

An alternative approach would be to do a homograft procedure where the anterior corneal surface was removed and a donor flap was used to replace the lost tissue and the anterior third of the cornea. Once the refraction has stabilized following this procedure, a LASIK enhancement could be performed to correct the residual refractive error. While this procedure could potentially have the best outcome, as it would remove the irregular anterior surface of the cornea, it also involves using donor tissue with the associated risks of graft rejection and the complexities of a more advanced procedure.

CASE B, LOSS OF FLAP REQUIRING PK

Michael Lawless, MBBS, FRACO, FRACS, FRCOphth, and Sue Webber, BSc(Hons), FRCOphth

Main Concern: Loss of Flap
Patient Age: 51

INITIAL PREOPERATIVE INFORMATION

	OD	OS	COMMENTS
Preoperative Refraction	+3.00/+0.75 X 95	+3.75 + 0.5 X 115	
BCVA	n/a	n/a	
Topography Details	mild irregularity	spherical cornea	Figure 10B-1
SimK Values	approx. 43 OU, values from topography		
Pachymetry	498 µm	496 µm	from Orbscan
Other	surgery performed elsewhere		

PROCEDURES PERFORMED

	OD	OS	COMMENTS
1. Date/type	9/9/97 LASIK	9/10/97 LASIK	
Laser/keratome/plate	n/a /Moria nonautomated keratome/160 µm footplate OU		right flap reposi-tioned after surgery
2. Date/type	9/14/97 removed epithelial ingrowth		
3. Date/type	9/16/97 sutured right flap due to movement epithelial defect persisting.		
4. Date/type	10/15/97 epithelial defect persists flap melt, flap removed		
5. Date/type	9/4/98 PK		

CURRENT POSTOPERATIVE INFORMATION

	OD	OS	COMMENTS
Time Postoperative	11 months post-LASIK	11 months post-LASIK	
Postoperative Refraction	+2.00 – 3.00 X 20	+2.00 – 0.50 X 160	
BCVA	6/45	6/12	left amblyopia
Topography Details	irregular astigmatism OU		
SimK Values	47.73@88, 45.24	45.00@48, 44.46	
Visual Complaints	poor visual acuity		
Medications	none	none	
Refractive Correction	balance	spectacles	intolerant of contact lenses

We feel that the fundamental problem with this case was the flap instability and epithelial defect. In his referral letter, the operating surgeon states that on day 1 postoperatively the right flap moved due to the contact lens, so it had to be repositioned. Five days postoperatively the patient was in a considerable amount of discomfort, so the flap was lifted and epithelial ingrowth was removed. The flap remained unstable and was sutured in position 2 days later. Throughout this period, the flap had failed to epithelialize. Both the repeated flap manipulations and persistent epithelial defect are likely to lead to corneal edema, which in itself delays epithelialization. As in other cases of chronic epithelial defect, the exposed corneal stroma is at risk of melting.

In addition, in this case the frequent instillation of topical medication is likely to have contributed to the epithelial fragility. On presentation to our practice (Figure 10B-2) this patient was using g. proxymetacaine hydrochloride 0.5% every 2 hours and Lacrilube hourly (Allergan Australia Pty, Ltd. Frenches Forest, NSW, Australia). In addition, she was also instilling chloramphenicol 0.5% and prednisolone sodium phosphate 0.5%. Topical anesthetic abuse is a recognized cause of stromal keratitis and in this case, Q2h application was probably a contributor to the demise of this flap. In addition to the topical anesthetic, the other medication (especially the preservative) may have served to exacerbate an already compromised cornea.

As with most problems, prevention is better than cure. It is not clear why some patients get perioperative epithelial defects and others not. It is our practice to wet the cornea thoroughly before the passage of the keratome to try to minimize the risk. However, once an epithelial defect has been created, quick closure must be the primary aim. Some surgeons would use a bandage contact lens at this stage, others just use copious ocular lubricants, preferably without preservatives.

The second problem in this case was the mobile flap. We do not yet fully understand flap stability, but it would seem likely that the thickness of the flap, the breadth of the hinge and the quality of the edge will all affect its positioning. Good initial adherence and position is likely to aid long term stability. Some surgeons feel that a period of relative dehydration immediately postoperatively helps flap adherence, allowing the lids to remain open for 30 to 60 seconds after flap positioning before removal of the speculum. We would also advocate checking the position of the flap 20 to 30 minutes postoperatively, because if it has moved it should be repositioned as soon as possible before any folds become too fixed. We feel that flaps can sometimes be dislodged by excessive eyelid squeezing, so if a patient is likely to do this (ie, those with epithelial defects) consideration should be given to applying a bandage contact lens to protect the flap. Our immediate management of this case was to stop all existing topical medication, prescribing just ofloxacin twice a day. The eye was padded and oral analgesia prescribed. Unfortunately, these measures were insufficient to prevent progression of the flap melt and finally, 5 weeks after surgery the flap was removed. This permitted healing of the stromal and epithelial defect. Unfortunately, the healing was accompanied by significant scarring (Figure 10B-3) as would have been expected with a deep PRK, though in this case it was probably increased in severity by the continuing inflammation. We have learned from our experience with PRK that haze and scarring can continue to reduce for up to 2 years after surgery and we would advocate waiting this long before considering it as the final result. However, this patient also developed a considerable degree of irregular astigmatism (Figure 10B-4), her BCVA was 6/45, and this improved to 6/12 with a rigid gas permeable contact lens. Unfortunately, she was unable to tolerate a contact lens. While the cornea is capable of a considerable degree of remodeling, in this patient it was thought that her cornea was not likely to improve to a satisfactory level. Therefore, 12 months after her original LASIK she underwent a PK to the right eye.

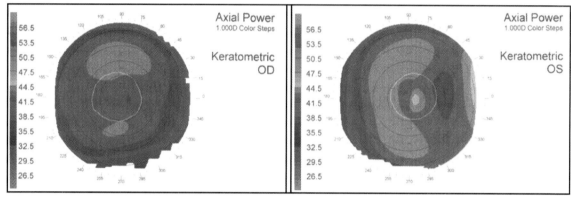

Figure 10B-1. Preoperative topography.

Figure 10B-2. The appearance of the right eye on presentation to our practice.

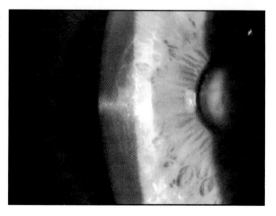

Figure 10B-3. Corneal appearance 8 weeks after LASIK. Note the high degree of corneal scarring.

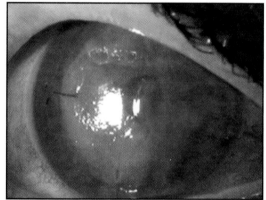

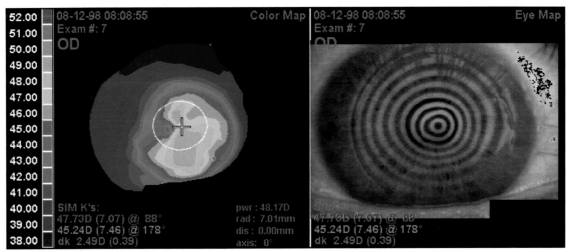

Figure 10B-4. Corneal topography 11 months after LASIK.

Editor's Notes

This case demonstrates how a relatively simple problem following LASIK such as epithelial defect can lead to a cascade of problems finally resulting in a PK. The authors have clearly described the possible etiologies for the decrease in the flap adherence and the eventual flap melt necessitating the removal of the flap. Thin flaps tend to be less adherent to the stromal bed and more prone to flap displacement. This may be because thin flaps become more edematous. In the case of a thin flap, it may be prudent to wait additional time for flap adhesion and monitor the patient more closely to ensure that there is no flap displacement in the early postoperative phase.

CASE C, PARTIAL LOSS OF FLAP

Roberto Zaldivar, MD, Susana Oscherow, MD, and Giselle Ricur, MD

Main concern: Loss of Flap
Patient age: 34

INITIAL PREOPERATIVE INFORMATION

	OD	OS	COMMENTS
Preoperative Refraction	-2.75 D		
UCVA	20/200		
BCVA	20/20		
Topography Details	symmetric 41.27 D		
SimK Values	41.82/40.95@4		
Pachymetry	565 µm		

PROCEDURES PERFORMED

	OD	OS	COMMENTS
1. Date/type	3/12/97 LASIK OU		striae
Laser/keratome/plate	NIDEK EC 5000/ ACS		
	(Chiron vision)/160		
2. Date/type	1 day post-LASIK		
	flap repositioned		
3. Date/type	3 months post-LASIK		
	flap removed		

CURRENT POSTOPERATIVE INFORMATION

	OD	OS	COMMENTS
Time Postoperative	1 year 9 months		awaiting PRK for
UCVA	20/30		residual astigmatism
Postoperative Refraction	-0.75 – 3.50 X 15		
BCVA	20/25		
Topography Details	symmetric 41.05 D		
SimK Values	41.46/39.24@5		
Pachymetry	467 µm		
Visual Complaints	none		
Medications	ocular lubricants, scheduled		
	for PRK in May, 1999		
Refractive Corrections	spectacles		
Other	slit lamp exam: very mild haze		

Flap loss is one of the potential intra- or early postoperative complications in LASIK surgery. Adequate treatment is essential in order to avoid vision-threatening complications.

Common examples of intraoperative causes are: decentrations, excessive ablation on very flat corneas, thin caps, fragile hinges, or lack of hinge protection during the ablation process. Early postoperative causes include traumatic eye rubbing, eye movement under pressure patch, excessive lid force on the corneal surface, epithelial abrasions, or accidental trauma.

Many surgeons tend to place bandage contact lens in the immediate postoperative of their LASIK procedures, mainly after flap repositioning. This case demonstrates the risk factor that bandage contact lens posed in the early postoperative LASIK.

The presence of striae in the immediate postoperative of a routine LASIK procedure led to the necessity of flap repositioning. The contact lens provided for the postoperative care resulted in the main cause of eye rubbing (which provoked a tear in the flap) with partial flap loss when the patient selfextracted the soft contact lens (Figures 10C-2 and 10C-3).

We decided to "wait-out" for spontaneous healing of the epithelial defect, with the aid of medication such as antibiotic-steroid ointments, topical steroids, and ocular lubricants.

Three months later, due to a very slow healing response and a rough evolution, the irregular remnant of flap tissue that extended over the corneal surface was removed and treated as if a surface PTK had been performed. Close follow-up and topical medication, which included thiotepa and Fluromethalone, was prescribed in order to avoid haze (Figure 10C-4 and 10C-5).

Follow-up controls performed during subsequent months revealed a marked improvement in UCVA and BCVA. Topography image changes were also favorable. Currently, the patient has been scheduled for PRK (Figures 10C-6 through 9).

Our experience with thiotepa, a radiomimetic drug that inhibits rapidly proliferating cells, has been encouraging. Local instillation of it has diminished dramatically the incidence of haze.

Over time, we've learned that adequate and immediate postoperative control (15 to 30 minutes) is essential in decreasing the incidence of flap anomalies such as striae, keratitis, etc. This in turn brings down the rate of retreatments (ie, repositioning, hydration) and contact lens are no longer indispensable for postoperative wear.

With prompt and adequate treatment, many cases of flap loss actually heal well and require no further treatment.

Suggested Reading

Buratto L, Brint S. *LASIK: Principles and Techniques.* Thorofare, NJ: SLACK Incorporated; 1998.

Machat JJ, Slade SG, Probst LE. *The Art of LASIK.* 2nd ed. Thorofare, NJ: SLACK Incorporated; 1999.

Zaldivar R, Davidorf J, Oscherow S, et al. Results and complications of laser in situ keratomileusis by experienced surgeons. *J Refract Surg.* March/April 1998;14(2).

Figure 10C-1. Preoperative topographic image OD.

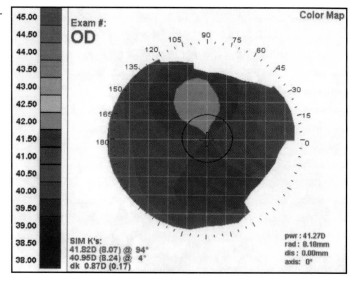

Figure 10C-2. Infrared image showing the partial loss of the flap.

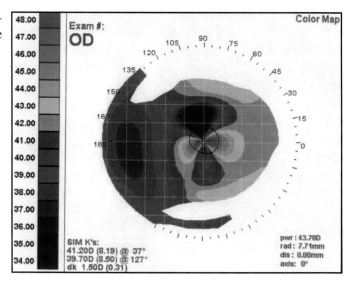

Figure 10C-3. Postoperative topographic image of the cornea with the remnant flap tissue.

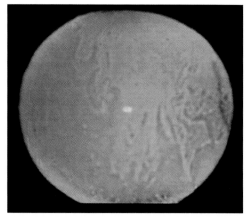

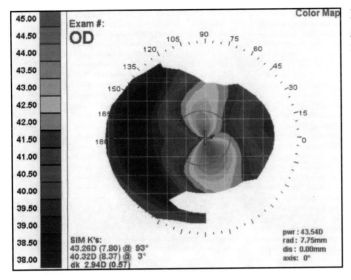

Figure 10C-4. Postoperative topographic image 4 months after treatment.

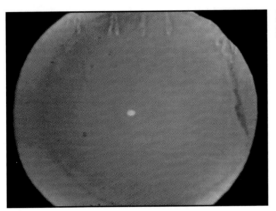

Figure 10C-5. Infrared image showing corneal healing after treatment.

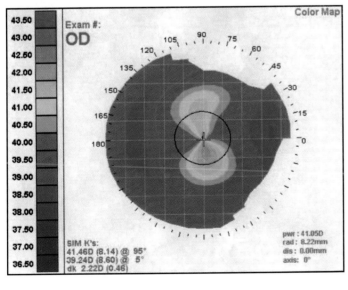

Figure 10C-6. Topographic image 19 months after the original procedure.

Figure 10C-7. Topographic image 24 months after the original procedure.

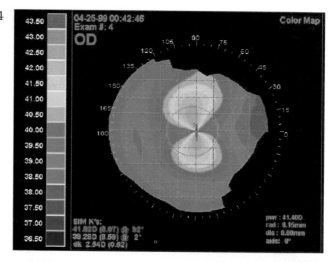

Figure 10C-8. Infrared image of the same cornea 1 year after the flap was lifted and the interface was scraped clean.

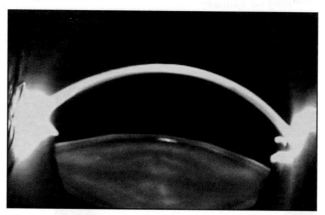

Figure 10C-9. Infrared image of the same cornea 1 year after the flap was lifted and the interface was scraped clean.

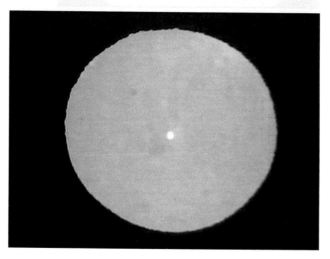

Editor's Notes

This case demonstrates how a small problem in LASIK can evolve into one of the worst outcomes, which involves complete loss of the cap. The initial problem of the flap striae was treated appropriately and a bandage contact lens was placed. Unfortunately the patient decided to remove the contact lens because it was uncomfortable, which removed part of the flap. It would generally be difficult to remove only part of the LASIK flap, which suggests that the flap was thin or friable. This could also explain why the flap striae occurred initially.

The slow healing and the irregular stromal bed created by the partial removal of the flap necessitated removal of the rest of the flap and the treatment of the patient as a PTK type of procedure. Roberto Zaldivar, MD, has pioneered the use of thiotepa for the control of haze following these types of cases where a large surface keratectomy has been performed. This case illustrates how this can be effective in the reduction of haze. Without its use, the risk of haze in this case would be very high, perhaps in the 25 to 50% range. Although the postoperative result in this case is encouraging, it can be seen that there is still some residual astigmatism and corneal irregularity induced by the loss of the cap. Further surface PRK procedures may also be able to correct some of this refractive error. The risk of haze following this PRK would be significant, so the patient would need close monitoring and the addition of antihaze medications. Given the multiple surface ablations and topical steroids used, there is the risk of developing posterior subcapsular cataracts. Therefore, the total dosage of topical steroid would need to be monitored closely. Nevertheless, after the additional PRK this patient could achieve an excellent outcome.

CASE D, BILATERAL DISPLACED FLAPS

Charlotte Burns, OD, MS, and Louis E. Probst, MD

Main Concern: Initial Pain
Patient Age: 43

INITIAL PREOPERATIVE INFORMATION

	OD	OS	COMMENTS
Preoperative Refraction	-11.75 – 0.50 X 095	-11.50 – 0.50 X 095	
BCVA	20/20	20/20	
Topography Details	normal	normal	
SimK Values	46.25/46.37 @ 180	46.50/46.75 X 180	
Pachymetry	560 μm	561 μm	

PROCEDURES PERFORMED

	OD	OS	COMMENTS
1. Date/type	1/31/97 LASIK	1/31/97 LASIK	bilateral dislodged
Laser/keratome/plate	Chiron 116/ACS/160	Chiron 116/ACS/160	flaps 1 hour post-LASIK

CURRENT POSTOPERATIVE INFORMATION

	OD	OS	COMMENTS
Time Postoperative	1 year	1 year	excellent outcome
Postoperative Refraction	pl – 0.25 X 095	pl – 0.75 X 090	
BCVA	20/15-2	20/20-1	
Topography Details	central flattening	central flattening	
SimK Values	39.75/40.37 X 124	39.37/39.62 X 180	
Visual Complaints	'star' effect while night driving	none	
Refractive Correction	none	none	

A 43-year-old white male presented for LASIK on January 31, 1997. The patient's preoperative refraction was -10.75 – 0.50 X 095 OD and -11.50 – 0.50 X 095. Topography was normal (Figure 10D-1), pachymetry readings were 576 μm OD and 574 μm OS. BCVA was 20/15-2 OU. For both eyes, the Chiron 116 was used, with the Chiron ACS microkeratome and a 160 μm plate. The zone diameter used was 6.6 mm in a multizone pattern.

Intraoperatively, there was a slight bleed OU from vascularization that stopped in 2 to 3 minutes. Approximately 30 minutes after surgery, the flaps were checked and they were in the correct position. The patient then walked out into the cold air as he left our center, and apparently squeezed his eyes. He immediately felt bilateral ocular discomfort and returned to the center.

He had dislodged both flaps significantly, so that a front office staff could see that the flaps were displaced without a biomicroscope. The surgeon had now traveled 2 hours away. The patient was transported to the surgeon, and en route both eyes were irrigated with BSS every 20 minutes. Upon arrival, both flaps were again irrigated with BSS, lifted and refloated into correct position. The interface was thoroughly irrigated OU. The left flap had to be refloated twice in order to perfectly align edges. The OD had some remaining striae due to folding of the flap, but edges were all aligned and the folds were nasal to the visual axis. There was also a small epithelial defect OD at the superior edge of the flap created by "ironing" the flap. At 20 minutes postoperatively the flaps were checked and all edges and flaps looked good. Ocuflox and Tobradex were used after the procedure. The patient left with the OD taped shut.

The next morning, approximately 12 hours later, the patient returned for follow-up. The patient reported that 'both eyes were 100% better,' although the OD was still a little scratchy. The UCVAs were 20/70 OD and 20/200 OS. Biomicroscopy showed flaps were stable with trace edema. There were no striae present, and there was good alignment with good adhesion.

One week later the patient was 20/40-2 OD and 20/40-1 OS uncorrected. The refraction was +0.75 - 1.25 X 035, best corrected to 20/25-2 OD, and the OS was -0.50 DS best corrected to 20/30-2. At 6 weeks the patient had improved to 20/20-2 OD, and 20/25-1 OS uncorrected, while refraction showed +0.25 - 0.25 X180 OD, -0.50 DS OS, with BCVAs of 20/20-1 OU.

At 1 year the patient's UCVAs were 20/15-2 OD, and 20/20-1 OS. Refraction revealed pl – 0.25 X 095 OD and pl – 0.75 X 090 OS. Topography showed central flattening (Figure 10D-2). The patient was extremely happy, and reported that his only problem was getting a 'star' effect while night driving. He was not wearing correction for distance or near.

Figure 10D-1. Preoperative topography OU demonstrates a regular pattern.

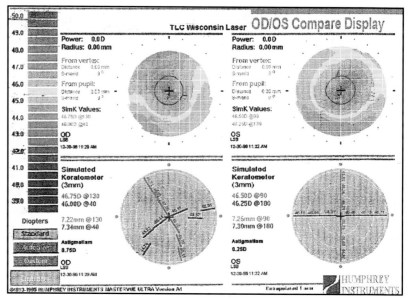

Figure 10D-2. Postoperative topography OU shows a well-centered ablation.

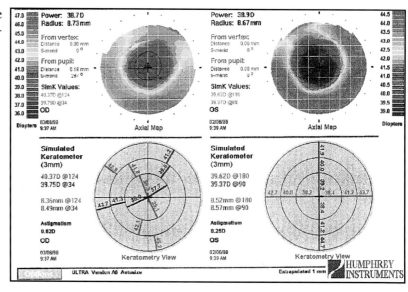

Editor's Notes

This is the most dramatic case of dislodged flap that I have experienced. Dislodged flaps tend to occur in approximately 1 in 1,000 LASIK cases. Generally they are associated with eyelid squeezing or rubbing that inadvertently occurs the first day following LASIK. When the displacement of the flap occurs, the patient will immediately experience intense ocular pain that surpasses the pain associated with a corneal abrasion. The vision will become blurred. The patient will be reluctant to open the eye. This is a surgical emergency and should be dealt with as soon as possible.

In this case, both flaps became dislodged and the patient was treated within 2 hours of this occurrence. Despite this relatively prompt treatment, the flaps had multiple folds due to their disfigured state after they displaced. Mucous debris was also present in the stromal bed. The treatment of this patient involved carefully cleaning the stromal bed and then replacing the flaps. Interface irrigation was performed and then the flaps were smoothed carefully in order to remove any of the wrinkles and folding that occurred during the displacement. This was a slow and careful procedure that took over 1 hour to perform for both eyes. Nevertheless, the procedure was quite successful with complete elimination of the striae and excellent final visual outcome.

The configuration of this patient's eye may have had some relationship to the occurrence of the bilaterally dislodged flaps. The patient had a very small corneas, so the 8.5 mm flap composed the entire cornea. The keratectomy edge occurred along the limbus in both eyes. The patient also had very wide palpebral apertures. Therefore, when the patient blinked, the lid would tend to come down over the limbus, which had the potential of catching the edge of the flap. In most LASIK cases, when the flap is well inside the limbus, the flap edge sits nicely in the groove of the stromal bed. In this case, the flap was not as well protected because of the large size of the flap relative to the small corneas. Finally, the patient was a tremendous eye squeezer, which was the reason he originally sought out LASIK to alleviate his difficulties with contact lens.

I now personally instruct each patient to keep their eyes closed during the first 24 hours after LASIK and to avoid any eyelid squeezing or rubbing. I tell the patients that this will help their eyes heal and keep their eyes protected. Since I have begun doing this I have had no further problems with flap displacement.

Case E, Dislodged Flap and Subsequent Interface Keratitis

Ted Smith, OD, Jeffery J. Machat, MD, and Louis E. Probst, MD

Main Concern: Dislodged Flap and Subsequent Sands
Patient Age: 46

Initial Preoperative Information

	OD	OS	Comments
Preoperative Refraction	+2.75 − 3.00 X 017		
UCVA	20/80		
BCVA	20/20		
Topography Details	46.00/43.12 X 014		
SimK Values	0.73		
Pachymetry	592 μm		

Procedures Performed

	OD	OS	Comments
1. Date/type	5/6/99 LASIK		dislodged flap
Laser/keratome/plate	Technolas 217/ACS/180		
2. Date/type	5/8/99 Lift		
Laser/keratome/plate	lift/replace dislodged flap		

Current Postoperative Information

	OD	OS	Comments
Time Postoperative	12 days		post-lift
Postoperative Refraction	-0.25 + 0.75 X 015		(5/19/99)
UCVA	20/25-		excellent final
BCVA	20/25+		outcome
Topography Details	46.25/43.62 X 014		
SimK Values	3.02		
Pachymetry	not done		
Visual Complaints	none		
Medications	Inflamase forte q.i.d		
Refractive Correction	none		

This patient was a 46-year-old white male. His surgical history consisted of bilateral LASIK performed on May 6, 1999 in attempt to correct refractions of OD +2.75 − 3.00 X 017 and OS +3.00 − 3.00 X 162. Topography showed a symmetrical, smooth astigmatic cornea within normal limits (Figure 10E-1). The procedure was uncomplicated OU, other than weak epithelial adhesion which resulted in bilateral epithelial defects which required bandage contact lens insertion OU. At 2 days postoperatively the patient went to his comanaging doctor to have the bandage contact lenses removed, at which time the right corneal flap became dislodged (Figure 10E-2).

The right flap was subsequently lifted and refloated on 2 days postoperative (10E-3 to 8) and the bandage contact lens was once again inserted due to an epithelial defect that reoccurred. At 3 days post flap lift the bandage contact lens was removed without complication and Ciloxan was prescribed q.i.d for the antibiotic coverage of the small residual epithelial defect. At 1 day post contact lens removal, the patient presented with UCVA OD of 20/25+ and a manifest *Rx* OD +0.75 + 1.00 X 015 with BCVA 20/20-. The superior cornea adjacent to the flap edge showed an area of epithelial ridge development with surrounding edema and grade 1 NSDIK (Figure 10E-9). Inflamase Forte was prescribed q.h for 2 days and tapered over the next week to q.i.d to encourage epithelial regrowth since the patient had exhibited poor epithelial adhesion. The left flap retained integrity, and at 1 week postoperatively showed faint striae inferior to the visual axis with UCVA 20/20- and a manifest Rx OS +0.50 + 0.50 X 020. It was not indicated to treat the striae.

On examination 1 week later, the patient presented with a similar UCVA of 20/25- and reduced manifest *Rx* of OD +0.50 − 0.75 X 105 with BCVA 20/25+. The NSDIK had cleared and there was only slight residual corneal edema. Topography showed significant central corneal asymmetric astigmatism with K values 46.25/43.62 X 014 and CIM 3.02; however, fortunately the topography did not reflect in the observed refraction and acuity (Figure 10E-10). The regimen of Inflamase Forte was maintained at q.i.d to encourage settling of the observed corneal edema.

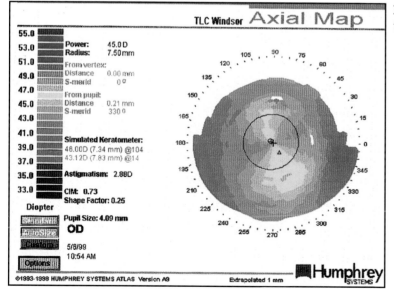

Figure 10E-1. Preoperative topography OD.

Figure 10E-2. Superiorly dislodged flap noted 2 days after LASIK.

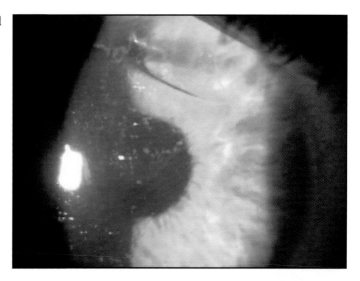

Figure 10E-3. Flap is dislodged superiorly on this intraoperative view.

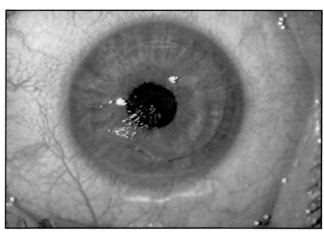

Figure 10E-4. Flap is lifted.

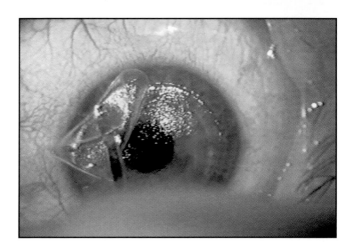

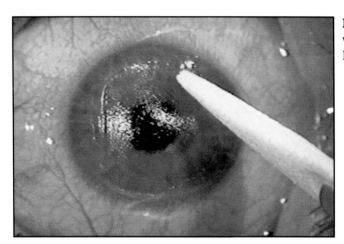

Figure 10E-5. Stromal bed is cleaned with a Murocel (Bausch and Lomb Pharmaceuticals, Inc. Tampa, Fla).

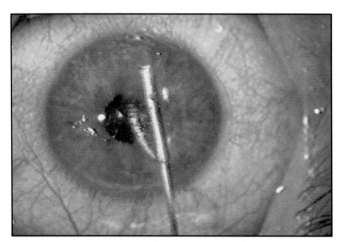

Figure 10E-6. Interface irrigation.

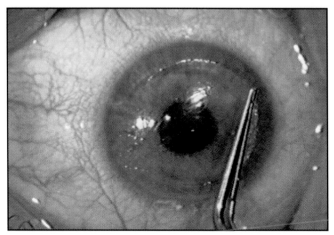

Figure 10E-7. Stretch and smooth the flap.

Figure 10E-8. Stretch and smooth out flap striae.

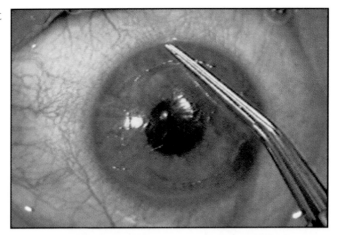

Figure 10E-9. Grade 1 sands OD in areas of superior epithelial defect.

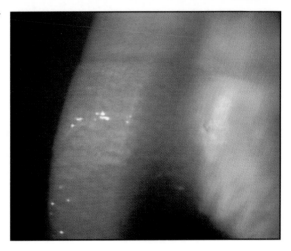

Figure 10E-10. Smooth topography OD 1 week following refloating and smoothing of flap.

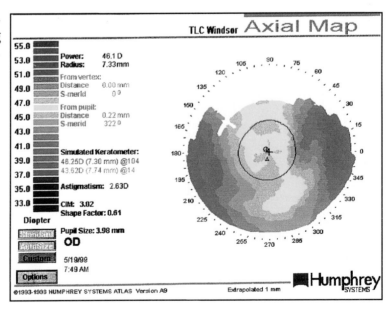

Editor's Notes

This patient was an intense individual who had very sensitive eyes and tended to squeeze them quite often. Although displacement of the flap could have occurred with the removal of the contact lens it is equally possible that he had squeezed his eyes in the postoperative period and caused the displacement to occur at that time. The patient called the center on the weekend because of extreme pain in his right eye and was immediately seen. He had this procedure performed 2 days previously. He was immediately assessed, as flap displacement was suspected. The flap was lifted, the stromal bed was cleaned, and the flap was refloated into place. The area of the flap displacement was stretched to ensure that no striae would persist in this area. The flap was left for 5 minutes to adhere and then a bandage contact lens was again placed on the eye because of the large epithelial defect that had occurred superiorly. The patient was instructed to try to keep his eyes closed for the next 24 hours.

It is interesting that this patient developed interface inflammation under the area of the epithelial defect. One of the causes of interface inflammation is known to be epithelial defects. This tends to be a more limited localized form of interface inflammation that occurs just under the epithelial defect. Because of the interface inflammation, this patient was placed on topical steroids. Because topical steroids will reduce epithelial healing, their use should be combined with the use of lubricants so that the interface inflammation is controlled and epithelial healing is not delayed.

COMPLEX LASIK ENHANCEMENTS

11

SUMMARY NOTES

COMPLEX LASIK ENHANCEMENTS - SUMMARY NOTES

Indications
- >1.00 D of myopia or hyperopia
- >1.00 D of astigmatism
- UCVA 20/40 or worse

Risks
- overcorrection
- epithelial ingrowth
- flap striae
- infection
- pain

Preoperative
- stable refraction
- adequate corneal thickness
- regular topography

Operative
- flap edge marked at slit lamp
- alignment marks placed on cornea
- lift flap before 6 months
- recut flap at a deeper depth after 6 months
- flap edge peeled back minimizing epithelial disruption
- excimer enhancement ablation performed
- flap refloated into position
- interface irrigation
- alignment marks and gutter checked for alignment
- wait 1 to 5 minutes for adhesion
- blink and/or striae test

Postoperative
- monitor for ingrowth
- check refractive outcome

CASE A, SECOND CUT COMPLICATED WITH CORNEAL RESECTION

Ioannis G. Pallikaris, MD, Theokliti Papadaki, MD, and Dimitrios S. Siganos, MD

Main Concern: Wedge Resection
Patient Age: 19

INITIAL PREOPERATIVE INFORMATION

	OD	OS	COMMENTS
Preoperative Refraction		-9.5 – 1.75 X 80	
BCVA		20/20	

PROCEDURES PERFORMED

	OD	OS	COMMENTS
1. Date/type		1995 M-LASIK	
Keratome/plate		ACS/160	
2. Date/type		6 months later enhancement	resection of wedge
Keratome/plate		ACS/200	

CURRENT POSTOPERATIVE INFORMATION

	OD	OS	COMMENTS
Time Postoperative		6 months	lateral cornea scan
Postoperative Refraction		n/a	
BCVA		20/20	
Topography Details		inferotemporal steepening	
SimK Values		n/a	
Pachymetry		n/a	
Visual Complaints		n/a	
Medications		none	

(Case and photographs reprinted with permission from Machat JJ, Slade SG, Probst LE. *The Art of Lasik*. 2nd ed. Thorofare, NJ: SLACK Incorporated; 1999.)

A 19-year-old woman underwent LASIK in OS for the correction of -9.5 – 1.75 X 80. Preoperative BCVA was 20/20. Although the attempted correction aimed at emmetropia, a shift to myopia had been detected throughout the first 3 postoperative months. By 6 months postoperatively, the refractive error had stabilized at -3.0 – 1 X 70. At the eighth month after the initial operation, the patient sought correction of the residual myopia.

Since retreatment was decided at a relatively late postoperative interval (later than the sixth month), we chose to perform a second flap instead of raising the primary one. Review of the operative data of the initial operation revealed that the ACS was used at that time to create an 8.5 mm wide, 133 μm thick, nasally based hinged flap. We decided to use the same microkeratome but to adjust the resection thickness to 200 μm.

The suction ring was placed slightly more nasally than the first time. Therefore, the microkeratome started cutting medially to the borders of the first flap. This resulted in resection of a sphenoid-shaped corneal meniscus approximately 0.5 mm wide (Figure 11A-1). A new hinged flap 8 mm wide and 192 μm thick was created. The operation was completed without any further complications. At the end of the procedure the flap was repositioned, but the corneal meniscus was too small to be sutured back. An elliptical area of exposed stroma, temporal to the flap borders, had to be left uncovered. A bandage soft contact lens was fitted and the standard postoperative LASIK regime was prescribed.

The contact lens was removed on the fourth postoperative day when reepithelialization of the exposed area was completed.

Six months after the operation, the patient was satisfied with an uncorrected visual acuity (UCVA) of 20/30. No loss in BCVA was detected. On slit lamp examination, three concentric lines were visible at the temporal corneal periphery. These were, laterally to medially, the scar within the borders of the two flaps corresponding to the area of exposed stroma, the mild punctuate scarring in the area of the sphenoidal corneal resection, and the borders of the ablation (Figure 11A-2). Upon narrowing the beam further, no noticeable corneal thinning was detected (Figure 11A-3), while on retroillumination, the central cornea showed a smooth, even surface (Figure 11A-4).

Computer-assisted corneal topography (Figure 11A-5) reveals a steepening of the inferotemporal paracentral zone, probably adjacent to a flatter zone corresponding to the area of corneal resection.

Unlike PRK, regression or undercorrection after LASIK cannot be reversed with steroids. In such cases, a second operation is required. Surgical intervention should be decided as soon as refractive stability is confirmed. The advantage of early retreatment (within 3 to 6 months from the initial operation) is that the flap can be easily raised and manipulated manually. In cases in which retreatment is undertaken later than the sixth postoperative month, we suggest that the most appropriate action is to perform a second thicker and wider cut.

Figure 11A-1. Schematic presentation of the intraoperative events. A second deeper, yet not wider, flap was created (see yellow area). The suction ring was slightly nasally decentered compared to the first time. The microkeratome started cutting medially to the borders of the first flap, which resulted in resection of a sphenoid-shaped corneal meniscus approximately 0.5 mm wide (see blue elliptical area). A = borders of the second flap. B = borders of the first flap. C = hinge of the first flap. D = hinge of the second flap.

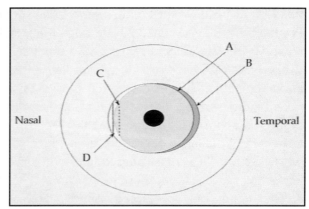

Figure 11A-2. Six months postoperatively. Slit lamp view of the temporal corneal periphery. Three distinct concentric areas are visible: the scar within the borders of the two flaps (see white arrow) corresponding to the area of exposed stroma, the mild punctate scarring in the area of the sphenoidal corneal resection (see black arrow), and he borders of the ablation (arrowheads).

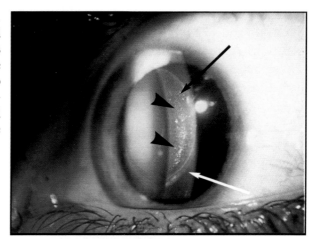

Figure 11A-3. Narrow slit view of the temporal corneal periphery. No noticeable corneal thinning is detected at the area corresponding to the resection.

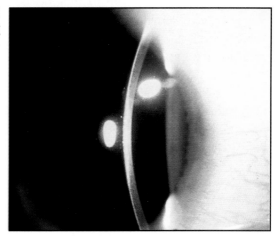

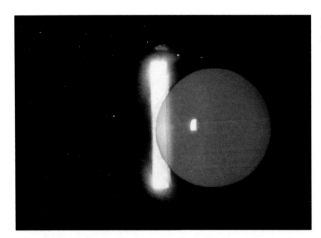

Figure 11A-4. The central cornea shows a smooth, even surface on retroillumination.

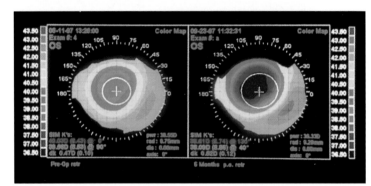

Figure 11A-5. Topographic appearance of the cornea prior to retreatment and at 6 months postoperatively.

Editor's Notes

LASIK enhancements can be performed prior to 6 months by lifting the corneal flap. When using this technique, great care must be made to minimize epithelial defects, as any epithelial defects will increase the chance of epithelial ingrowth following the enhancement. When an enhancement is done on an eye with reasonably adherent epithelium and a careful technique, the epithelial defects are no more significant than with primary LASIK.

After 6 months, it is generally appropriate to recut the flap as the flap is generally quite adherent to the stromal bed. In this case, however, the second cut was decentered slightly more nasally than the previous cut with the ACS. This nasal decentration resulted in the crescent-shaped wedge of tissue being cut free from the peripheral edge of the flap. In general it is preferable to position the microkeratome *less* nasally so the cut will start more peripherally. The second adjustment is that the flap cut would be made deeper, as it was done in this case. Interestingly, the loss of this peripheral wedge of tissue did not seem to affect the postoperative result, as the visual axis remains clear. This removal of peripheral tissue will result in prolonged healing with a peripheral ring of corneal haze.

CASE B, ENHANCEMENT OF MYOPIC LASIK OVERCORRECTION

James D. Ferguson, OD, and Louis E. Probst, MD

Main Concern: Overcorrection
Patient Age: 43

INITIAL PREOPERATIVE INFORMATION

	OD	OS	COMMENTS
Preoperative Refraction	-7.75 – 3.25 X 098	-7.75 – 3.00 X 074	
BCVA	20/20	20/20	
Topography Details	bow-tie astigmatism OU		
SimK Values	45.54/43.39	45.16/43.44	
Pachymetry	626 μm	633 μm	

PROCEDURES PERFORMED

	OD	OS	COMMENTS
1. Date/type	1/27/99 bilateral LASIK		significant
Laser/keratome/plate	VISX S2/Chiron ACS/180 OU		overcorrection
2. Date/type	3/5/99 bilateral enhancement		
Laser/keratome/plate	VISX S2/Chiron ACS/Flap lifted		

CURRENT POSTOPERATIVE INFORMATION

	OD	OS	COMMENTS
Time Postoperative	4/20/99		requested SI mono OS
Postoperative Refraction	+0.25 – 0.75 X 012	-0.50 – 1.00 X 174	
BCVA	20/20	20/20@16ft	
Topography Details	central flattening OU		
SimK Values	37.68/37.07	39.02/38.29	
Visual Complaints	none		
Medications	none		
Refractive Correction	none		

This 43-year-old male underwent bilateral LASIK without intraoperative complications. Preoperative refractive error was measured without cycloplegia. Refractions were OD -7.75 – 3.25 X 098 20/20 and OS -7.75 – 3.00 X 074 20/20. Habitual spectacle *Rx* was OD -6.25 – 2.75 X 085 20/30 and OS -6.75 – 2.25 X 076 20/30. Topographical analysis revealed a normal astigmatic bow-tie configuration with a corneal cylindrical component of OD -2.06 and OS -1.72 (Figure 11B-1). A newly installed updated software package was used to fully correct the right and a correction of +1.00 in the left eye.

On day 1 postoperative, the patient was complaining of blur and was quite anxious. The comanaging doctor's staff measured a significant amount of hyperopia, which was then immediately discussed with the patient. Further anxiety ensued and the patient returned to TLC for follow-up.

Postoperative *Rx* was measured OD +4.00 – 0.50 X 035 20/40, OS +3.50 – 050 X 060 20/60. Topographical analysis revealed a centrally flattened cornea OU with a flattening of 14.00 D (Figure 11B-2). Patient reassurance was given and reinforced.

On day 6 postoperative, refraction was stable at OD +3.50 – 1.25 X 015, OS +2.50 – 1.00 X 010. Topographical analysis was essentially unchanged. Spectacle and contact lenses were given and the patient was reassured.

On week 6, refractive error and topography was essentially stable, with OD +4.00 – 1.00 X 004 20/20, OS +2.50 – 1.25 X 007 20/20. Topography was unchanged. Enhancement was performed without complications. Monovision was attempted again.

The spherical component only was addressed in this case. The amount of programmed correction in myopic overcorrections used is one half of the spherical equivalent. We programmed for OD +1.69 and OS +0.94 on the VISX S2 laser.

On day 1 post-enhancement, the patient was extremely happy as visual acuities had improved at both distance and near. OD +0.25 – 0.75 X 012 20/20, OS -0.50 – 1.00 X 174 (giving 20/20 at 16 inches). Topographical analysis showed a typical the flattened central cornea to have steepened from 35.00 D to 39.00 D in both eyes (Figure 11B-3).

The importance of a cycloplegic refraction and patient education is demonstrated in this case. This patient was found to have been slightly overaccommodating. In combination with his accommodative status he also overresponded to the laser correction. This case also demonstrates the necessity of monitoring nomograms carefully when changing any of the software/hardware components of your laser. Although the possibility of overcorrection was explained to the patient, his response demonstrated that he was not prepared for this sort of outcome. Also, patient reassurance should be on the forefront of the comanaging doctor's mind in the case of any postoperative complication. Overcorrection is a complication in which many surgeons and comanaging doctors tend to minimize. As in this case, reassurance and proper enhancement techniques can overcome the anxieties patients may experience.

Enhancements of overcorrections can be done once the patient's refractive error is stable. Stabilization can range from 6 to 36 weeks. During this period of time patient reassurance becomes paramount.

Figure 11B-1. Preoperative topography.

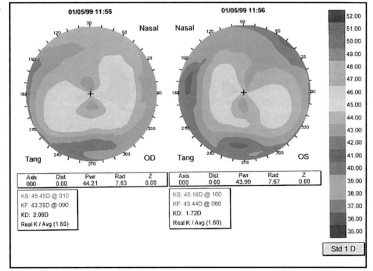

Figure 11B-2. Bilateral central flattening with slightly decentered ablations OU.

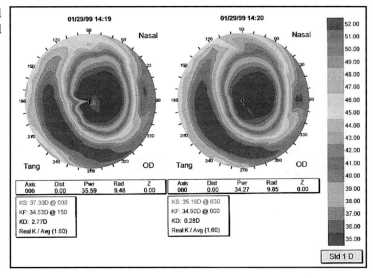

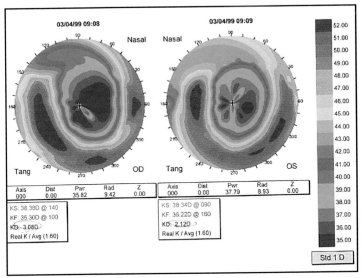

Figure 11B-3. Postenhancement topographies continue to show decentration and irregularity. However, UCVA has been restored.

Editor's Notes

This racing car driver was not pleased when he discovered that he was hyperopic the day following his LASIK. His main motivation for LASIK had been to drive his car without glasses. He now found that he needed to wear hyperopic correction, along with a bifocal add in order to read. He came to our office weekly for the full 3 month stabilization period in order to inquire about his condition and to have his refraction checked. Since he was quite intense, these visits tended to have a humbling effect on the atmosphere of our center. Despite tremendous pressure from the patient to correct his refractive error as soon as possible, we waited for full regression prior to performing an enhancement procedure.

The hyperopic overcorrection was treated by programming only 50% of the refraction. For overcorrections following myopic PRK, LASIK, or RK, only 50% of the hyperopic correction needs to be programmed. Using this nomogram in this case, the patient achieved a perfect result with distance vision in the right eye and monovision in the left eye as he had originally requested.

12

LASIK AFTER PENETRATING KERATOPLASTY

LASIK AFTER PENETRATING KERATOPLASTY - SUMMARY NOTES

Indications
- residual myopia and astigmatism after PK
- at least 1 year after sutures removed
- stable refraction
- regular astigmatism on topography
- adequate corneal thickness

Risks
- unstable postoperative refraction
- decreased postoperative refractive predictability
- epithelial ingrowth
- dehiscence along graft edge
- induction of graft rejection
- greater enhancement rate

Preoperative
- wait 12 months after sutures are out
- stable refraction
- ensure regular astigmatism on topography

Procedure
- center suction ring on graft
- minimize suction time
- wait 2 weeks before performing ablation

Postoperative
- topical steroids for 1 to 2 weeks to prevent rejection
- watch for ingrowth
- wait 4 months for enhancement
- lift flap for enhancement

CASE A, LASIK FOR PK ASTIGMATISM

Eric J. Linebarger, MD, David R. Hardten, MD, and Nelson Preschel, MD

Main Concern: Astigmatism
Patient Age: 72

INITIAL PREOPERATIVE INFORMATION

	OD	OS	COMMENTS
Preoperative Refraction	-5.25 + 4.00 X 25		rigid gas permeable
BCVA	20/40		contact lenses 20/30
Topography Details	irregular astigmatism		
SimK Values	43.6/50.0		
Pachymetry	n/a		

PROCEDURES PERFORMED

	OD	OS	COMMENTS
1. Date/type			no complications
Laser/keratome/plate	VISX S2/Hansatome/180		

CURRENT POSTOPERATIVE INFORMATION

	OD	OS	COMMENTS
Time Postoperative	1 month		excellent result
Postoperative Refraction	-0.75 + 1.00 X 123		
BCVA	20/25		
Topography Details	irregular		
SimK Values	n/a		
Pachymetry	n/a		
Visual Complaints	none		
Medications	none		

A 72-year-old male underwent PK in the right eye approximately 15 years ago for treatment of keratoconus. He has become increasingly intolerant of contact lens wear for correction of high astigmatism, and was interested in other options for improving vision.

UCVA OD was 9/200. Manifest refraction in the right eye was -5.25 + 4.00 X 025 giving a BCVA of 20/40. A rigid gas permeable contact lens fit to the above refraction yielded a BCVA of 20/30-.

Slit lamp examination revealed a clear, well-centered, corneal graft with no remaining suture fragments, and no graft/host override (Figure 12A-1). A sector iridectomy was present, along with a well-positioned posterior chamber lens. IOP by applanation tonometry was 10 mmHg, and fundoscopic exam was unremarkable.

TMS corneal topography (Computed Anatomy System, Inc) demonstrated high astigmatism with a SimK of 43.6 @ 114/ 50.0 @ 024, with SRI and SAI values of 1.41 and 1.34 respectively (Figure 12A-2).

With over 30,000 transplants performed each year, corneal transplant surgery is the most successful and most frequently performed surgical organ transplant procedure throughout North America. Improved eye banking, surgical techniques, and postoperative antibiotic and immunosuppressive agents have made long term graft survival the rule, rather than the exception.

However, many eyes with clear, healthy grafts will experience compromised acuity from extreme astigmatic refractive errors. Options for treating this induced ammetropia have included rigid gas permeable contact lenses, astigmatic keratotomy (AK), radial keratotomy (RK), and automated lamellar keratoplasty (ALK). While many patients are successful with contact lens fitting, a significant portion are either intolerant to rigid gas permeable lenses, or unable to adhere to the daily regimen of cleaning and maintenance that is required. AK can successfully treat simple astigmatism, but does not correct the residual spherical myopia or hyperopia. RK and ALK have been attempted on postcorneal graft eyes, but have met with only limited success.

Over the last few years, the application of the 193 nm excimer laser has shown promise in treating high refractive errors in this population. While PRK initially met with mixed enthusiasm as a result of visually disabling corneal haze, early reports of LASIK have shown much more positive results.

The LASIK technique is employed in much the same way as in conventional nontransplanted eyes, with a few areas requiring special attention. The transplant should be at least 24 months old with good wound approximation in order to withstand the increased IOP generated by the suction ring., Anecdotal reports of wound dehiscence after suction ring application confirm what has long been known regarding wound strength of the graft/host interface. Careful inspection of the graft/host interface to identify any areas of override or weakness will identify eyes that may be at risk. Microkeratome complications such as free flaps, partial flaps, and buttonholes are also more common in eyes with graft/host interface irregularities, and discretion is certainly warranted in these cases. Meticulous attention to suture placement at the time of PK will optimize graft outcomes and allow for successful management of postoperative ammetropia with the LASIK technique.

The eye should be free of any recent signs of rejection, and all suture material that could potentially jam the microkeratome blade must be removed. Pachymetry measurement should be taken on all eyes prior to surgery and after the microkeratome cut to ensure an adequate amount of remaining stroma prior to performing the ablation.

After performing the ablation, the flap is refloated in position and allowed to dry in place for several minutes undisturbed. The adherence of the flap is directly related to the pumping and deturgescence provided by the corneal endothelium, which may be reduced in transplanted eyes.

The patient underwent LASIK surgery OD with the VISX Star S2 excimer laser and the Bausch and Lomb Hansatome. On postoperative day 1, his UCVA in the right eye was 20/30. At his 1 month visit, his UCVA remained stable, with a manifest refraction of -0.75 + 1.00 X 123 yielding a BCVA of 20/25. His 1 month corneal topography demonstrates a significant reduction in corneal astigmatism (Figure 12B-3).

Suggested Reading

Arenas E, Maglione A. Laser in situ keratomileusis for astigmatism and myopia after penetrating keratoplasty. *J Cataract Refract Surg.* 1997;13:27-32.

Lam DS, Leung AT, Wu JT, Tham CC, Fan DS. How long should one wait to perform LASIK after PKP (letter, comment). *J Cataract Refract. Surg.* 1997;24:6-7.

Parisi A, Salchow DJ, Zirm ME, Stieldorf C. Laser in-situ keratomileusis after automated lamellar keratoplasty and penetrating keratoplasty. *J Cataract Refract Surg.* 1997;23:1114-8.

Zaldivar R, Davidorf J. LASIK for myopia and astigmatism after penetrating keratoplasty (letter, comment). *J Cataract Refract Surg.* 1997;13:501-2.

Figure 12A-1. Preoperative appearance of corneal graft.

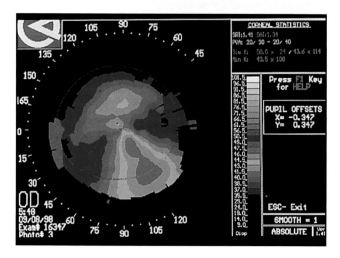

Figure 12A-2. Preoperative topography.

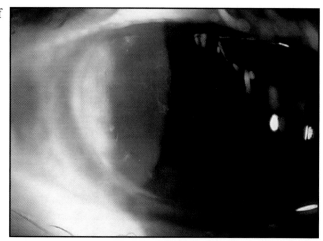

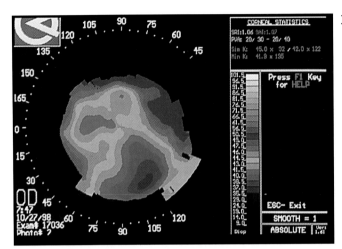

Figure 12A-3. Postoperative topography.

Editor's Notes

Although PK is an extremely successful procedure, it is plagued by large residual refractive errors that are very difficult to treat, and many of these patients are contact lens intolerant. LASIK is the first procedure that really offers a precise and successful method of dealing with residual refractive errors following penetrating keratoplasty.

It is generally recommended that LASIK not be performed for at least 12 months after the original transplant procedure and some surgeons have suggested that we should wait for 12 months after all the sutures have been removed. Close attention to the wound edge is critical as wound dehiscence can occur if the graft/host interface is thin.

Preoperative topical steroids have been suggested by Jose Güell, MD, as a means of reducing the incidence of graft rejection with LASIK after penetrating keratoplasty. Since simple suture removal can induce graft rejection, it would seem reasonable to use preoperative topical steroid drops for several weeks prior to LASIK to reduce the incidence of this potential complication. Michiel Kritzinger, MD, has suggested that the LASIK flap be cut first and then laid back down to allow the eye to settle and the residual refractive error and astigmatism to adjust. Once the eye is stable, the refractive error is reassessed and then the corrective LASIK ablation is performed. Dr. Kritzinger has performed this technique with over 100 post-PK patients and he has found it improved the accuracy of his results.

While this technique may improve results, it also requires two procedures (each with potential complications including graft rejection). If the correction is performed with the first keratectomy, the patient has the chance of needing only one procedure.

Case B, Corneal Perforation Following LASIK and AK after PK

Michael Lawless, MBBS, FRACO, FRACS, FRCOphth

Main Concern: Astigmatism
Patient Age: 72

Initial Preoperative Information

	OD	OS	Comments
Preoperative Refraction		+2.0 – 12.0 X 120	previous PK
BCVA		20/50	

Procedures Performed

	OD	OS	Comments
1. Date/type		PRK and AK	previous PK
Laser/keratome/plate		Summit Apex Plus	
2. Date/type		2 years later, LASIK	
Laser/keratome/plate		Summit Apex/ACS/180	
		and AK perforation	
3. Date/type		next day, wound sutured	
4. Date/type		next day, wound sutured	
5. Date/type		next day, wound sutured	

Current Postoperative Information

	OD	OS	Comments
Time Postoperative		6 days	dramatic loss of BCVA
Postoperative Refraction		n/a	
BCVA		cf	
Topography Details		irregular astigmatism	
SimK Values		n/a	
Pachymetry		n/a	
Visual Complaints		n/a	

A 40-year-old man in good health had bilateral corneal transplants for keratoconus in 1976. Both grafts were of a small 7.25 mm diameter. When first assessed in March 1995, the BCVA was 20/30 OD and 20/200 OS; both eyes were contact lens intolerant. The grafts, although of small diameter, were healthy, but the left had a combination of regular and irregular astigmatism. With a BCVA of +2.0 − 12.0 X 120, the vision could be improved to 20/50 OS. The vision with pinhole was 20/40.

In August 1995, I performed a surface ablation using a disposable disk with a Summit Apex Plus system of -5 at axis 120° using a transepithelial approach. This was combined with two relaxing incisions in the steep axis at 30° just inside the graft/host scar at a depth of 450 μm. This improved his unaided vision to 20/200 and gave a BCVA of 20/30 with a refraction of -2.0 − 6.0 X 120.

In October 1997, nearly 2 years later, the patient presented again requesting further surgery to his left eye. The UCVA was count fingers, and with -2.0 − 7.0 X 120 he could achieve 20/30. The cornea was still healthy with no haze from the previous surface ablation and endothelial cell count was good. His topography (Figure 12B-1) demonstrated a steep axis on SimK at 24° and 11 D of topographic astigmatism with significant irregularity.

The decision was made to proceed with a left toric LASIK in combination with arc incisions in the steep refractive axis at 30°. This was performed in December 1997. A 180 μm plate was used with the Chiron ACS microkeratome to create a flap with a nasal hinge. The laser portion of the procedure was then performed without difficulty with an ablatable disk. The two arcuate incisions were to be at a depth of 450 μm and axis 30° for a length of 45° just inside the old graft/host scar. The first incision was placed without difficulty in the steep axis superotemporally. On placing the blade for the inferonasal incision, a microperforation occurred. The blade was immediately withdrawn. The anterior chamber shallowed with the microperforation and then formed over approximately 1 minute. The incision was not completed, but the bed and undersurface of the cap were irrigated, and the cap was repositioned without difficulty. A disposable contact lens was applied because of the microperforation. No patch was used and a shield was placed on the eye overnight.

The next morning the anterior chamber was flat with the iris and lens touching against the cornea. The patient was returned to the operating room, the flap was lifted, and viscoelastic was placed through the microperforation to reform the anterior chamber. Three interrupted sutures were placed in the area of the microperforation, which was just inside the graft/host scar inferonasally. There was no residual leak and the cap was repositioned without difficulty. One hour later, the anterior chamber was formed and there was no leak, so a shield was applied and follow-up was arranged for the next day. The next day, the anterior chamber was formed but slightly shallow; however, there was no detectable leak around the cap.

Two days later, the anterior chamber was flat with no obvious leakage of aqueous. The patient was returned to the operating room that evening. The cap was lifted and again viscoelastic was placed through the previous microperforation. It was not obvious where the leak was occurring. The old graft/host scar was tending to split with an area of ectasia beyond the three interrupted sutures. There was no leak from this area, but because of the ectasia, four more interrupted sutures were placed at either end of the previously sutured microperforation. The anterior chamber remained formed for more than 5 minutes, and the cap was repositioned and secured with two interrupted sutures. The patient was checked 1 hour later showing a deep anterior chamber and no sign of a leak.

The next morning, the anterior chamber was once again flat with the lens and iris touch against the cornea. The patient was taken back to the operating room, the cap sutures were removed and the cap lifted. At this stage, the anterior chamber was reformed with BSS through the previous microperforation. Once formed, a paracentisis was performed in the host cornea. BSS was then placed through the host cornea and fluorescein applied to detect the area of leakage. There was no obvious leak in the old graft/host scar nor at the site of microperforation. There was a slight suture track leak from one of the interrupted sutures. It was again noted that the area of graft/host scar seemed to have split and was ectatic for about 6 clock hours—more so than it had been on the previous day.

The interrupted suture with the track leak was removed and two overlay cross sutures were placed in this area. Additional interrupted sutures were placed in the area of graft/host scar ectasia. The anterior chamber was formed with BSS through the paracentisis. No leak was observed and the cap was repositioned and again resutured with two interrupted sutures. After a further 5 minutes of observation, there was no obvious leak from beneath the cap.

The next day, the anterior chamber was formed with no leak. The patient was next seen 6 days later. The UCVA was count fingers and did not improve with pinhole. Corneal topography (Figure 12B-2) showed significant vertical steepening and irregular astigmatism. The cornea was remarkably clear considering the tumultuous week of four operative procedures. The cap was well-positioned and the anterior chamber was deep (Figure 12B-3).

What started out as a relatively minor refractive LASIK procedure with arc incisions in a post-graft setting turned into a series of serious consequences requiring multiple surgeries to restore the corneal integrity. It is not certain that this corneal graft will survive, and even if it does, it may have intolerable regular and irregular astigmatism.

Figure 12B-1. Topographic astigmatism with significant irregularity is present after PRk, and AK was used to treat residual astigmatism following a PK.

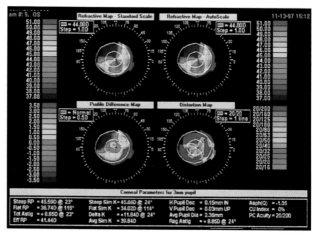

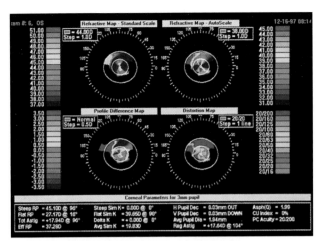

Figure 12B-2. Corneal topography illustrates the significant irregular astigmatism after corneal perforation and multiple corneal sutures.

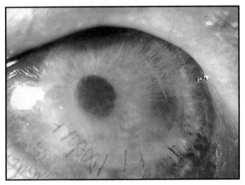

Figure 12B-3. Despite the four operative procedures over 1 week, the cap was well-positioned and the anterior chamber deep. The previous AK is visible supranasally. The multiple sutures were required to arrest the wound leak.

Editor's Notes

This case demonstrates that performing LASIK after previous ocular surgery, particularly PK, is not always easy. In this case, perforation occurred due to the AK incision. A similar perforation could occur because of thinning along the graft/host junction. If this perforation occurred while the suction was activated, it is possible to have extrusion of the intraocular contents. The graft/host interface should be carefully examined before LASIK to ensure that the interface is of normal thickness and stable.

This case also demonstrates that the combination of AK and LASIK can lead to undesirable consequences. Incision keratotomy is known to be associated with microperforations, which are generally not a problem when the procedure is done alone. When a corneal flap is created, fluid leakage from the microperforation can occur underneath the flap, decrease flap adherence, and cause interface flap edema.

If extremely high amounts of astigmatism are present, AK can be done prior to LASIK. The cornea should be left to heal for 6 months to ensure there is no risk of aqueous fluid leak through the astigmatic cut once the LASIK flap has been performed. A better technique may be cross cylinder LASIK, which allows correction of high cylinder. This steepens the flat axis in one meridian and flattens the steep axis in the opposite meridian. Using this technique, high degrees of astigmatism (up to 8.0 D) can be corrected with LASIK. Large amounts of tissue are ablated, so the corneal thickness should be closely monitored.

Case C, LASIK for Post-PK Astigmatism

Michael Lawless, MBBS, FRACO, FRACS, FRCOphth, and Sue Webber, BSc(Hons), FRCOphth

Main Concern: Post-Graft Astigmatism
Patient Age: 64

Initial Preoperative Information

	OD	OS	Comments
Preoperative Refraction		+8/-10 X 165	
BCVA		6/7.5	
Topography Details		regular and some irregular astigmatism	
SimK Values		44.17/55.78@71	
Pachymetry		not performed	
Other		PKP 2 years previously for keratoconus	

Procedures Performed

	OD	OS	Comments
1. Date/type		11/20/97	
Laser/keratome/plate		Summit Apex Plus/ ACS/180 µm Arc T-cuts in the stromal bed	

Current Postoperative Information

	OD	OS	Comments
Time Postoperative		7 months	
Postoperative Refraction		+2.25/-2.00 X 003	
BCVA		6/6	
Topography Details		small amount regular astigmatism	
SimK Values		49.70@46, 44.58	
Pachymetry		not performed	
Visual Complaints		none	
Medications		none	
Refractive Correction		spectacles	

This patient has a fairly common postoperative problem following a PK, namely, that of high astigmatism (Figure 12C-1). According to the Australian Corneal Graft Registry[1] 35% of patients undergoing a PKP in whom a value was recorded, have a postoperative astigmatism of 5 D or more. Since three-quarters of patients undergoing corneal transplantation do so for reasons of improved visual acuity, it is therefore disappointing if an anatomically successful graft has limited visual use due to high astigmatism. Various techniques have been used to correct high ametropia and astigmatism after PKP, but LASIK with or without adjunctive Arc T-cut seems to be particularly promising[2].

Most previous refractive surgery performed after PK has been for the correction of astigmatism. Techniques used include arcuate T-cuts, Troutman Wedges, compression sutures, or a combination of these. However, while these techniques may correct the astigmatism, they do little to correct any myopia or hypermetropia that may coexist. On the other hand, PRK has been used on corneal transplants to correct myopia and hypermetropia, with some degree of success. The use of toric PRK has been generally disappointing.

While our previous report[2] focuses on the correction of myopic errors and astigmatism after PK, the case presented here illustrates that the technique may also be applied to hypermetropic eyes. These cases demonstrate that we can address both the ametropia and astigmatism at the same surgical event.

When considering these procedures one must ensure refractive stability and adequate wound strength. It is generally agreed that a minimum period of 12 months should elapse after graft suture removal before LASIK may be performed, though this period may be shorter in young patients in whom healing occurs at a faster rate. No adjustment is made to our usual LASIK procedure when operating on corneal transplants. Although there is a theoretical risk to the graft/host junction, especially on application of the suction ring, this has not caused any problems in practice.

We use an 8.5 mm diameter LASIK flap and a laser ablation zone that extends to 6.5 mm. Arcuate cuts are performed after laser ablation at the 7 mm zone with the blade set to a depth of 350 μm. Some surgeons perform the lamellar keratectomy and refractive correction as two separate surgical stages, recognizing that a keratectomy alone may correct a significant amount of astigmatism. However, this approach necessitates two surgical interventions to a corneal transplant, increasing the theoretical risk of rejection. We have not encountered an allograft reaction in the 35 procedures we have performed, but postoperative prednisolone is always prescribed. We have encountered one surgical complication in our series of patients. One eye sustained a full thickness perforation at the time of T-cut which required resuturing.

The preoperative spherical equivalent in this patient was +3 D. Bearing in mind a tendency towards undercorrection and the acceptability of slight overcorrection, we treated this patient for +3.5 D. The postoperative spherical equivalent is +1.25 demonstrating less correction than anticipated, but nonetheless a useful change. The decrease in astigmatism was achieved solely with the Arc T-cuts, which have no effect on the spherical equivalent (Figure 12C-2). In other cases where the astigmatism has been a less prominent component of the postoperative refractive error, cylindrical correction may be performed with toric laser ablation. The astigmatism that may be corrected depends on the laser and treatment algorithms. With the Summit Apex Plus we are able to correct up to 5 D of astigmatism, depending on the spherical component of the correction.

This patient now has an unaided acuity of 6/15, having improved from CF pre-operatively and with her spectacle correction she sees 6/6. This is now her better eye (Figure 12C-3).

References

1. Ed Williams KA, Muehlberg SM, Lewis RF, Giles LC, Coster DJ. *The Australian Corneal Graft Registry 1996 Report.*
2. Webber SK, Lawless MA, Sutton GL, Rogers CM. *LASIK for Post-PK Astigmatism and Myopia.* Submitted to the BJO.

Figure 12C-1. Preoperative topography showing approximately 11.5 D of regular astigmatism.

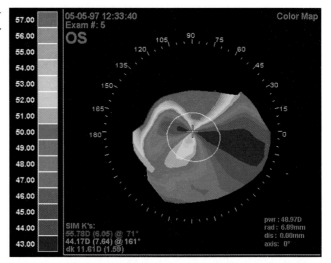

Figure 12C-2. Postoperative topography showing markedly decreased astigmatism.

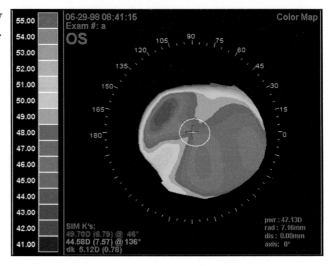

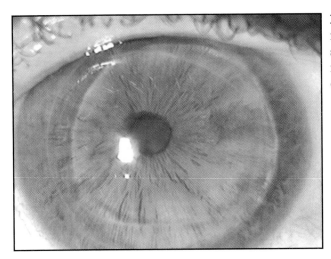

Figure 12C-3. Clinical photograph 7 months postoperatively. The arcuate incisions can be seen top and bottom extending for almost 3 clock hours, just inside the corneal graft/host junction.

Editor's Notes

This case demonstrates how LASIK can be combined with incisional keratotomy to reduce a significant amount of graft astigmatism with LASIK. The -10.0 D correction would be difficult to treat with the toric ablation with LASIK alone.

Performing the T cuts in the stromal bed to a depth of 350 μm at the 7 mm zone is one effective method of reducing astigmatism. However, the surgeon must be careful that microperforations do not occur as any leakage underneath the LASIK flap would lead to a decrease in adherence of the flap and further healing problems. Microperforations with AK alone are not usually a major issue as the incisions do seal on their own and simply require topical antibiotic drops during the healing process.

The risk of graft rejection must be considered whenever manipulation of a corneal transplant occurs. It is known that graft rejection can be induced by a procedure as simple as removing a corneal suture so graft rejection induced by the lamellar keratectomy of LASIK is certainly not inconceivable. These patients should be treated with postoperative steroids and perhaps preoperative steroids as suggested by Jose Güell, MD.

Other options for treating the astigmatism in this case would include a two step procedure where an AK is carried out to first reduce the astigmatism and a toric LASIK ablation is performed 6 months later for the residual astigmatic refractive errors. The cross cylinder technique of LASIK for correcting high refractive errors could also be used. Finally topography assisted LASIK may be useful in these situations when it is more developed in the future.

CASE D, LASIK FOR AMMETROPIA AFTER PK

Lucio Buratto, MD, and Remato Valeri, MD

Main Concern: Astigmatism
Patient Age: 30

INITIAL PREOPERATIVE INFORMATION

	OD	OS	COMMENTS
Preoperative Refraction	-1.00 – 6.00 X 75	-3.50 – 4.50 X 50	PK OS
BCVA	20/25	20/30	keratoconus OD
Topography Details	regular	irregular	
SimK Values	49.7 - 43.7	45.7 - 39.9	
Pachymetry	495 µm	480 µm	

PROCEDURES PERFORMED

	OD	OS	COMMENTS
1. Date/type		6/3/98 LASIK	uncomplicated
Laser/keratome/plate		117/Hansatome/160	
2. Date/type		10/13/98	
Laser/keratome/plate		217/Lift	

CURRENT POSTOPERATIVE INFORMATION

	OD	OS	COMMENTS
Time Postoperative		6 months	excellent result
Postoperative Refraction		+1.00 – 1.00 X 50	
BCVA		20/22	
UCVA		20/30	
Topography Details		more regular	
SimK Values		37.2 - 38.9	
Pachymetry		370 µm	
Refractive Correction		none	

A 30-year-old male patient had bilateral keratoconus diagnosed in 1988. In 1995, at another surgical center, he had a to PK OS with a running suture. When the suture was removed 12 months later, severe, partially irregular astigmatism remained that could not be corrected with spectacles. The patient wears gas permeable contact lenses OU, which is tolerated for just a few hours per day.

When he was visited at our center, the following Rx was observed:

Va OD = 20/25 –1.00 –6.00 @ 75 (Stage II keratoconus)

Va OS = 20/30 –3.50 –4.50 @ 50 (cycloplegia -3.00 –6.00 @ 45, PK)

The left eye demonstrated a PK with a centered flap, well-positioned edges, flap diameter 7.5 mm, central pachymetry 480 μm (Figure 12D-1). The endothelium showed good vitality of the transplant (1500 cells/mm²). Topography (Figure 12D-2) showed severe, slightly irregular astigmatism (dK = 5.79 D) with the most refractive axis at 143°.

It was decided to perform a primary LASIK in OS. The operation was performed with a lamellar cut with the Hansatome down-up microkeratome and the Keracor 117 laser with a 50 Hz ceramic chamber. A 160 μm plate was used with a 10 mm flap. The flap raised easily showing wound healing from the PK. The treatment OS was set at -4.00 – 4.50 X 50 with a minimum optic zone of 4.00 mm for the total ablation of 96 μm.

The postoperative course was uneventful and one month post-operatively, the UCVA OS was 20/200 and the BCVA was 20/25 (-3.50 cyl @ 50, cycloplegia: -4.50 cyl @ 50). The topography (Figure 12D-3) showed good symmetry and good centering of the treatment while confirming high residual astigmatism (dK 3.73 D), the axis and the endothelium were unchanged.

Three months later, it was observed that the BCVA was 20/22.5 (-4.00 cyl @ 50, cycloplegia + 0.50 sph – 4.75 cyl @ 50); the topography was basically unchanged. An enhancement was programmed.

Using a lens hook, the epithelium was perforated at the flap edge and the flap is raised from down upwards using a corneal forceps. The enhancement was performed using the Keracor 217 laser for -5.00 cyl @ 50 with minimum optic zone 4.00 mm

The postoperative course was uneventful. One month after the enhancement, the UCVA OS was 20/30 and the BCVA was 20/22.5 (+1.00 – 1.00 @ 50). Topography confirmed the good refractive result with residual astigmatism of 1.71 D (in the 0 to 3 mm zone) (Figure 12D-4); the central pachymetry is 370 μm.

Kritzinger prefers to perform the lamellar cut initially and only at a later stage perform the ablative treatment because the cut with the microkeratome can modify the patient's refraction.

We feel that a primary LASIK is always advisable (a corneal cut followed by the refractive treatment performed during the same surgical session) because we often obtain a reasonably good results with one operation which involves less stress for the patient. And in the event the patient has to be retreated, the refractive defect to be corrected will be lower with greater guarantees for an excellent final outcome. One of the risks of performing LASIK following PK is that of rejection; reducing the number of surgical sessions certainly contributes to reducing the risk of rejection and infection.

It would be useful to be able to use the TopoLink system in order to reduce the astigmatic asymmetries; but at the moment, the system is not able to manage complex situations with severe astigmatism or large irregularities.

Figure 12D-1. Well-centered clear corneal transplant.

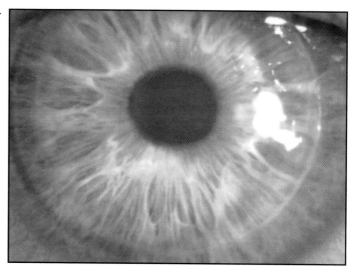

Figure 12D-2. Pre-LASIK topography showing slightly irregular astigmatism.

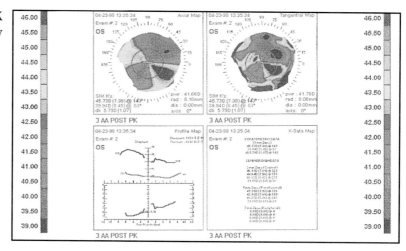

Figure 12D-3. Post-LASIK topography indicating a well-centered ablation with significant residual astigmatism.

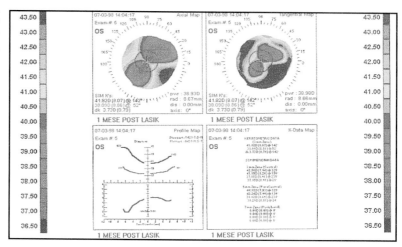

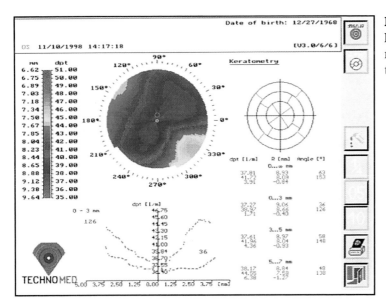

Figure 12D-4. One month after LASIK enhancement OU the topography shows less corneal astigmatism.

Editor's Notes

The Hansatome was used to perform the keratectomy cut following the PK in this case, however, the suction ring size was not specified. The large ring with the Hansatome generally produces a flap 9.5 mm in size and the size of the penetrating keratoplasty donor tends to be between 7.5 and 8 mm. This would mean that the flap would extend beyond the edges of the penetrating keratoplasty. With the ACS microkeratome or the small ring (8.5 mm) of the Hansatome, the corneal flap will be approximately 8 to 8.5 mm in size and therefore it tends to cut exactly along the donor/host edge of the PK. This can help minimize the risk the occurrence of a free wedge of tissue when the flap extends outside of the edges of the PK.

In this case, primary LASIK was used along with enhancement to successfully remove the astigmatism from the patient's left eye. The authors point out that performing the excimer ablation on the primary procedure reduces the correction needed for the secondary procedure. However, it should be noted that in the primary procedure, the corneal thickness was 480 μm and with the enhancement procedure, the cornea was left to be 370 μm. Performing two excimer ablations will generally ablate more tissue as opposed to one ablation. Therefore, close attention needs to be paid to the corneal thickness prior to performing any primary excimer ablation as well as any enhancement procedure.

It would be possible to reduce the astigmatism prior to LASIK with relaxing incisions along the previous graft/host junction, AK incisions, or limbal relaxing incisions. The cross cylinder technique of LASIK involving steepening the flat axis and flattening the steep axis may be more successful in reducing high levels of astigmatism. Finally, topography-assisted LASIK should offer new and more successful methods of treating these high degrees of irregular astigmatism following PK in the future.

Case E, LASIK after PK with High Astigmatism

Lucio Buratto, MD, and Sergio Belloni, MD

Main Concern: Astigmatism
Patient Age: 30

Initial Preoperative Information

	OD	OS	Comments
Preoperative Refraction	-3.0 – 12.0 X 20		keratoconus OS
BCVA	n/a		PK OD
Topography Details	regular		
SimK Values	52.89 X 37.41		
Pachymetry	580 μm		
Other	dk 15.48		

Procedures Performed

	OD	OS	Comments
1. Date/type	3/27/98 LASIK		
Laser/keratome/plate	117/Hansatome/180		
2. Date/type	5/18/98 enhancement		
Laser/keratome/plate	117		

Current Postoperative Information

	OD	OS	Comments
Time Postoperative	5 months		residual astigmatism
Postoperative Refraction	pl – 4.0 X 10		
BCVA	20/40		
Topography Details	regular		
SimK Values	33.59/44.66		
Pachymetry	401 μm		

A 45-year-old female patient had bilateral keratoconus diagnosed in 1976. In 1979, at another surgical center, she had a PK OD with a continuous suture. The suture was removed 1 year after the transplant and residual astigmatism was 15.5 D with efficacious correction impossible.

The patient was intolerant to contact lenses.

The patient was referred to us in November 1997.

     OD Va: 20/400 with plano − 7.0 X 30

     OS Va: 20/20 with -4.0 − 1.5 X 160 (Stage II keratoconus)

Cycloplegic Refraction

     OD: -3.0 − 12 X 20

     OS: -5.0 − 2.0 X 160

Biomicroscopic examination of the right eye found signs of the penetrating keratoplasty with a centered flap, smooth edges, diameter of the flap 8.5 mm, central pachymetry 580 µm, endothelial cell count 1000 c/mm^2.

The preoperative keratometric map showed significant with the rule astigmatism of 15 D with an irregular hourglass and most of the refractive axis at 103° (Figure 12E-1).

LASIK was suggested for OD, which was performed on March 27, 1998. A corneal cut was performed with the Bausch & Lomb Hansatome; the down-up technique was used with a 180 plate and a 10 mm ring. An excimer laser treatment was performed using the Keracor 117 Technolas laser with a 50 Hz ceramic cavity. The treatment set for OD was -10 cyl X 20 with a minimal optical zone of 4.5, maximum 6.0 for a total ablation of 70 µm.

PROGRAMMED CORRECTION	OPTICAL ZONE	DEPTH (µM)
-4.50 cyl X 20	4.50 to 6 mm	32
-3.70 cyl X 20	4.80 to 6 mm	22
-1,80 cyl X 20	5 to 6 mm	16

On the fourth postoperative day the UCVA was 20/200 and the BCVA was 20/100 was a refraction of -6 X 10. The cycloplegic refraction was 10 cyl at axis 10. Biomicroscopic examination found that the flap of the transplant was still crystal clear with no variations in the endothelial cell count. The epithelium was intact with subepithelial and stromal haze and the interface was clean. The analysis of the keratometric map shows a high degree of with-the-rule astigmatism (12 D, dK 12.62) with the most refractive axis at 95 (Figure 12E-2) The pachymetric analysis gave a thickness of 458 µm. On day 16 after LASIK, the exam and the topography were unchanged (Figure 12E-3). Since the astigmatism had remained unchanged, we decided on an enhancement procedure.

The surgical enhancement was performed on May 18, 1998. With a lens hook, the epithelium is cut along the incision line of the previous cut. Using a corneal forceps and Buratto's spatula the flap is raised from down upwards. An enhancement treatment is performed with the Keracor 117 Technolas excimer laser. The treatment set was performed with multiple zones.

PROGRAMMED CORRECTION	OPTICAL ZONE	DEPTH (µM)
-2.50 cyl X 10	4.50 to 6 mm	27
-1.90 cyl X 10	4.80 to 6 mm	22
-1.60 cyl X 10	5 to 6 mm	20

On the first postoperative day, the BCVA was 20/40 with a refraction of plano − 4.0 X 10, The cycloplegic refraction was -1.0 − 8.0 X 10. Biomicroscopic examination shows a good condition of flap with a clean interface, intact epithelium, and slight corneal edema. Analysis of the keratometric map shows astigmatism of 9 D (dk 9.81) with the most refractive axis at 95° (Figure 12E-4) The central pachymetry was 400 μm. After 2 weeks the keratometric map (Figure 12E-5) shows astigmatism of 10 D (dK 10,40) with the most refractive axis at 97°. After 5 months, the keratometric map showed astigmatism of 11 D (dK 11.1) with the most refractive axis at 101°. (Figure 12E-6). The central pachymetry was now 401 μm.

This clinical case highlights how the LASIK technique on transplanted corneas can also create problems with reduced predictability in the refractive result. Nevertheless the visual performance was better and there was a reduction in the astigmatism. In this clinical case, there was obvious difficulty in obtaining even a minimal correction of the high astigmatic error. Enhancement was necessary, which is not optimal in view of the surgical stress on the corneal transplant (graft dehiscence, shift in the astigmatism, endothelial cell loss, peripheral corneal neovascularization). The possibility of performing topography-assisted LASIK to reduce the astigmatic errors is unquestionably a valid contribution, but at present this system is not able to resolve complex refractive situations.

Figure 12E-1. PK with well-healed wound edge.

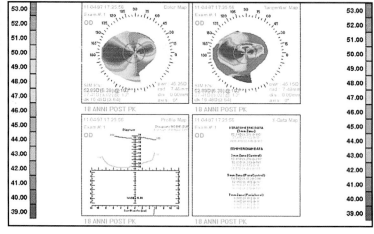

Figure 12E-2. The preoperative keratometric map highlights with-the-rule astigmatism of 15 D (dk 15.48) in a regular hourglass configuration with the most refractive axis at 103°.

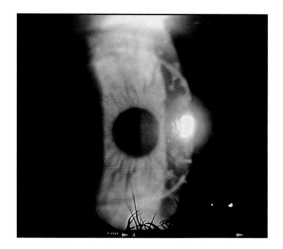

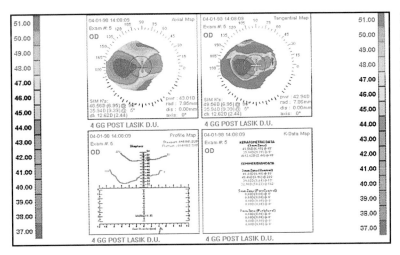

Figure 12E-3. The keratometric map on day 4 highlights with-the-rule astigmatism of 12 D (dk 12.62), with the most refractive axis at 95°.

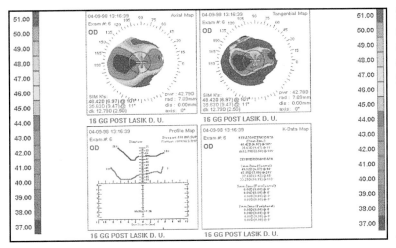

Figure 12E-4. The keratometric map on day 16 highlights serious with-the-rule astigmatism of 12.79 D, with the most refractive axis at 101°.

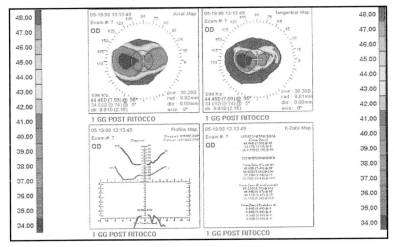

Figure 12E-5. The keratometric map on day 1 postenhancement highlights with-the-rule astigmatism of 9 D (dk 9.81), with the most refractive axis at 95°.

Figure 12E-6. The keratometric map on day 15 postenhancement highlights with-the-rule astigmatism of 10 D (dk 10.40), with the most refractive axis at 97°.

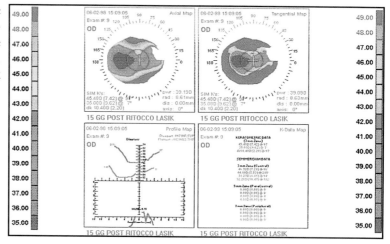

Figure 12E-7. The keratometric map 5 months postenhancement highlights with-the-rule astigmatism of 11 D (dk 11.1), with the most refractive axis at 101°.

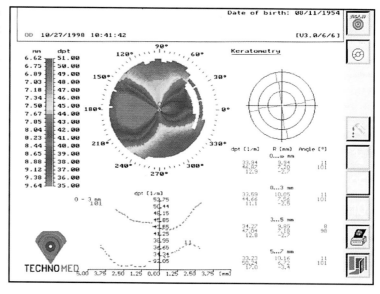

Editor's Notes

This case demonstrates the difficulties with a high degree of astigmatism following PK. This patient originally had a PK almost 20 years ago when the graft used was likely quite small (7.0 mm) and a high level of postoperative astigmatism was more common. Despite two valiant attempts at correcting the cylinder using multiple optical zones, the patient still has 5 D of astigmatism, which is a significant improvement over the preoperative level.

In this case, the arcuate incisions performed prior to the LASIK may have provided some assistance with the astigmatism. These AK incisions would need to be performed at least 6 months prior to the LASIK procedure. They would be placed in the steep axis and could be expected to reduce the astigmatism by approximately one-half to one-third. A cross cylinder LASIK technique could also be used. Finally topography-assisted LASIK should offer some solution for these corrections in the future.

13

LASIK after Radial Keratotomy

LASIK AFTER RADIAL KERATOTOMY - SUMMARY NOTES

Indications
- myopia or hyperopia following radial keratotomy (RK)
- post-RK at least 1 year
- stable refraction
- regular astigmatism on topography

Risks
- unstable postoperative refraction
- decreased postoperative refractive predictability
- flap fragmentation
- epithelial ingrowth
- persistent starbursts and night glare
- persistent diurnal variation
- potential increase in corneal anatomical instability

Preoperative
- refractive stability
- early morning refraction
- eight or less radial incisions
- optical zone at least 3.0 mm
- radial incisions well healed
- no epithelial cysts
- no reduction in BCVA

Procedure
- 200 µm depth plate with ACS
- target slight myopia
- monocular treatment
- use extreme care with flap manipulation
- careful alignment of flap and radial incisions

Postoperative
- expect greater refractive fluctuations initially
- watch for epithelial ingrowth
- flap must be *lifted at 1 week* for enhancements
- *recut at 1 year* for later enhancements

Case A, LASIK for Correction of Secondary Hyperopia Following RK

Eric J. Linebarger, MD, David R. Hardten, MD, and Richard L. Lindstrom, MD

Main Concern: Hyperopia Following RK
Patient Age: 42

Initial Preoperative Information

	OD	OS	Comments
Preoperative Refraction	+1.50 + 075 X 010		progressive hyperopia
BCVA	20/20		following RK
Topography Details	n/a		
SimK Values	n/a		
Pachymetry	n/a		

Procedures Performed

	OD	OS	Comments
1. Date/type	110% correction		no flap problems
Laser/keratome/plate	VISX S2/Hansatome 9.5 mm/180		

Current Postoperative Information

	OD	OS	Comments
Time Postoperative	1 month		excellent result
Postoperative Refraction	-0.25		
BCVA	20/20		
Topography Details	steepening		
SimK Values	n/a		
Pachymetry	n/a		
Visual Complaints	none		
Medications	none		

A 42-year-old female presented for a second opinion regarding refractive surgery. She previously underwent RK in 1990 for correction of moderate myopia. She had notice progressive blurring of vision in the right eye at both distance and near over the last 2 years.

Distance UCVA OD was 20/50-. Manifest refraction revealed a correction of +1.50 + 0.75 X 010, yielding a BCVA of 20/20.

Slit lamp examination revealed a previous eight-cut radial keratotomy treatment with a 3 mm clear zone (Figure 13A-1). All incisions were well healed with no evidence of wound gape or persistent epithelial plugs. The remainder of the anterior segment and fundoscopic exam was normal.

This patient presents with consecutive hyperopia after previous radial keratotomy surgery. Estimates from the PERK study suggest that approximately 1.2 million patients were treated with RK in the United States between 1980 and 1990, and upwards of 20% to 30% of these eyes are now hyperopic.[1]

These patients can pose a unique and difficult challenge to the refractive surgeon. Treatment options have focused on steepening the central cornea with placement of a variety of peripheral circumfrential compression sutures. Several techniques have been described, the most popular being the "lasso" suture described by R. Bruce Grene (Figure 13A-2).[2] However, enthusiasm for these techniques has been tempered by several factors. The technique is meticulous and challenging, and refractive results are often unpredictable and difficult to titrate. In addition, the steepening effect may be lost over time, and problems such as suture erosion and stromal melting can occur (Figure 13A-3).

These and other concerns have led to a search for alternative options to offer this growing number of patients. Hyperopic photorefractive keratectomy (H-PRK) has shown success in treating eyes with primary hyperopia. However, early reports of its use in post RK eyes have suggested an increased risk of postoperative haze and scarring.[3] Anecdotal use of noncontact Holmium/Yag thermokeratoplasty (LTK) in post-RK patients with hyperopia has been associated with unpredictable results and irregular astigmatism.

The role of LASIK in addressing hyperopia after radial keratotomy is currently being explored. Concerns exist over the possible dehiscence and separation of RK incisions while creating the lamellar flap (the so-called "pizza pie" complication). However, a recent study by the authors looking at initial results in a series of ten patients showed encouraging results and avoidance of any flap complications.[4]

Successful treatment of the post-RK patient with LASIK relies on meticulous inspection of all incisions during preoperative evaluation. The radial incisions should be well healed with no evidence of persistent epithelial plugs. While early healing after RK surgery involves epithelium migration into the wound, this "plug" of epithelium eventually retracts after several months to allow collagen remodeling and crosslinking (Figures 13A-4a through d). The strength of the RK incision relies on this new collagen formation. Persistent epithelium in the RK incision suggests tenuous wound integrity. LASIK should be avoided in these eyes until all epithelial cell remnants have cleared. While no consensus exists on when LASIK can safely be performed after RK, the authors found no intraoperative or postoperative flap complications in those patients at least 24 months post-RK with no epithelial cell plugging.

The patient underwent hyperopic LASIK surgery on the right eye using the VISX Star S2 excimer laser, and the Bausch and Lomb Hansatome with a 9.5 mm ring and 180 μm blade depth. Treatment parameters were adapted from hyperopic PRK nomograms and consisted of 110% spherical correction and full cylinder correction.

On postoperative day 1, the patient's distance UCVA was 20/25 with an *Rx* of -0.25 sph. Slit lamp examination revealed a well-positioned, clear LASIK flap with no complications. At 1 month postoperative, the patient's distance UCVA was 20/20 with a stable refraction of -0.25 sph. Postoperative topography demonstrates central corneal steepening after hyperopic LASIK (Figure 13A-5).

References

1. Waring GO, Lynn MJ, McDonnell PJ, et al. Results of the prospective evaluation of radial keratotomy (PERK) study ten years after surgery. *Arch Ophthalmol.* 1994; 112:1298-1308.

2. Grene RB. How to reduce induced hyperopia. *Rev Ophthalmol.* 1995 (Mar): 86-89.

3. Meza J, Perez-Santonja JJ, Moreno E, Zato MA. Photorefractive keratectomy after radial keratotomy. *J Cataract Refract Surg.* 1995; 11:165-69.

4. Linebarger EJ, Hardten DR, Chu YR, Lindstrom RL. *The Role of LASIK in the Treatment of Hyperopia After Previous Radial Keratotomy.* Presented at International Society of Refractive Surgery (ISRS) meeting. New Orleans, November 7, 1998.

Figure 13A-1. Pre-LASIK photo of well-healed RK incisions.

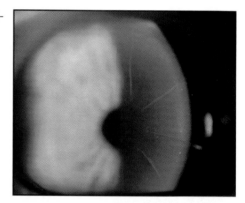

Figure 13A-2. Lasso compression suture.

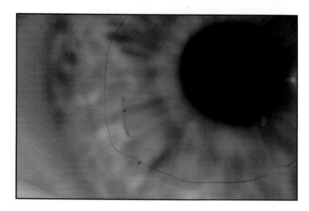

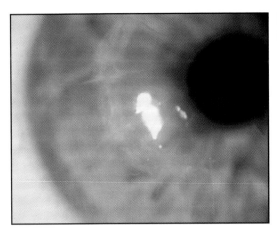

Figure 13A-3. Erosion and stromal melt associated with a compression suture.

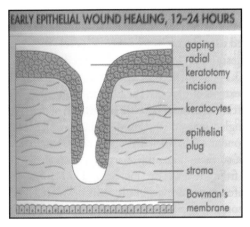

Figure 13A-4a. Early epithelial wound healing, 12 to 24 hours. After an incisional wound to the epithelium and stroma, the epithelial cells migrate and replicate, and move down into the groove during the 12 to 24 hour postincision period. (Reprinted with permission from Assil KK. Radial and Astigmatic Keratometry. In: Yanoff M, Duker JS. *Ophthalmology.* St. Louis: Mosby; 199;3:3.30.)

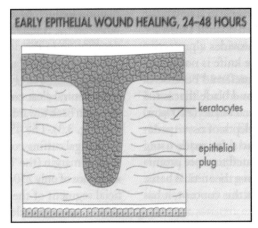

Figure 13A-4b. Early epithelial wound healing, 24 to 48 hours. The formation of a complete epithelial plug within the wound 24 to 48 hours postincision. (Reprinted with permission from Assil KK. Radial and Astigmatic Keratometry. In: Yanoff M, Duker JS. *Ophthalmology.* St. Louis: Mosby; 199;3:3.30.)

Figure 13A-4c. Stromal phase of wound healing, 2 to 6 weeks. Keratocytes migrate into the wound cavity and then transform into myofibroblasts that help to pull the wound closed while collagen is deposited and the epithelial plug displaced. (Reprinted with permission from Assil KK. Radial and Astigmatic Keratometry. In: Yanoff M, Duker JS. *Ophthalmology.* St. Louis: Mosby; 199;3:3.30.)

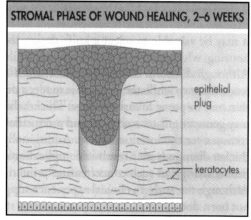

Figure 13A-4d. Remodeling phase of wound healing, 2 to 6 months. This late phase of stromal healing includes the synthesis, breakdown, and crosslinking of collagen, which results in overall wound remodeling and strengthening. (Reprinted with permission from Assil KK. Radial and Astigmatic Keratometry. In: Yanoff M, Duker JS. *Ophthalmology.* St. Louis: Mosby; 199;3:3.30.)

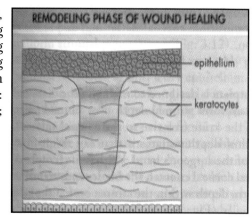

Figure 13A-5. Postoperative topography demonstrating central steepening with hyperopic LASIK to treat RK overcorrection.

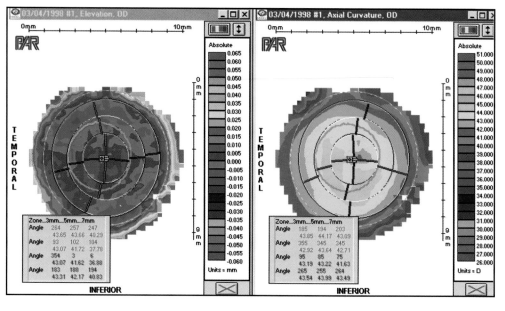

Editor's Notes

As the authors of this case point out, there are a large number of patients with residual refractive errors following RK who will be seeking LASIK in the near future. Some of these patients will be hyperopic and this certainly does pose a complex situation.

It is important to evaluate the post RK cornea to ensure that there are 8 or less radial incisions, that the optical zone is adequate to provide good vision (3 or greater mm) and that the refraction is truly stable. Topography should also be evaluated as grossly irregular patterns would likely lead to unpredictable results. As the authors mention, looking for epithelial plugs in the incision is also helpful to identify the risk of epithelial ingrowth.

When performing a procedure, it is useful to use the deepest cut possible as this will provide the most integrity for the flap and reduce the incidence of flap fragmentation during the procedure. In this case performing 110% of the hyperopic treatment, it was very effective in correcting the entire refractive error. I have found that in many of these cases of overcorrection, it is often helpful to form only 50% of the refractive correction, both for overcorrected RK patients as well as overcorrected PRK and LASIK patients. If there is a residual refractive error after LASIK has been performed with previous RK, it is important to recognize that the flap must lifted within 1 week after the original LASIK procedure so there is no additional trauma provided to the flap. If more than this time has elapsed, it is best to leave the flap to heal and perhaps consider recutting another flap at some time in the distant future.

CASE B, LASIK FOR RESIDUAL MYOPIA AFTER RK

Amar Agarwal, MD, Sunita Agarwal, MD, and Athiya Agarwal, MD

Main Concern: Residual Myopia Following RK
Patient Age: 42

INITIAL PREOPERATIVE INFORMATION

	OD	OS	COMMENTS
Preoperative Refraction	-2.75 D spherical		
BCVA	20/20		
Topography Details	Figure 13B-1		
SimK Values	42.61/42.24@162		
Pachymetry	550 μm		

PROCEDURES PERFORMED

	OD	OS	COMMENTS
1. Date/type	12/19/96 LASIK after RK		no flap fragmentation
Laser/keratome/plate	Chiron 217/ACS/160		

CURRENT POSTOPERATIVE INFORMATION

	OD	OS	COMMENTS
Time Postoperative	28 months		excellent result
Postoperative Refraction	plano		
BCVA	20/20		
Topography Details	Figure 13B-2		
SimK Values	41.99/41.24@180		
Pachymetry	not performed		
Visual Complaints	none		
Medications	none		
Refractive Correction	none		

RK has been done in many cases. When the refractive power is not fully corrected, LASIK is the best alternative to correct such cases in which residual power is still present after RK. One should be careful that not to tear the flap at the areas of the RK cuts when using the microkeratome.

This patient came to the hospital in 1994 with a refraction of -4.5 D spherical. On October 22, 1994 RK was done. Postoperatively the power was -3.25 D spherical. Then on January 21, 1995, a RK enhancement was done. The postoperative refraction was -2.75 D spherical. The visual acuity was still 20/20. Then on December 12, 1996, LASIK was performed.

The Chiron 217 was used with the ACS microkeratome. One should be careful when creating the flap as the RK cuts can get torn off. The pachymetry preoperatively was 550 μm. The preoperative topography (Figure 13B-1) was taken. The postoperative topography (Figure 13B-2) showed a good result. The patient was plano 20/20 post-LASIK.

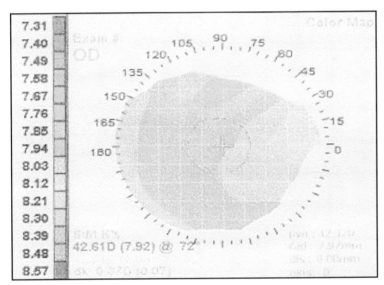

Figure 13B-1. Preoperative topography in which RK was done.

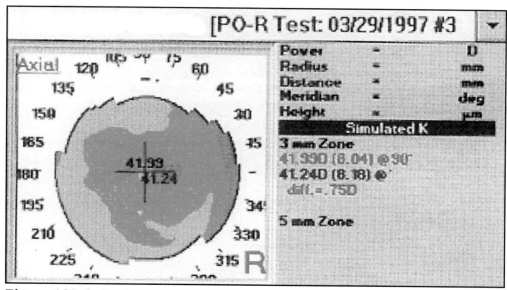

Figure 13B-2. Postoperative topography in which LASIK was done after RK.

Editor's Notes

Patients who have had previous RK with residual refractive error can often be excellent candidates for LASIK. However, because of the previous RK incisions a number of precautions should be made. Patients should be told that the starbursts phenomenon at night, the diurnal refractive fluctuations, and the gradual hyperopic shift in their vision with age cannot be corrected as the RK incisions will remain in the cornea.

RK patients should be evaluated for the number of cuts on the cornea, the size of the optical zone and the stability of their refraction as well as the regularity of their topography. Patients with more than eight radial cuts have an increased chance of flap fragmentation and should be discouraged from a LASIK enhancement procedure. Patients with an optical zone of less than 3 mm can experience interface haze because of the fibrotic reaction at the interface from the previous RK cuts and LASIK should be avoided. Any epithelial plugs or splitting of the incisions will increase the chance of epithelial ingrowth after LASIK. Finally there is usually greater variation in the refractive outcome of the procedure so undercorrections are desirable. I generally program only 50% of the amount of the measured myopia.

Hyperopic RK patients should be approached with more caution as the results are even less predictable and the hyperopic shift post-RK will continue. When selecting the flap depth for LASIK after previous RK, it is best to use a deeper cut such as a 200 µm plate with the ACS or a 180 µm plate with the Hansatome in order to ensure that adequate flap thickness is achieved. This will decrease the chance of flap fragmentation and a central buttonhole caused by the corneal attenuation and the corneal flattening from the previous refractive procedure.

CASE C, LASIK AFTER UNEFFECTIVE RK

Lucio Buratto, MD, and Remato Valeri, MD

Patient Age: 42

INITIAL PREOPERATIVE INFORMATION

	OD	OS	COMMENTS
Preoperative Refraction	-8.50		post-RK
BCVA	20/25		
Topography Details	central flattening		
SimK Values	n/a		
Pachymetry	518 μm		

PROCEDURES PERFORMED

	OD	OS	COMMENTS
1. Date/type	1998 M-LASIK OU		no complication
Laser/keratome/plate	Keracor 117/Hansatome/180		

CURRENT POSTOPERATIVE INFORMATION

	OD	OS	COMMENTS
Time Postoperative	40 days		excellent result
Postoperative Refraction	-0.50		
BCVA	20/20		
Topography Details	mean K 31.87		
SimK Values	n/a		
Pachymetry	n/a		
Visual Complaints	n/a		
Medications	none		

A 26-year-old male patient was operated in 1995 with RK OD. The preoperative refraction in OD was -10.50 sphere. Following the incisional operation, the patient had poor refractive result. Our evaluations found a BCVA OD of 20/25 with -8.50 sph (cycloplegia -8.50 – 1.00 X 5 and a BCVA OS of 20/25 with -7.50 sph. The topography map (Figure 13C-1) showed a modest central flattening which did not affect the tectonic structure of the cornea and did not produce the desired refractive result. Under slit lamp examination, we observed eight radial cuts that reached about 60% of the stromal depth and touches the 4 mm optic zone. The low depth of the cuts could be the cause of the incomplete refractive result. We measured a central pachymetry of 518 μm, and the pupil diameter as measured with the Colvard pupillometer under mesopic light, was 6.00 mm in OU. The OS has not been subjected to any previous refractive treatment and showed a cycloplegic refraction of -7.75 – 1.00 X 170 and central pachymetry was 519 μm. The topography OS (Figure 13C-2) showed an absence of central flattening present in OD (profile map). The echobiometry in OD was 30.88 mm and 29.28 mm in OS.

We decided to proceed with a bilateral LASIK. In this case, a comparison between OD and OS may provide an evaluation between the 'virgin' eye and the right eye that had already been subjected to RK. In both eyes, (operated in the same surgical session) a Hansatome down-up microkeratome was used with a 180 μm plate in OD and a 160 μm plate in OS. (The 180 μm plate was used in OD because the flap was thicker and therefore greater hold of the scars from the radial cuts).

The diameter of the flap in OU was 9.5 mm. The flap was raised with a spatula inserted through the temporal side and was a straightforward procedure in both eyes. After RK, it is important not to use forceps to raise the flap as the radial incisions may open. No tendency of a 'daisy-petal opening' of the flap OD was observed demonstrating the good hold of the RK scars and the low level of trauma caused by the microkeratome. The Keracor 117 laser with a ceramic 50 Hz chamber is set for OD as -11.50 sph (minimal optic zone 4.7 mm) and for OS -9.5° sph (minimal optic zone 4.7 mm).

The postoperative course was regular. No epithelial proliferation was observed at the interface (this risk is accentuated by the possibility of residual epithelial cells inside the radial incisions that can be dispersed at the interface by the lamellar cut). Forty days after the cut UCVA was 20/25 OD and 20/27 OS with a refraction of -0.50 sphere. The mean keratometric value was 31.87 in OD (Figure 13C-3) and 35.29 in OS (in the 0 to 3 mm zone) (Figure 13C-4). In both eyes the treatment was centered with no impurities in the interface (Figure 13C-5).

The symmetrical refractive result observed in both eyes would suggest that LASIK is a safe efficacious method for enhancement of RK, even though in this particular case none of the possible complications associated with previous RK were observed.

Figure 13C-1. PreLASIK topography OD show modest central flattening following RK.

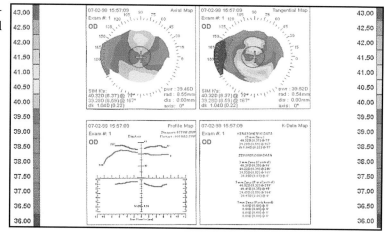

Figure 13C-2. Topography OS shows absence of mild central flattening when compared to Figure 13C-1.

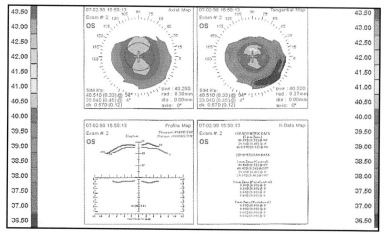

Figure 13C-3. PostLASIK topography demonstrated a well-centered ablation OD.

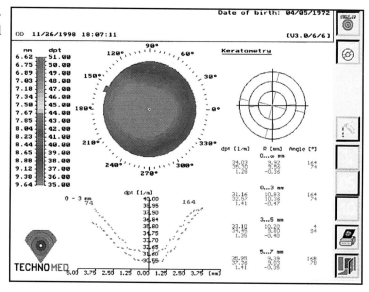

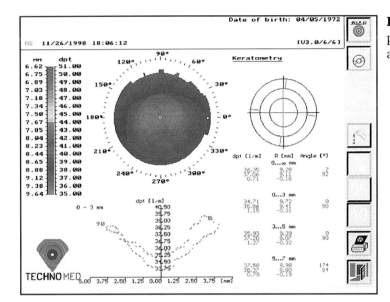

Figure 13C-4. PostLASIK topography demonstrated a well-centered ablation OS.

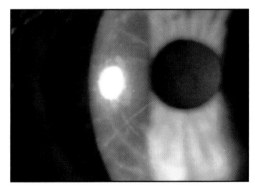

Figure 13C-5. LASIK flap incision can be seen along with previous RK incisions.

Editor's Notes

The patient had an excellent result with LASIK following RK OD. To create the flap in the right eye, a 180 μm flap was used which will improve the integrity of the flap and guard against the incision splitting when the flap is lifted.

It is important to note that it is best to undercorrect eyes that have had previous RK. The hyperopic shift shown in the PERK study tends to occur at approximately 0.1 D per year. This means that a young patient should be ideally undercorrected by approximately -0.50 to -0.75 D to account for the hyperopic shift for the next 10 years. The patient corrected to plano could be expected to be approximately +1 D in 10 years. In this particular case, the under correction may not be as necessary, as the RK incisions were not felt to be full thickness and hence the hyperopic shift would likely not be as significant.

14

LASIK AFTER PHOTOREFRACTIVE KERATOMETRY

SUMMARY NOTES

LASIK AFTER PHOTOREFRACTIVE KERATOMETRY - SUMMARY NOTES

Indications
- myopia or hyperopia following PRK
- no corneal haze
- corneal thickness at least 450 μm

Risks
- persistence of superficial corneal haze
- epithelial defects
- epithelial ingrowth
- reduction in corneal anatomic integrity

Preoperative
- refractive stability
- adequate corneal thickness
- no corneal haze
- no history of recurrent erosion after PRK
- well-centered ablation on topography
- no loss of BCVA

Procedure
- 200 μm depth plate with ACS
- minimal topical anesthetic
- lubrication to protect epithelium

Postoperative
- watch for epithelial ingrowth

CASE A, LASIK AFTER PRK REGRESSION

*Amar Agarwal, MS, FRCS, FRCOphth(Lon), Sunita Agarwal, MS, FSVH(Germ), DO,
and Athiya Agarwal, MD, FRSH(Lon), DO*

Main Concern: Avoiding Corneal Haze
Patient Age: 27

INITIAL PREOPERATIVE INFORMATION

	OD	OS	COMMENTS
Preoperative Refraction	-4.75 – 0.5 D X 180		post-PRK
BCVA	20/20		
Topography Details	Figure 14A-1		
SimK Values	41.81@90; 40.14@180		
Pachymetry	490 μm		

PROCEDURES PERFORMED

	OD	OS	COMMENTS
1. Date/type	3/30/98 LASIK		no complication
Laser/keratome/plate	Chiron 217/ACS/160		

CURRENT POSTOPERATIVE INFORMATION

	OD	OS	COMMENTS
Time Postoperative	13 months		excellent result
Postoperative Refraction	plano		
BCVA	20/20		
Topography Details	Figure 14A-2		
SimK Values	37.70@91; 35.64@1		
Pachymetry	431 μm		
Visual Complaints	none		
Medications	none		
Refractive Correction	none		

Many patients have had PRK done. Many of these patients still have residual power and are not happy with their visual acuity. The solution to these complex cases is to perform LASIK. This patient had PRK done elsewhere. The postoperative refraction after PRK was -4.75 – 0.5 X 180. The pachymetry was 490 µm. The cornea was thin, as PRK had already been done.

The Chiron 217 excimer laser machine was used with the ACS microkeratome. A 6 mm zone diameter was selected. The preoperative topography (Figure 14A-1) showed ablation centrally. Once the flap was created, the laser ablation was performed. The postoperative topography (Figure 14A-2) showed a good centralized ablation. The postoperative visual acuity was 20/20 without glasses. The patient never had any corneal haze either pre- or postoperatively.

This case shows one can perform LASIK after PRK with good results. If the patient has a corneal haze after PRK, then things get a bit more complicated. In such cases, if the haze is not very bad then one can continue LASIK.

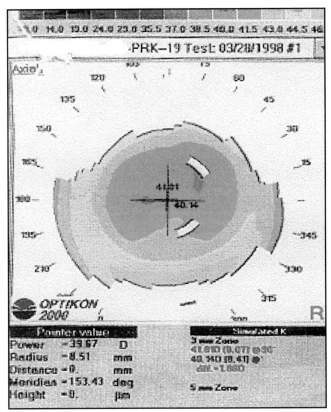

Figure 14A-1. Preoperative topography in which PRK was done previously.

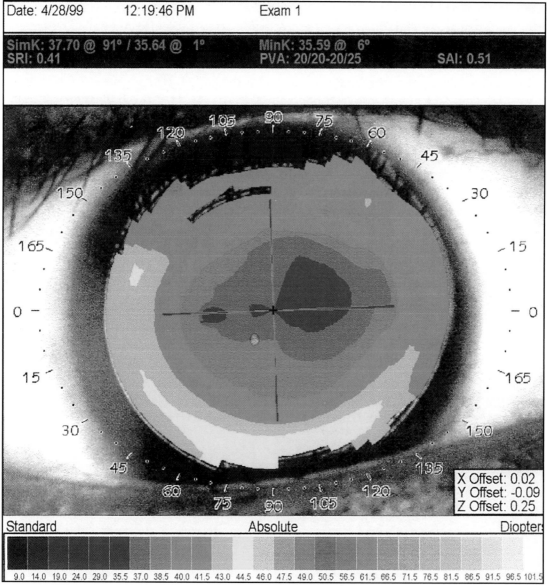

Figure 14A-2. Postoperative topography in which LASIK was done after PRK.

Editor's Notes

In many cases, LASIK after PRK is a preferable option than to perform repeat PRK. When performing PRK enhancements, it is often more difficult to pick the endpoint of the epithelial removal as the stromal surface is irregular. The transepithelial techniques as described by Don Johnson, MD, may be preferable, however this algorithm has not be widely distributed. If the patient does have significant central corneal haze affecting the BCVA, a PRK/PTK type of procedure is required to remove the haze and restore the BCVA.

If there is no haze and the BCVA can be refracted to the preoperative level, then a LASIK enhancement is an excellent option for patients with previous PRK. There is usually less regression after LASIK and the patients enjoy the increased postoperative comfort. Because the epithelium is often less adherent after a PRK procedure, there is a greater chance of having epithelial defects with LASIK and therefore great care should be taken with the topical anaesthetic drops and lubrication during the LASIK procedure. Since these eyes have already had one ablative procedure, the corneal thickness must be carefully monitored with the goal to preserve at least 400 μm of total corneal thickness.

It is important to note that performing PRK *after* LASIK generally does not result in a favorable outcome. If the PRK ablation transcends below the epithelium it can result in significant haze which is very difficult to treat. In general, any LASIK enhancement should be treated by intrastromal ablation by lifting or recutting the flap as opposed to a PRK procedure on top of the flap.

Finally, the central keratometry values of corneas with previous refractive surgery such as PRK, LASIK or RK will be very flat but this does not mean that the flap cannot be successfully created as the peripheral K readings, where the microkeratome engages, are usually still sufficiently steep. Nevertheless, it is probably best to use a thicker cut (180 to 200 μm) because of the potential danger of the flap being thinner in the center or having a buttonhole from central flattening from the previous refractive procedure.

15

TOPOGRAPHY-ASSISTED LASIK

SUMMARY NOTES

TOPOGRAPHY-ASSISTED LASIK - SUMMARY NOTES

Indications
- irregular astigmatism with primary LASIK
- decentered ablation zone after LASIK
- small optical zone after LASIK

Risks
- reduction in corneal thickness
- increase in irregular astigmatism
- misalignment of centration or axis of custom ablation
- poor results with central islands

Preoperative
- pachymetry
- estimate central K reading
- multiple high quality topography
- send data to Technolas in Germany

Operative
- Hansatome flap to gain full effect of custom ablation
- centration critical
- axis alignment critical

Postoperative
- longer visual rehabilitation

CASE A, TOPOLINK FOR IRREGULAR ASTIGMATISM AFTER CORNEAL GRAFT

Michael Knorz, MD

Main Concern: Uncorrectable Astigmatism
Patient Age: 58

INITIAL PREOPERATIVE INFORMATION

	OD	OS	COMMENTS
Preoperative Refraction	-2.5 – 4.0 X 165		post-PK
BCVA	20/60		irregular astigmatism
Topography Details	irregular astigmatism		
SimK Values	50.00/132, 44.94/42		
Pachymetry	610 μm		

PROCEDURES PERFORMED

	OD	OS	COMMENTS
1. Date/type	1992 corneal graft		
2. Date/type	1994 AK		
3. Date/type	August 1996 TopoLink LASIK		
Laser/keratome/plate	Keracor 117C/ACS/160		

CURRENT POSTOPERATIVE INFORMATION

	OD	OS	COMMENTS
Time Postoperative	1 year		improved BCVA
Postoperative Refraction	+1.0 – 2.0 X 10		
BCVA	20/25		
Topography Details	astigmatism		
SimK Values	40.81/148, 37.87/58		
Pachymetry	n/a		
Visual Complaints	none		
Medications	none		
Refractive Correction	spectacles		
Other	patient very happy		

The patient, a judge at a local court, had a penetrating corneal graft because of recurring stromal herpetic keratitis in 1992. He was first referred in 1993. Manifest refraction was +0.25 − 6.0 X 135. Corneal astigmatism was -8 D axis 135 and slightly asymmetric. I performed AK to reduce the astigmatism in 1994. After AK, manifest refraction was -2.5 − 4.0 X 165. UCVA was 20/400 and BCVA was 20/60. Corneal topography 2 years later showed marked irregularity and axis shift (Figure 15A-1). We therefore decided to perform TopoLink LASIK.

A 5.4 mm optical zone was used, and ablation depth was 150 µm. Corneal thickness was 610 µm centrally, and both the internal and external margins of the graft were aligned with the host cornea. It is very important to check alignment prior to the lamellar cut. In poor alignment or localized ectasia at the edge, corneal thickness might be reduced. The keratome cut may cause further weakening of the cornea, inducing more ectasia or even a penetration of the anterior chamber.

In this patient, alignment was perfect and the LASIK procedure performed in August 1996 was uneventful. A 160 µm flap was used. Five days after topography-assisted LASIK, UCVA had improved to 20/30, and BCVA was 20/25 (correction: +0.75 sphere). Corneal topography showed an almost perfectly spherical cornea (Figure 15A-2).

After 4 months, UCVA was 20/30 and BCVA was 20/25, but manifest refraction had changed slightly to +1.0 − 2.0 X 10. Corneal topography 4 months after topography-assisted LASIK showed marked improvement of irregularity, but also some regression of astigmatism (Figure 15A-3).

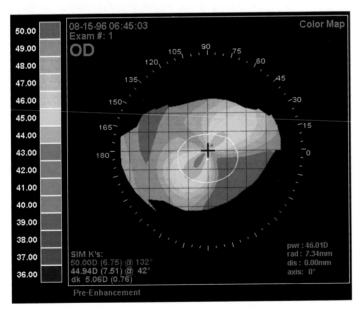

Figure 15A-1. Topographic map prior to TopoLink LASIK.

Figure 15A-2.
Differential map
5 days after
TopoLink LASIK.

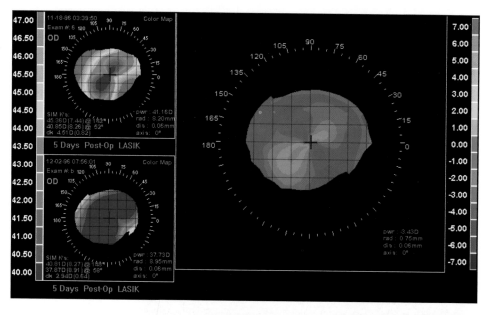

Figure 15A-3. Topographic map 4 months after TopoLink LASIK.

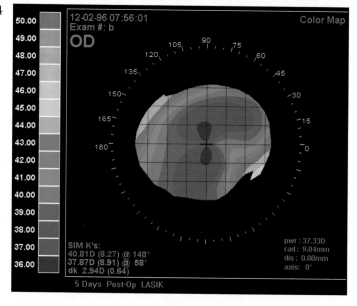

Editor's Notes

While the excimer laser been very useful for the correction of the regular astigmatism associated with myopia and hyperopia, it has been less successful in the treatment of irregular astigmatism. With the current excimer lasers, corrections of an irregular cornea will result in an unpredictable result. Topography-assisted LASIK allows a customized ablation in which the patient's topography is used to create a specific ablation pattern designed to improve the contour of the cornea. Initially this will provide a method of correcting irregular corneas after refractive surgery, PK, or ocular trauma. Taken to its full potential however, topography-assisted LASIK could allow us to achieve "super vision" where even the slightest irregularity of the corneal contour is corrected yielding an improved BCVA.

Most cases of PK have residual astigmatism that ranges from 4 to 6 D. Despite improvement in our microsurgical techniques, it seems impossible to reduce the astigmatism to a lower level for all cases on a consistent basis. This patient demonstrates a slightly irregular pattern of a high degree of astigmatism in the oblique axis. While this topographic and refractive pattern could be treated with a standard excimer laser ablation, it would likely result in an asymmetrical result.

Since the preoperative central corneal pachymetry in this case was 610 µm and the depth of the ablation used for the topography-assisted LASIK at 5.4 mm was 150 µm, the total corneal thickness at the end of this procedure should be at least 460 µm. This patient is fortunate that he had a large amount of corneal tissue to ablate. Otherwise, this large amount of excimer ablation may not have been possible while still leaving 400 µm of total stromal tissue.

CASE B, TOPOLINK TO TREAT A DECENTERED MYOPIC ABLATION

Michael Knorz, MD

Main Concern: Halos and Double Vision
Patient Age: 36 years

INITIAL PREOPERATIVE INFORMATION

	OD	OS	COMMENTS
Preoperative Refraction		+1.0 + 1.0 X 1	previous LASIK
BCVA		20/40	halos and double
Topography Details		decentered ablation	vision
SimK Values		n/a	
Pachymetry		485 μm	

PROCEDURES PERFORMED

	OD	OS	COMMENTS
1. Date/type		3/18/99 LASIK TopoLink	
Laser/keratome/plate		Keracor 117 C/Hansatome	
		160 μm, 8.5 mm ring	
		max. ablation 69 μm	

CURRENT POSTOPERATIVE INFORMATION

	OD	OS	COMMENTS
Time Postoperative		1 day	excellent result
Postoperative Refraction		plano	
BCVA		20/25	
Topography Details		improved centration	
SimK Values		n/a	
Pachymetry		n/a	
Visual Complaints		none	
Medications		Dexamethasone and Gentamicin	

This 36-year-old lady had LASIK in both eyes in 1998 and was referred to me because of a decentered ablation. The right eye was perfect, but she complained bitterly about permanent monocular diplopia and distorted halos in her left eye. A TopoLink LASIK was planned.

The corneal topography taken prior to the TopoLink LASIK is shown in Figure 15B-1, lower left, and Figure 15B-2, lower right. A decentered myopic ablation is visible. The ablation is decentered about 1.5 mm downwards and 1 mm temporally. We calculated a customized ablation based on the topographic map described. The planned ablation pattern is shown in Figure 1, upper right. The scale is in µm. The predicted outcome of corneal topography is shown in Figure 1, lower right. The scale is in diopters. I used the Hansatome to create a new flap with a thickness of 160 µm and a diameter of 8.5 mm (8.5 mm suction ring).

The surgery was uneventful. The ablation was centered on the center of the entrance pupil, and the eye tracker was used. Figure 15B-2 shows the pre- and postoperative maps as well as the differential map, taken 1 day after surgery. The postoperative map, upper right, shows significantly improved centration and no residual astigmatism. The differential map, left, shows the asymmetric ablation pattern, customized to this individual eye. Visual acuity improved to 20/25 uncorrected, and even more important, monocular double vision and halos were no longer visible. This case confirms again that TopoLink LASIK is a valuable tool in the treatment of decentered ablations.

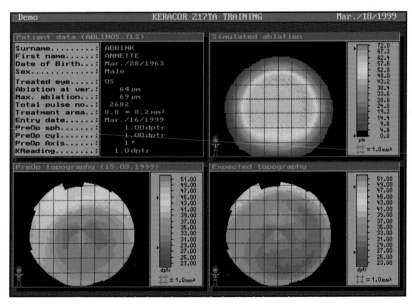

Figure 15B-1: Treatment plan in TopoLink LASIK. This plan is shown on the screen of the Keracor 117C/217 excimer lasers when the treatment is loaded. It features patient data, upper left, preoperative topography, lower left, the simulated ablation pattern, upper right, and the expected postoperative topography, lower right.

Figure 15B-2: Differential map after treatment. The preoperative map, lower right, shows a decentered ablation, the postoperative map, upper right, shows improved centration. The differential map is shown on the left.

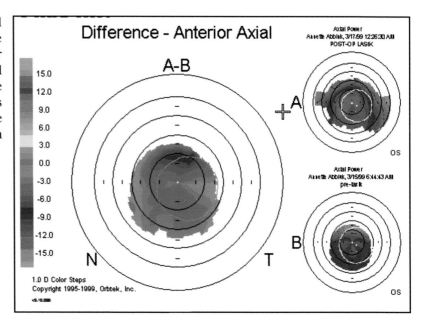

Editor's Notes

This case demonstrates a decentered ablation following myopic LASIK. The preoperative topography in Figure 15B-1, shows that the ablation is inferior to the visual axis. There is a bow-tie pattern that extends through the visual axis, which will cause astigmatism and explains the diplopia. The patient has also become slightly hyperopic, which has caused further visual difficulties. Using a conventional excimer laser, it would be extremely difficult to treat this type of situation.

The correction of decentered ablations with conventional excimer lasers has been attempted by several methods. An ablation pattern decentered in the opposite direction, PTK with a masking agent to protect the previously ablated area, and simply correcting the resultant refractive error with the hope that the flap will provide a masking effect and smooth out the contour of the cornea have all been used. While these methods have had some degree of success, the advantages of the customized ablation of topography-assisted LASIK is obvious.

Pachymetry is also crucial in this case. The preoperative corneal pachymetry was thin at 485 μm because of the previous excimer ablation. The planned topography-assisted LASIK ablation removed another 69 μm of central corneal tissue. This means the patient had over 400 μm of final total central corneal thickness, which should be adequate to maintain the long-term corneal integrity.

CASE C, TOPOLINK FOR DECENTERED HYPEROPIC LASIK

Michael Knorz, MD

Main Concern: Halos and monocular diplopia
Patient Age: 36

INITIAL PREOPERATIVE INFORMATION

	OD	OS	COMMENTS
Preoperative Refraction	-1 sph		post-H-LASIK halos
BCVA	20/25		and diplopia
Topography Details	asymmetric astigmatism		
SimK Values	40.91/177, 42.11/87		
Pachymetry	625 µm		

PROCEDURES PERFORMED

	OD	OS	COMMENTS
1. Date/type	October 1998 LASIK		uncomplicated
2. Date/type	April 1999 TopoLink LASIK		
Laser/keratome/plate	Keracor 117C/Hansatome/180		

CURRENT POSTOPERATIVE INFORMATION

	OD	OS	COMMENTS
Time Postoperative	4 weeks		excellent result
Postoperative Refraction	plano		
BCVA	20/25		
Topography Details	well-centered ablation zone, no astigmatism		
SimK Values	41.13/135, 41.79/45		
Pachymetry	n/a		
Visual Complaints	none		
Medications	none		
Refractive Correction	none		
Other	patient very happy		

This patient had LASIK OD at our center in October 1998. His preoperative refraction was +1.75 cyl A 15°. He was treated using the Hansatome with a 9.5 mm suction ring and a 180 µm thickness plate. Surgery was uneventful. On day 1, visual acuity was 20/100 uncorrected and 20/30 with -1.00 D sphere. The patient complained about blurred vision and monocular diplopia. Corneal topography showed asymmetric astigmatism (Figure 15C-1, left). We decided to retreat using TopoLink in April 1999. The flap was lifted without problems, and the ablation was performed. After retreatment, a well-centered ablation zone is visible, with no residual astigmatism (Figure 15C-1, right). The subjective complaints also disappeared.

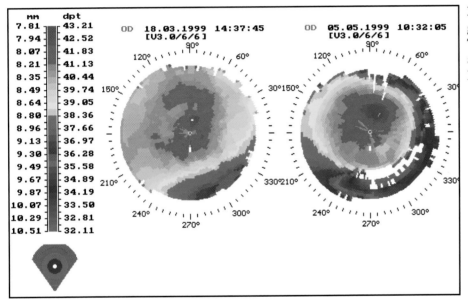

Figure 15C-1. Topographic map prior to TopoLink LASIK (left) and after TopoLink LASIK (right).

Editor's Notes

Decentered ablations with hyperopic LASIK are perhaps one of the most difficult problems to treat. Hyperopic LASIK enhancements frequently do not improve the visual acuity and can result in a loss of BCVA. The symptoms of double vision and distorted vision often persist. Topography-assisted LASIK offers the ideal solution for the correction of these decentered ablations. Since the Hansatome was used, the flap could be easily lifted and the topography-assisted LASIK ablation performed. There is little doubt that this procedure will offer great therapeutic benefit for many patients in the future.

Case D, TopoLink PRK for Induced Hyperopia after PTK

Michael Knorz, MD

Main Concern: Significant Hyperopia
Patient Age: 63

Initial Preoperative Information

	OD	OS	Comments
Preoperative Refraction	+8.00 – 1.50 X 175		central superficial
BCVA	20/25		corneal scar
Topography Details	asymmetric flattening		
SimK Values	35.75/37.49@134°		
Pachymetry	n/a		

Procedures Performed

	OD	OS	Comments
1. Date/type	October 1998 PTK		PRK for corneal scar
2. Date/type	January 1999 TopoLink PRK		PRK as corneal thin
Laser	Keracor 117C (PRK)		

Current Postoperative Information

	OD	OS	Comments
Time Postoperative	3 months		excellent result
Postoperative Refraction	+1.25 – 1.5 X 160		
BCVA	20/25		
Topography Details	well-centered ablation zone, no astigmatism		
SimK Values	39.67/40. 40.73/130		
Pachymetry	n/a		
Visual Complaints	none		
Medications	none		
Refractive Correction	none		
Other	patient happy		

This patient had a central superficial scar following nonspecific keratitis in 1961. Visual acuity was UCVA 20/100 and BCVA 20/30 with +1.00 – 4.00 X 170. In October 1997, transepithelial PTK was performed with a scanning-beam excimer laser (Keracor 117 C). The so-called PC-controlled ablation mode was used, which allows the surgeon to perform a surface-parallel ablation of a pre-selected depth. A 5 mm central zone and a transition zone up to 8 mm were used. Central ablation was approximately 145 μm. Two months later, refraction was +8.00 – 1.50 X 75, and BCVA was 20/25. Corneal topography showed significant flattening of the cornea, especially on the temporal half-meridian (Figure 15D-1, left), which explained the induced hyperopia. Because of the asymmetry, we decided to perform a TopoLink retreatment. As PTK had been performed, we choose PRK instead of LASIK. TopoLink PRK was performed in January 1999. Surgery was uneventful. Three months after surgery, refraction was +1.25 – 1.5 X 160, and visual acuity was 20/25. The patient was happy with the result. Corneal topography showed a symmetrical central steepening, representing the hyperopic correction performed (Figure 1, right).

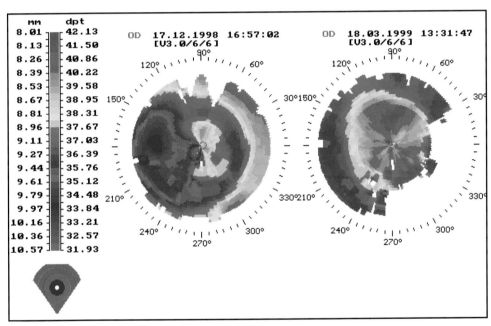

Figure 15D-1. Topographic map prior to TopoLink LASIK (left) and after TopoLink PRK (right).

Editor's Notes

While PTK can be a very useful modality for removing anterior stromal scars, it will also induce a hyperopic shift in the cornea. In this case, a PTK procedure was performed down to 145 μm or approximately one-third of the corneal thickness. This induced a substantial hyperopic shift of +8 D. Unfortunately pachymetry values are not available, however, we can estimate what the pachymetry values would be after the PTK procedure. The average corneal thickness is 540 μm so the PTK ablation of 145 μm would leave us with 395 μm of total corneal tissue. This unfortunately does not allow the creation of a LASIK flap or further ablation while leaving sufficient total stromal thickness to preserve the corneal integrity.

For this reason topography-assisted PRK was performed rather than LASIK. The risk of performing a large surface ablation of this nature would be the development of postoperative corneal haze. This patient was fortunate in that haze did not develop and the postoperative result was excellent.

CASE E, POST-LASIK CENTRAL CORNEAL IRREGULAR ASTIGMATISM

Michiel S. Kritzinger, MD

Main Concern: Irregular Astigmatism

INITIAL PREOPERATIVE INFORMATION

	OD	OS	COMMENTS
Preoperative Refraction	+1.25 – 4.0 X 88	-050 – 450 X 4	post-LASIK
BCVA	20/30	20/25	referring center
UCVA	20/100	20/100	
Topography Details	irregular astigmatism OU (Figures 15E-1a and b)		
SimK Values	42.7/41.3	45.6/42.9	
Pachymetry	584 µm	597 µm	

PROCEDURES PERFORMED

	OD	OS	COMMENTS
1. Date/type	M-LASIK	M-LASIK	referral center
2. Date/type	topography-assisted LASIK OU		see text
Laser/keratome/plate	Technolas 217/Technomed		

CURRENT POSTOPERATIVE INFORMATION

	OD	OS	COMMENTS
Time Postoperative	4 days	4 days	excellent results
Postoperative Refraction	+1.00 – 1.25 X 129	pl – 175 X 23	
BCVA	20/30	20/25	
Topography Details	irregular/island OU (Figures 15E-2a and b)		
SimK Values	43.1/40.3	44.4/42.7	
Pachymetry	520 µm	525 µm	
Refractive Correction	none	none	

This patient had LASIK done 1 year prior to consulting me for the first time. The patient was not wearing any form of spectacle or contact lens correction, but was not satisfied with either the quantity or quality of the vision. This case was made complex by the severe degree of irregular astigmatism present. Preoperative information was unfortunately not available.

A Technomed topography was done for a Technolas 217 Topolink customized ablation. A new LASIK flap was cut because previous surgery was performed more than 1 year ago. The latest infrared eye tracker was used during laser ablation. Topolink treatment was calculated and sent electronically to my offices. The proposed treatment was programmed into the Technolas 217.

Planoscan topolink eye tracker treatment:

	OD	OS
Sphere	+1.25	-0.50
Cylinder	-4.00	-4.50
Cylinder Axis	88	4
Treatment area	9.4 mm x 10.2 mm	9.9 mm x 9.5 mm
Ablation/total pulses	40 µm/2099 pulses	50 µm/2188 pulses
Spot size	1 and 2 mm	1 and 2 mm

Surgery was uneventful. Four days postoperatively a dramatic reduction in astigmatism was apparent with improved quality and quantity of vision.

Patient satisfaction was particularly positive. The option of further customized ablation has not been excluded entirely. The patient will be reevaluated 6 to 9 months after surgery to explore options of further customized ablation.

Figure 15E-1a. Irregular astigmatism OD after primary LASIK.

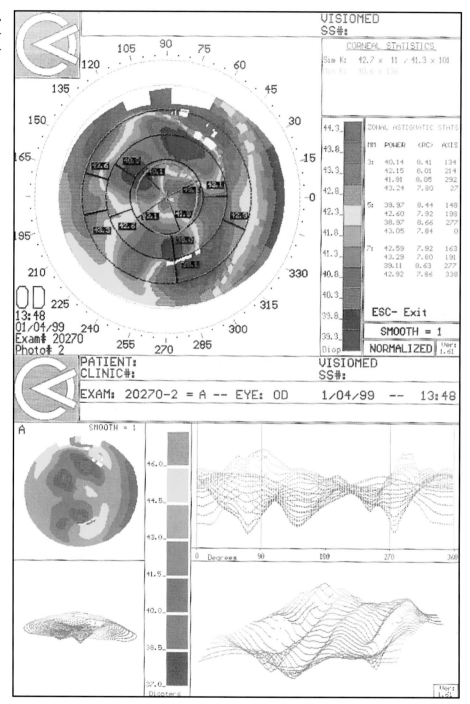

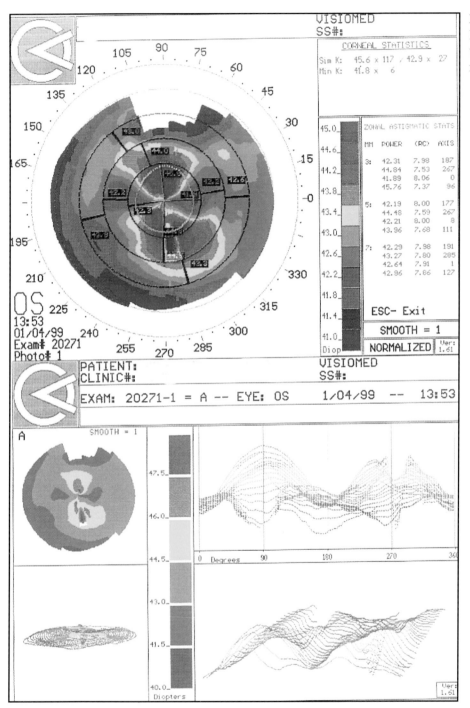

Figure 15E-1b. Irregular astigmatism OS after primary LASIK.

Figure 15E-2a. Persistent irregular pattern with central island OD 4 days after TopoLink LASIK.

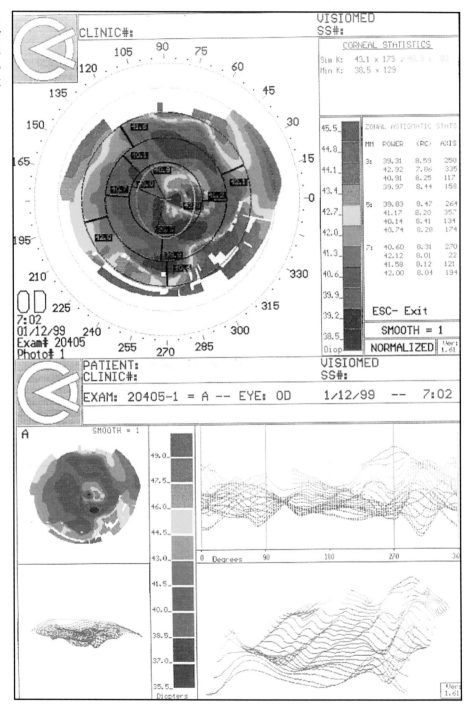

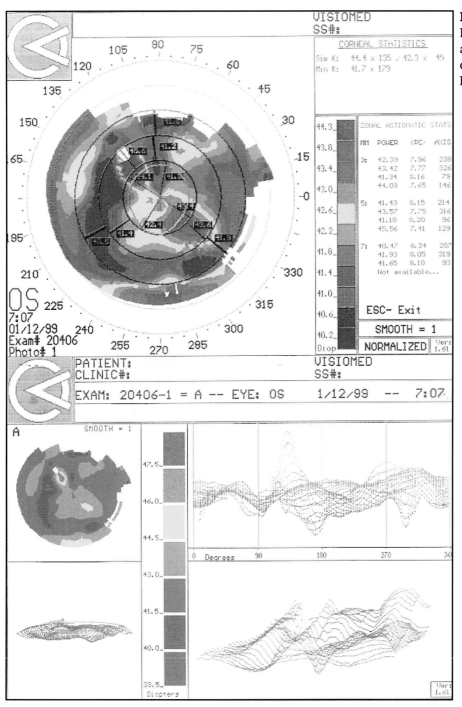

Figure 15E-2b. Persistent irregular astigmatism OS 4 days after TopoLink LASIK.

Editor's Notes

The reduced BCVA OD is related to the extremely irregular topography demonstrated prior to the enhancement procedure OD. The high degree of residual astigmatism and the central island pattern OD suggests some error in the referring doctor's technique such as incorrect programming of the laser or poor attention to stromal fluid control resulting in inadequate treatment of the central cornea.

In this case topography-assisted LASIK was used on the Technolas 217 laser in order to correct this irregular ablation pattern. Since a large number of pulses over a large area are required for topography-assisted ablation, the corneal thickness is crucial when making these calculations in order to ensure that the adequate corneal thickness is available in order to perform this correction. The final visual result, while improved in the right eye still demonstrates a reduction in the BCVA and indicates a reduced BCVA in the 20/30 range in association with a small central island on topography. The BCVA OS also did not improve, and areas of central corneal steepening are still evident.

This case demonstrates the utility and limitations of topography-assisted LASIK. This procedure allows us to correct irregular ablations and therefore customize the treatment for patients, such as this case, with irregular corneal patterns. This can significantly improve their quality of vision and therefore improve their refractive results. Because the topography is done prior to the procedure, the correct centering and orientation of the axis of the customized ablation is essential in order to get the desired outcome. Since this cannot be perfectly controlled using the present techniques for laser correction, the results of this procedure will be limited until real-time topography is possible during the excimer laser ablation.

CASE F, PSYCHOLOGICAL EFFECTS ON VISUAL RESULTS

Michiel S. Kritzinger, MD

Main concern: Lack of Patient Cooperation

INITIAL PREOPERATIVE INFORMATION

	OD	OS	COMMENTS
Preoperative Refraction	+1.00 – 1.75 X 124	+1.00	post-M-LASIK OU
BCVA	20/30	20/30	
Topography Details	small zone		
SimK Values	40.3/39.2	36.6/36.3	
Pachymetry	517 µm	479 µm	

PROCEDURES PERFORMED

	OD	OS	COMMENTS
1. Date/type	LASIK enhancement OU		
Laser/keratome/plate	Technolas 217/ACS	Technolas 217/ACS	
2. Date/type	8 months later, topography-assisted LASIK OU		

CURRENT POSTOPERATIVE INFORMATION

	OD	OS	COMMENTS
Time Postoperative	n/a	n/a	reduced BCVA OU
Postoperative Refraction	+0.50	+2.25 – 0.50 X 84	thin corneas
BCVA	20/70	20/70	
Topography Details	symmetrical island OU		
SimK Values	37.1/36.3	41.5/39.5	
Pachymetry	361 µm	328 µm	
Visual Complaints	poor vision OU		
Medications	none		

This case illustrates how a patient's state of mind can eventually influence the visual outcome of a surgical procedure. Persistent complaints of visual aberrations, can and will intimidate the surgeon. This can lead to unnecessary surgery with further, sometimes more disastrous, visual effects!

This patient's first LASIK operation was done elsewhere by a competent LASIK surgeon, but he finally became discouraged and referred the patient to me. The patient's main complaint was that he was experiencing multi-images at night after his first LASIK operation. (Figure 15F-1).

Original prescription (Figures 15F-2 and 3):

OD: -4.50/-2.75 X 280
OS: -10.25 D

The patient was treated with the Technolas 217 Planoscan. His results were as follows:

	OD	OS
Sphere	+1.45	+1.15
Cylinder	-1.50	0
Cylinder Axis	124	
Zone diameter	5 mm	5 mm
Ablation/Total pulses	27 μm/917	0 μm/448

LASIK was performed on both eyes with visual outcome of:

	OD	OS
UCVA	20/30	20/80
BCVA	20/30	20/30
Refraction	+0.50/-0.50 X 5	-0.50
Topography	Figure 15F-4a and b	

This patient insisted on having more surgery done, and continued complaining about prevailing multi-images. Slit lamp biomicroscopy revealed clear ocular media. Three months later, refractions were +0.50 DS (20/25) OD and -0.25 DS (20/25) OS. Multi-images were reduced subjectively as well, but the patient remained dissatisfied. Vision continued to fluctuate for the following months, ranging from 20/200 on one assessment to 20/25 on the next.

As a last resort I tried a customized ablation with Technolas 217 on both eyes, eight months after initial surgery, purely to reduce the multi-images the patient was experiencing.

Preoperative Planoscan TopoLink Eyetracker

	OD	OS
Sphere	+0.25	+0.50
Cylinder	-1.25	0
Cylinder Axis	135	0
Treatment area	8.8 x 8.9 mm	9.1 x 8.8 mm

Patient postoperative cooperation was now worse than ever. Postoperative refraction was now +0.50 (20/70) OD and +2.25/-0.50 X 84 (20/70) OS. Postoperative topography was good OU, but there was a central island on the right eye. (Figures 15F-5a and b). I decided to terminate further surgical treatment and let the eye progress naturally.

After 3 months, a dramatic change of the central island (for the better) was apparent (Figures 15F6a and b). This patient ended up with:

- huge ablations OD and OS
- still experiencing the same glare and halos
- slightly overcorrected due to topolink treatment (but this will improve with time)
- scarred, thin corneas after all the unnecessary treatment
  - OD 361 µm with slight posterior surface ectasia
  - OS 328 µm with slight posterior surface ectasia

There is a fine line to be drawn between satisfying the patient's real visual needs and satisfying a patient's psychological needs. We as ophthalmologists need to combine the two. If patients do not give their full cooperation, accurate measurements and visual and psychological satisfaction are impossible.

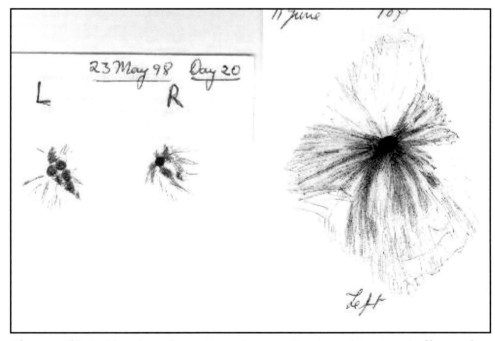

Figure 15F-1. Sketches the patient drew to illustrate his visual effects after the first LASIK procedure.

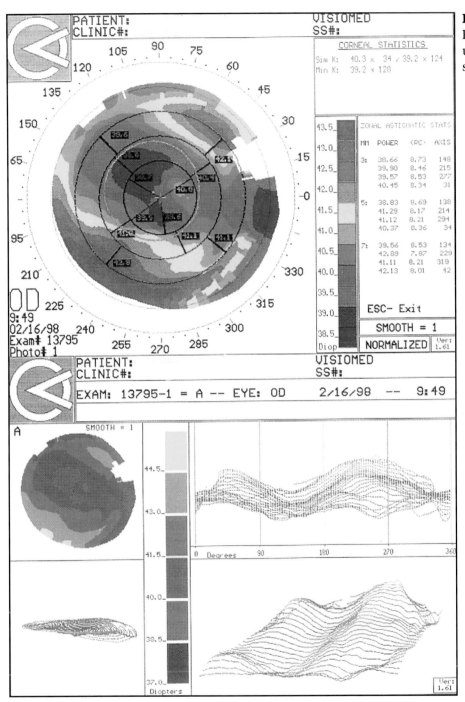

Figure 15F-2. Preoperative irregular pattern OD with small optical zone.

Figure 15F-3.
Preoperative well-centered ablation with a small optical zone OS.

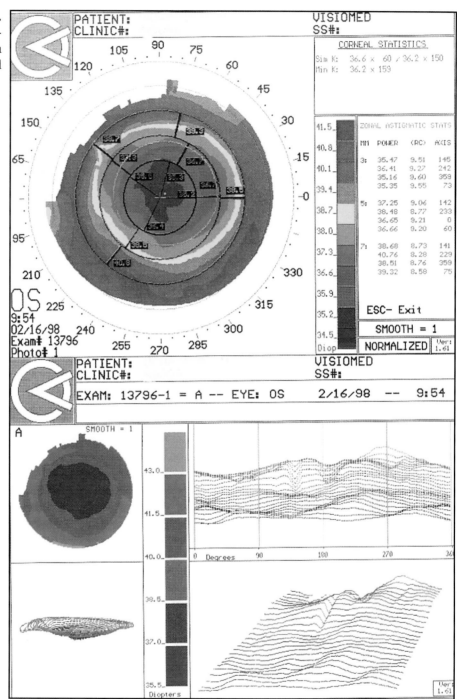

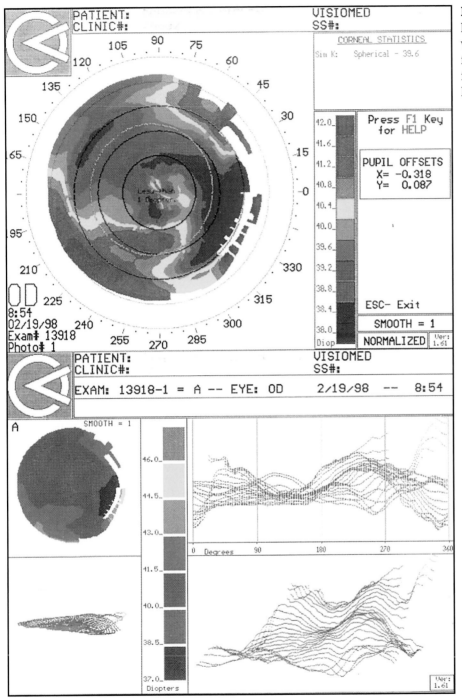

Figure 15F-4a. Enlarged optical zone with small central island and persistent irregularity OD after LASIK enhancement.

Figure 15F-4b. Enlarged optical zone with mild central irregularity OS after LASIK enhancement.

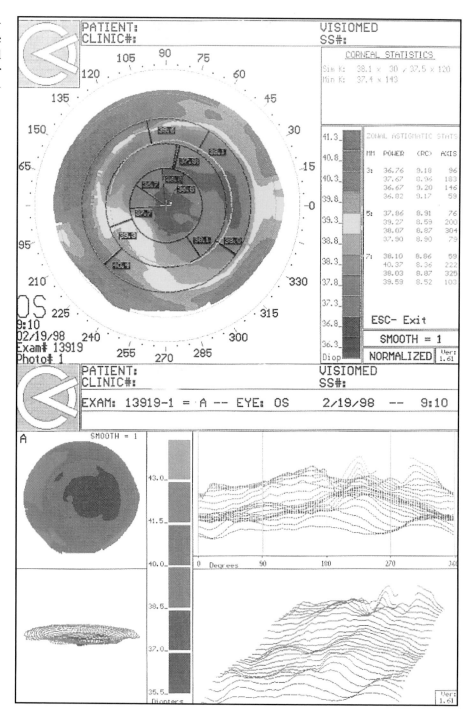

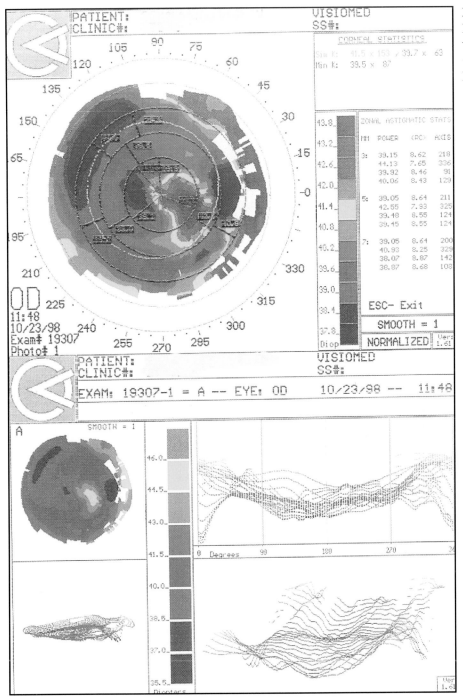

Figure 15F-5a. Enlarged optical zone with central island OD following Topo-Link.

Figure 15F-5b. Extensively enlarged optical zone with dramatic increase in surface regularity OS following Topo-Link.

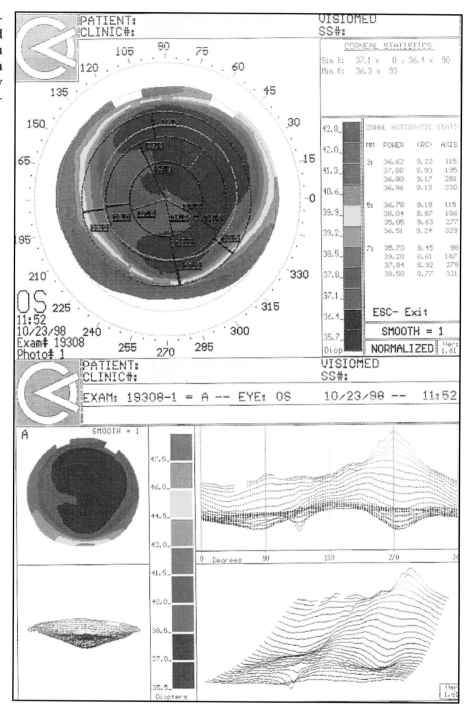

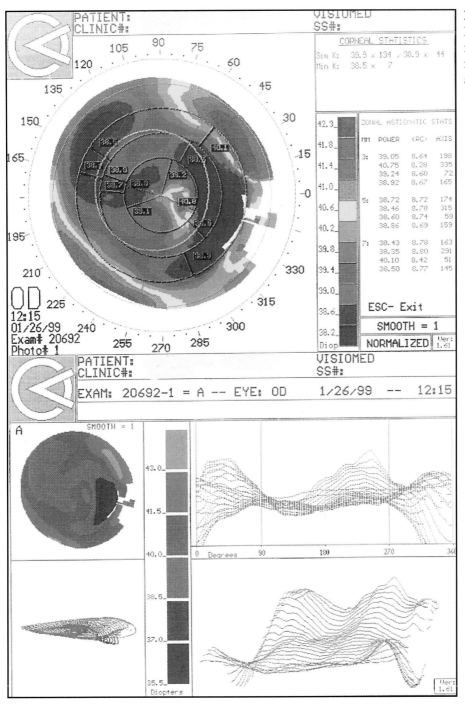

Figure 15F-6a. Dramatic improvement in central island OD, 6 months after TopoLink.

Figure 15F-6b. Smooth, large, well-centered optical zone OS, 6 months after TopoLink.

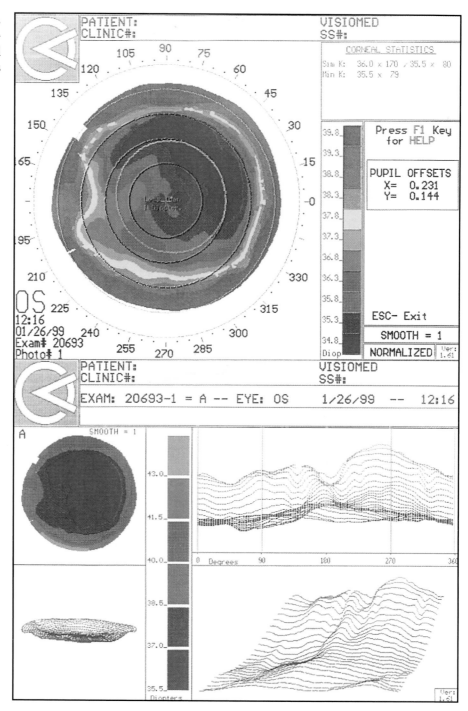

Editor's Notes

The variation in satisfaction with LASIK can truly be remarkable. While over 99% of patients receive an excellent result and are extremely satisfied with their outcome, there will be unhappy patients, despite having what we generally consider to be a successful result. These patients are perhaps the greatest challenge for the LASIK surgeon as our desire to help them and improve their vision must be balanced with our concerns with making their vision worse. I try to give the patient an honest appraisal as to my prediction of their final visual result. In this case, I would tell the patient from the initial topography and refractive information that there is a 50% chance their vision will improve and a 50% chance it could be worse. This way the patient accepts some responsibility for the final refractive outcome.

Evaluation of the initial topography indicates that the optical zone in both eyes is small which could be causing some of the distortion and night vision problems. The pattern in the right eye is only moderately irregular, however it is possible this is also causing some of the visual distortions. Following the enhancement procedure, the topography pattern in the right eye is more irregular with a small area of central steepening. The treatment in the left eye results in a larger zone but a slightly more irregular central cornea. The final refractive outcome, however, in both eyes after the first enhancement procedure indicates virtually no refractive error. Nevertheless, the patient continued to experience fluctuations in vision with large variations in measured visual acuity.

At this point in the management of a difficult patient, the psychology of LASIK becomes more difficult than the surgery. All patients initially undergo LASIK with the expectation that they will have perfect vision following the procedure. While they certainly understand that complications are possible no one would undergo an elective procedure expecting to have a complication. When they end up with a visual result that does not meet their level of satisfaction most patients can adapt and will do well with enhancement procedures. There are some patients however, who do not adapt well and become extremely emotional and frustrated with this situation. These patients will often become so focused on their visual function that it can disrupt their general day to day functioning and even their work performance. In this case, this patient appears to be truly experiencing visual distortion given the appearance of the topography, however a psychological component has likely contributed to the widely fluctuating visual refractive errors on a day to day basis.

The patient's final outcome after the topography assisted LASIK indicates a smooth ablation pattern now in the left eye with central island pattern in the right eye. Three months later, the central island pattern in the right eye has dramatically improved and the ablation pattern in the left eye continues to appear symmetrical. The Orbscan results also confirm the relatively regular central corneal flattening now. Despite these heroic attempts to improve the patient's vision, the patient has now become slightly hyperopic and has a BCVA of 20/70 in both eyes. In retrospect it would appear that no treatment would have been the best choice in this patient as in fact the BCVA has continued to decrease with each further treatment. Finally, this case illustrates the importance of paying attention to the central corneal pachymetry thickness prior to considering any corneal ablation procedure. This patient now has a corneal thickness of 361 µm OD and 328 µm OS. There have been several case reports indicating that corneal ectasia can occur when the corneal thickness drops below 400 µm. This patient now has a greater chance of losing corneal stability. Extreme care therefore must be exercised when using topography-assisted LASIK in order to ensure that adequate tissue of the cornea is preserved.

16

HOMOGRAFT LAMELLAR KERATOPLASTY

SUMMARY NOTES

HOMOGRAFT LAMELLAR KERATOPLASTY - SUMMARY NOTES

Indications
- irregular anterior cornea surface
- anterior corneal scar
- minimal corneal thickness

Risks
- graft rejection
- irregular astigmatism
- reduction in BCVA

Preoperative
- slit lamp examination
- pachymetry
- topography

Operative
- preparation of stromal bed
- keratome
- PTK with laser
- preparation of the donor button
- cut with anterior chamber maintainer
- cut from globe at eye bank
- sutured versus sutureless

Postoperative
- longer visual rehabilitation
- refractive enhancement when stable

CASE A, SURFACE ABLATION INFINITUM
John F. Doane, MD

Main Concern: Recurrent Corneal Haze after PRK
Patient Age: 27

INITIAL PREOPERATIVE INFORMATION

	OD	OS	COMMENTS
Preoperative Refraction	-6.0 sph	-6.0 sph	prior to original PRK
BCVA	20/15	20/15	
Topography Details	regular	regular	
SimK Values	45.12/43.6@168	44.7/43.54@164	
Pachymetry	490 µm		

PROCEDURES PERFORMED

	OD	OS	COMMENTS
1. Date/type	6/6/96 PRK	6/6/96 PRK	
Laser/keratome/plate	VISX Star	VISX Star	
2-8. Date/type	7 subsequent PRK's OU		recurrent haze
9. Date/type	host 7.2/65 µm	host 7.2/65 µm	
Laser/keratome/plate	ACS 7.1 mm/180	ACS 7.1 mm/180	
		Nylon 8-bite	
		antitorque suture	

CURRENT POSTOPERATIVE INFORMATION

	OD	OS	COMMENTS
Time Postoperative	3 months	2 1/2 months	photokeratoscopy,
Postoperative Refraction	-0.50 + 0.75 X 055	-1.5 + 1.75 X 110	smooth mires OU
BCVA	20/30	20/25	
Topography Details	n/a	n/a	
SimK Values	40.75/36.87@040	43.37/41.25@008	
Visual Complaints	none	slight blur	
Medications	none	none	
Refractive Correction	none	none	

This 23-year-old male presented with recurrent haze formation after PRK for 6 D of myopia bilaterally. At the time of his initial bilateral PRK surgery he was 20 years of age. On physical presentation this young man seemed very happy and normal He then revealed a remarkable surgical history. In our first meeting he stated he had undergone eight laser surgeries for nearsightedness. I was taken aback by this first statement, but even more so when he revealed that he meant eight surgeries per eye! After initial PRK, haze formation and regression occurred bilaterally so the treating surgeon elected to retreat on seven additional occasions by PTK to remove corneal haze.

UCVA revealed 20/100 OD and 20/70 OS. Retinoscopy revealed +2.50 + 2.0 X 090, OD and +2.25 + 2.5 X 100, OS Retinoscopy reflexes were moderately poor OU. Manifest refraction revealed +3.0 + 2.25 X 093 for 20/30 BCVA and +1.0 + 3.0 X 085 for 20/30- BCVA. The endpoint refraction was not precise in either eye. It was obvious this patient was functioning via use of marked accommodative exertion. Slit lamp examination revealed moderate central corneal haze OU. (Figures 16A-1 and 2) and thin central corneas. Central pachymetry readings were 273 and 258 μm for the right and left corneas, respectively. Corneal topography revealed flat central corneal curvature values of 35.0 and 38.7 D, respectively, for the right and left eyes (Figures 16A-3 and 4). The crystalline lens, retina and optic nerve were without pathology.

Due to the recurrent nature of his haze formation that the referring doctor stated was progressing similar to all previous occasions. Induced hyperopia, surgical intervention was entertained since the patient was contact lens intolerant and resistant to spectacle wear due to active life style. Repeat surface ablation was not considered as an option due to his history of aggressive healing. Because of the iatrogenically induced hyperopic astigmatism, restoration of corneal stromal thickness was considered paramount.

Two corneal surgical options existed: PK or lamellar keratoplasty. Some might advocate clear lens or intraocular surgery, but this does not rid the patient of the probable risk of progressive corneal haze formation. The patient underwent bilateral lamellar keratoplasty. This is a rather unique case in that maximal preservation of patient stroma was necessary to maintain ocular integrity and avoid a keratoconus-like ectasia. I planned a 7.2 mm keratectomy with a 65 plate with the ACS of Ruiz. I simply wanted to remove the epithelium and a few microns of anterior stroma in this pass. One could have done epithelial removal only via mechanical means, but the mild to moderate anterior corneal haze would have persisted. Computation of donor tissue required an understanding of what had been removed from previous surgeries. Pre-PRK pachymetry was not available. The goal was to overshoot thickness by 15 to 30 μm in case re-LASIK would be required for refractive purposes. I postulated that the patient had 10.25 D of correction on the central cornea OD (6 D to reduce myopia and 4.25 D of overcorrection). I then calculated 11 D x 14 μm of tissue removal per diopter of treatment for a grand total of 154 μm of stromal tissue removal that would need to be replaced. I selected a 180 μm plate for the donor lenticule. From prior subtraction pachymetry calculations in my hands, the ACS on average gave a flap of 75% of predicted value centrally. I was hoping for as close to 180 μm as possible. Another large variable in final effect is that the corneal/scleral rim in all likelihood was somewhat swollen compared to the natural state and thus, when whatever I obtained came to equilibrium, it would likely be thinner.

The lamellar keratoplasty OD went as planned and the lenticule was replaced without sutures. At 24 hours postoperative, the lenticule was in good position with intact epithelium. UCVA at 24 hours was 20/25-2. Manifest refraction revealed -0.25 + 0.50 X 126 for 20/25-2 BCVA. Corneal topography was obtained (Figure 16A-5). At 1 month postoperatively the uncorrected vision was 20/25+1. Manifest refraction was -1.0 + 1.25 X 151 for 20/25+3 BCVA. An epithelial rejection line was noted (Figure 16A-6) and the patient was initiated on Lotemax (Bausch and Lomb Pharmaceuticals, Inc. Tampa, Fla) q.i.d. to minimize white cell activation and potential tissue melting. At 6 weeks postoperative the UCVA had dropped to 20/100 with pinhole improvement to 20/30. Manifest refraction of -2.0 provided 20/40+2 visual acuity. Corneal topography revealed irregular corneal astigmatism near the visual axis (Figure 16A-7). Three months postoperatively the corneal surface had improved dramatically (Figure 16A-8) and the patient had 20/30 UCVA. Manifest refraction was -0.50 + 0.75 X 055 for a 20/30 BCVA.

The left eye underwent lamellar graft 2 weeks after the right eye. Due to poor epithelial integrity an 8-bite antitorque suture was placed (Figure 16A-9). On postoperative day 5 the suture was removed. Prior to suture removal the UCVA was 20/200. Corneal topography was obtained and revealed irregular astigmatism on the photokeratoscope view peripherally associated with suture placement (Figure 16A-10). At this time the 5 to 8 o'clock meridian was lifted to remove suspected epithelial ingrowth that was not present on direct observation. Three weeks postoperatively the uncorrected vision was 20/30-2 and his refraction was -0.75 + 3.50 X 905 for 20/20 vision. Two and a half months later his UCVA was 20/40. On manifest refraction of -1.5 + 1.75 X 110 his acuity was 20/25. Note on topography that his central axis was smooth and there is essentially no irregularity (Figure 16A-11). Slit lamp examination revealed a clear cornea. (Figure 16A-12).

Figure 16A-1. Slit lamp view of right cornea revealing moderate corneal haze after eight surface excimer laser ablations in each eye.

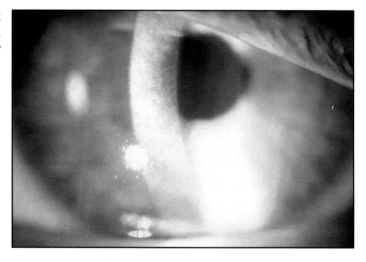

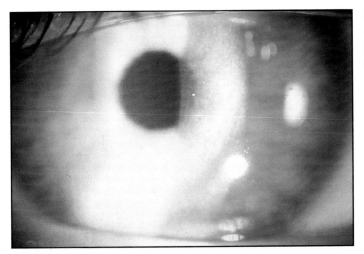

Figures 16A-2. Slit lamp view of left cornea revealing moderate corneal haze after eight surface excimer laser ablations in each eye.

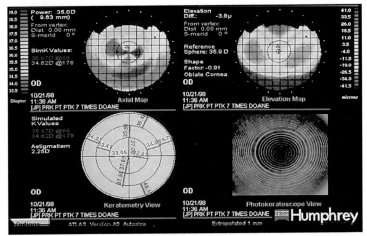

Figure 16A-3. Corneal topographies of the right eye prior to lamellar grafting.

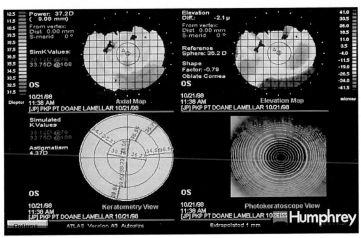

Figure 16A-4. Corneal topographies of the left eye prior to lamellar grafting.

Figure 16A-5. Corneal topography of the right eye 24 hours after sutureless lamellar graft completed.

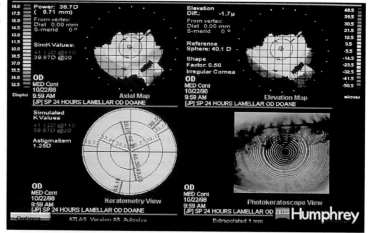

Figure 16A-6. Slit lamp view of an epithelial rejection line that complicated the postoperative course of the right eye at 1 month.

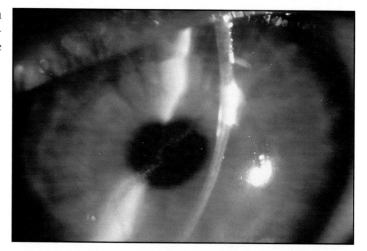

Figure 16A-7. Corneal topography revealing surface irregular astigmatism of the right cornea related to the epithelial rejection line.

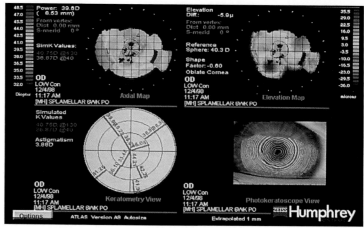

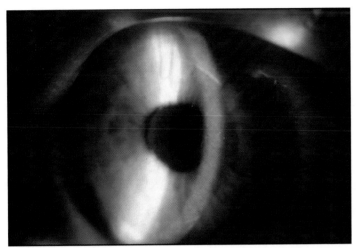

Figure 16A-8. Slit lamp view of the right cornea revealing clarity and complete resolution of the epithelial irregularity. See gutter fibrosis superiorly.

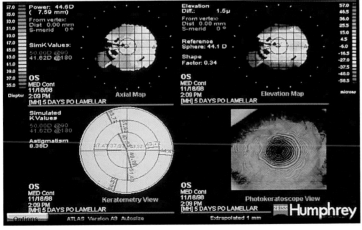

Figure 16A-9. Eight-bite antitorque suture of lamellar graft of the left eye. Suture was placed due to poor epithelial integrity. Excellent epithelium is required for the lamellar cap to be left sutureless.

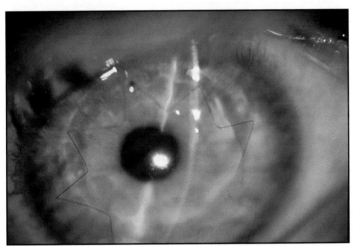

Figure 16A-10. Corneal topography 5 days after sutured lamellar grafting. Irregular astigmatism is noted on the photokeratoscope view peripherally in location of suture placement.

Figure 16A-11. Corneal topography 6 weeks postoperatively reveals minimal to no irregularity (see photokeratoscope view).

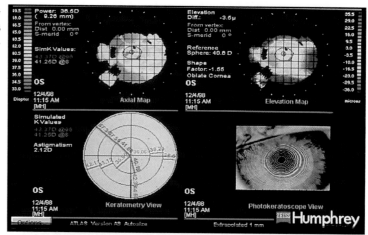

Figure 16A-12. Clear cornea noted on slit lamp examination. See gutter fibrosis superiorly.

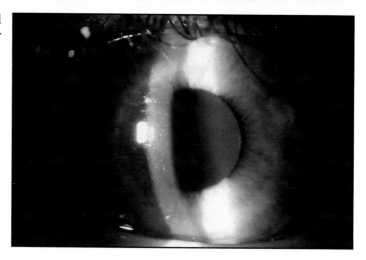

Editor's Notes

This is a dramatic illustration of the problems with repeat PRK. The patient had eight PRK/PTK procedures for regression and haze resulting in bilateral hyperopia. The pachymetry revealed a corneal thickness less than 300 μm in both eyes, which would place the patient at risk for ectasia.

This case illustrates the importance of pachymetry even with PRK. Despite the need for surface ablation to remove the recurrent haze, the corneal thickness must be monitored to ensure that adequate thickness is preserved. For PRK, at least 300 μm of total corneal thickness should remain.

The success of the homoplastic grafting technique in this case is truly remarkable. The method of removing the anterior stromal scar with the maximum preservation of stromal tissue along with the calculations used for the thickness of the lamellar graft illustrates the precision that can be achieved with these techniques. Even if this patient did have a refractive error that required further refinement, this could perhaps be performed with an enhancement procedure in the stromal bed or on the undersurface of the cap.

Case B, Recurrent Visually Significant Haze after PRK

John F. Doane, MD

Main Concern: Recurrent Haze after PRK
Patient Age: 42

Initial Preoperative Information

	OD	OS	Comments
Preoperative Refraction	-9.00	-9.00	
BCVA	20/20	20/20	

Procedures Performed

	OD	OS	Comments
1. Date/type	September 1995	September 1995	severe haze OD
Laser	PRK	PRK	
2. Date/type	12 months later		
	lamellar keratoplasty		

Current Postoperative Information

	OD	OS	Comments
Time Postoperative	6 months		excellent result
Postoperative Refraction	+0.25 + 0.25 X 135		
BCVA	20/20-		
Topography Details	n/a		
SimK Values	n/a		
Visual Complaints	none		
Medications	none		

This case represents that of a 42-year-old male who had recurrent anterior corneal haze after excimer laser PRK for myopia. The patient is a computer software programmer who underwent refractive surgery due to contact lens intolerance and a stated desire to be less dependent on spectacles and certainly contact lenses. His preoperative refraction was -9.0 D OU and BCVA was 20/20 in each eye. He underwent his initial uncomplicated PRK procedures in September 1995 with target plano OD and -1.00 sphere OS. Six months later his UCVA was 20/200 OD and 20/60 OS. Refraction revealed -3.5 +1.25 X 120 OD for 20/40 acuity and -1.0 + 1.0 X 075 OS for 20/30 acuity. Slit lamp examination revealed 2+ central corneal haze OD and 1+ paracentral haze OS. Due to his undercorrection and haze, the patient elected to undergo enhancement OD.

Twelve months after the enhancement surgery of the right eye, examination revealed UCVA of 20/200 O.D. and 20/40 O.S. Manifest refraction was -5.0 + 1.0 X 115 for 20/70 acuity OD and -1.00 + 0.25 X 87 for 20/40 acuity OS. Slit lamp examination revealed 3+ central corneal haze OD (Figures 16B-1a and b) and 1+ paracentral haze OS. Central pachymetry was 568 µm OD and 521 µm OS. The patient had been on aggressive topical corticosteroids after the enhancement. Despite this regimen, the patient had recurrent haze that was significantly worse than after the initial operation. He was quite dissatisfied with his situation since his dominant eye had poor best-corrected acuity that made driving a car difficult. He also noted significant scotopic visual symptoms (glare and haloes). He felt he was unable to satisfactorily complete the tasks of his occupation and wanted active intervention to be considered. He was instructed that his three options would be expectant observation for resolution, repeat PRK, or homoplastic lamellar grafting. The patient strongly opposed repeat PRK or expectant observation.

Therefore, the patient underwent sutureless homoplastic lamellar grafting of the right eye. A 180 µm thick, 7 mm diameter keratectomy was completed with the ACS. The host tissue was harvested from a donor corneoscleral rim with an anterior chamber maintainer (Figures 16B-2a through d). This device is unique in that it has a geared track analogous to the geared suction ring that allows for a constant speed of microkeratome passage for donor lenticle harvesting. Postoperatively, a clear shield was placed over the orbit and the patient was prescribed Tobradex (Alcon Laboratories, Ft. Worth, Texas) q.i.d. for 5 days. One day postoperatively, the patient was comfortable with 20/200 UCVA. Manifest refraction revealed -6.75 + 0.25 X 130 for 20/30 acuity. Slit lamp examination revealed a clear cornea and well positioned sutureless graft (Figure 16B-3a and b). Four months post lamellar grafting the patient's refraction was -7.50 sphere. LASIK was performed using a standard nomogram with a target refraction of plano. Six months status post-LASIK his uncorrected vision is 20/20 minus and with refraction of +0.25 + 0.25 X 135 his vision is 20/15. He is fully functional with no visual complaints.

This case highlights several points pertinent to the differences in excimer laser surgical techniques, the utility of lamellar corneal surgical techniques, excimer laser complications management and unmet patient expectations. This patient's personality characteristics and lifestyle are quite typical for an elective self-pay surgical procedure. The patient was a classical "type A" personality that wanted an excellent UCVA. In the end, these became the guiding factors for clinical decision making. Visual loss secondary to corneal haze formation with surface PRK tends to be more likely with larger refractive errors treated; although, significant visual loss can occur with PRK for low myopia (<3 D). Visual loss due to haze with lamellar refractive surgical techniques, especially LASIK, is exceedingly uncommon and this is one factor favoring a lamellar technique over PRK. Once visually significant haze has formed with PRK, it is quite common for retreatment with surface excimer laser treatment to be recommended. This approach requires that the patient instill topical corticosteroids for several months. After the initial surgery, the medical regimen is rigorous. To go through this a second time it can be physically, if not mentally, exhausting for the typical patient that has a very busy family and professional life. Additionally, since the patient is subject to several more months of topical corticosteroids, there is potential risk of significant IOP elevation and cataract formation. If haze recurs after the second operation, the patient will be utterly disappointed with what he or she perceived preoperatively to be a relatively hassle-free "high-tech" laser refractive surgical technique that was going to be lifestyle enhancing.

The final point to be made for this case study is that the visual rehabilitation plan (lamellar graft followed by LASIK for residual refractive error) may not be something the majority of surgeons have experience or comfort in performing. From the patient's standpoint, his preoperative expectations of excellent uncorrected vision have been met. With expectant observation of the visually significant haze he had after PRK, resolution could take years and the significant refractive error the patient had would not endear him to this approach. Surface retreatment of haze after PRK is relatively simple but requires considerable effort for the patient to adhere to the postoperative regimen and inherently has a certain level of risk related to intraocular pressure elevation and cataract formation. The plan that ultimately was taken does require additional surgical instrumentation and surgical skill, but if done correctly, the patient can have an excellent result by using lamellar corneal surgical techniques that allow for quick visual rehabilitation without risk inherent to long-term topical corticosteroid usage.

Figure 16B-1a. Slit lamp biomicroscope view OD prior to lamellar keratectomy revealing dense central corneal haze after two excimer laser PRK procedures.

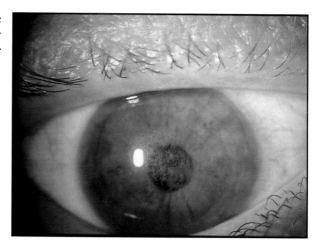

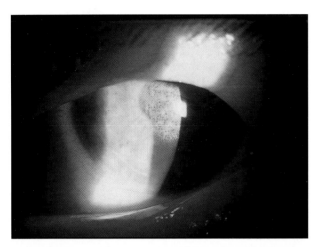

Figure 16B-1b. Slit lamp biomicroscope view OD prior to lamellar keratectomy revealing dense central corneal haze after two excimer laser PRK procedures.

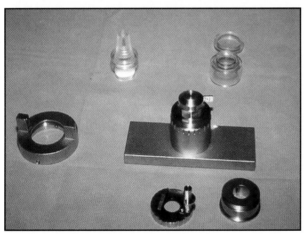

Figure 16B-2a. Four-piece anterior chamber maintainer set for the ACS. Antidesiccation chamber (left) and Barraquer tonometer (right) are also pictured.

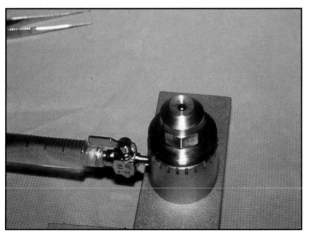

Figure 16B-2b. Fluid-filled syringe is placed on stopcock and fluid is filling reservoir.

Figure 16B-2c. Corneoscleral rim is placed over anterior chamber maintainer reservoir.

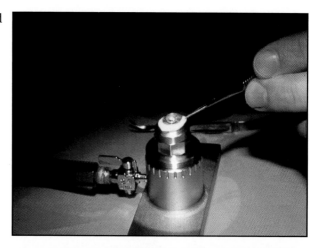

Figure 16B-2d. The lamellar cap is harvested with the ACS.

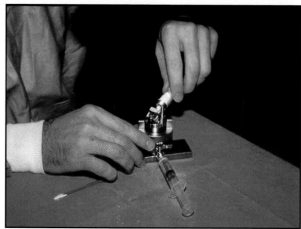

Figure 16B-3a. ACS loaded on geared-track stage of anterior chamber maintainer in preparation of lamellar cap harvesting.

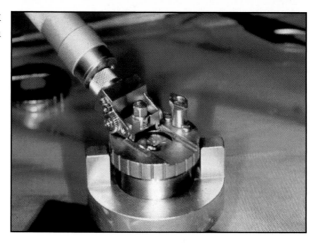

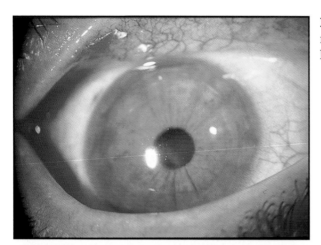

Figure 16B-3b. Comparative slit lamp biomicroscope views OD 1 day after sutureless homoplastic lamellar graft.

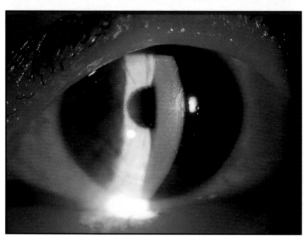

Figures 16B-4. Comparative slit lamp biomicroscope views OD 1 day after sutureless homoplastic lamellar graft. Noted marked clarity of visual axis in both views compared to the preoperative figures.

Editor's Notes

Recurrent corneal haze following PRK may be one of the greatest motivations to perform LASIK for the corrections of moderate to high myopia. While haze is not a common concern following PRK it certainly is not uncommon when performing corrections over 6 D. When haze is recurrent it involves multiple procedures with reduced predictability, and increased exposure to topical steroids. This can be one of then most frustrating and difficult situations both for the patient and the refractive surgeon.

While we tend to focus on the haze, the refractive error, and the BCVA, one of the most insidious problems in this situation is the development of a posterior subcapsular cataract. After the original PRK for high myopia, patients are often on topical steroids for 4 months. Following the enhancement procedure, this maybe extended for another 4 months. Following another procedure such as PTK or a PRK enhancement, another four months of topical steroids may be used. It is not uncommon for patients with haze formation to end up being on topical steroids for over 12 months, which places them at significant risk for developing a posterior subcapsular cataract. These cataracts may take several years to develop. Nevertheless, my PRK experience from 5 to 6 years ago has indicated that a number of these patients can develop cataracts. For this reason, if a patient regresses after a PRK enhancement and the cornea is clear, we now perform a LASIK enhancement in order to reduce the total steroid exposure to that eye.

If cataract formation does occur in a post-PRK or post-LASIK eye, it is important to recognize that the current third generation IOL calculation formulas are not accurate. Excimer ablations of the cornea result in more flattening of the central cornea compared to the peripheral cornea. This means that the standard K readings that are taken at the 3.0 mm diameter optical zone to calculate the IOL power will overestimate the K value and therefore underestimate of the IOL power. Jack Holladay, MD, has suggested obtaining the preexcimer K measurements or using the contact lens overrefraction method, however these methods are inconvenient and difficult to organize. Generally if 3.0 D is added to the IOL power the patient will achieve the adequate correction. Alternatively, 1 D of power can be added to the IOL for each diopter of myopic correction with PRK or LASIK. Any residual refractive error can be treated with a small LASIK enhancement.

CASE C, CORNEAL SCAR FOLLOWING COMPLICATED PRK

Lucio Buratto, MD, and Remato Valeri, MD

Main Concern: Corneal Scar Following PRK
Patient Age: 43

INITIAL PREOPERATIVE INFORMATION

	OD	OS	COMMENTS
Preoperative Refraction	-2.00 – 2.00 x 165	-8.00 – 0.75 x 45	post-PRK
BCVA	20/40	20/200	severe haze
SimK Values	38.6/40.7	44.5/45.6	
Pachymetry	362 μm	470 μm	

PROCEDURES PERFORMED

	OD	OS	COMMENTS
1. Date/type		10/27/98 ELLK	see text
Laser/keratome/plate		Chiron 117	
2. Date/type		1 month later	
		continuous suture	
		placed	

CURRENT POSTOPERATIVE INFORMATION

	OD	OS	COMMENTS
Time Postoperative		3 weeks	with continuous
Postoperative Refraction		-1.00 – 3.50 X 0.50	suture
BCVA		20/40	
SimK Values		43.57	
Refractive Correction		spectacles	

A 43-year-old male patient had severe myopia of -11.00 – 2.5 @ 145 OD and -9.00 – 1.5 cyl @ 60 OS with a BCVA of 20/25 OU. In 1996, in another surgical center, the patient had been subjected to PRK OU. Seven months after treatment, there was regression of about 7 D in OD and 6 D OS with ++Haze in OU. Enhancement PRK was performed in both eyes.

At the initial visit to our center in September 1998, the situation was as follows:

Va OD = 20/200 UCVA; 20/40 BCVA with -2.00 – 2.00 X 165

Va OS < 20/200 UCVA; 20/200 BCVA with -8.00 – 0.75 X 45;

20/80 with the stenopeic foramen

Reticular haze was observed (++ in OD and +++ in OS) for an extension for about 5 mm centrally (Figure 16C-1). Central pachymetry was 362 μm OD and 470 μm OS. Using the Colvard pupillometer, the pupil diameter under mesopic light was 5.5 mm in OU.

The crystalline was crystal clear and the retina intact. Echobiometry in OD was 26.70 mm and in OS was 25.73 mm. Topography (Figure 16C-2a and b) showed a nonsymmetrical corneal profile that created irregular astigmatism OU.

It was decided to subject the patient to lamellar keratoplasty in order to remove the anterior stromal haze using the technique of Excimer Laser Lamellar Keratoplasty (ELLK). PTK was performed with the Keracor 117 laser with a 50 Hz ceramic chamber, with an optic zone of 6 mm that produces an ablation of 170 μm in order to obtain regular removal of a corneal disk with smooth edges and desired thickness and diameter (not obtainable with the same results, neither manually nor with the microkeratome). The donor cornea can then be inserted following the creation of a stromal pouch using a disk knife. The pouch measures about 2 mm and is positioned at the edge of the ablation. The donor cornea was provided by the Eye Bank Foundation of the Veneto Region and was preserved in the dehydrated state in silica gel. It had the following characteristics: thickness = 340 microns, diameter 9.0 mm. A refractive treatment of -8.00 D was performed on the stromal side of the lamella with the same laser with an optic zone of 5.5 mm following moderate rehydration with BSS. The lamella was then inserted in the corneal pouch without sutures. The reepithelialization was complete by day 4.

One month after treatment the BCVA OD was 20/40 with an refraction of +6.50 + 1.00 X 130. The insertion edge of the lamella inside the corneal pouch appeared to be raised and some semicircular folds were observed at the external extremity.

The transparency of the cornea was good, ocular pressure was 8 mmHg, central pachymetry was 380 μm; pachymetry at 12 o'clock, 3 o'clock, 6 o'clock and 9 o'clock was 600, 570, 580, 560 μm respectively.

The overcorrection following this treatment created concerns about the excessive flattening of the cornea (Figure 16C-3). This may have been due to the absence of the suture resulting in flattening on the cornea, the flattening effect of the PTK, or the removal of the haze causing regressive myopia combined with the refractive correction on the lamellar cap. Finally, it is possible that the overcorrection resulted from a greater than expected response from the refractive ablation on the lamella due to the partial rehydration of the donor cornea. This latter theory is justified by an evaluation of the pachymetric parameters: preoperative thicknesses – cornea = 470, lens = 340; removal PTK = 170, refractive treatment -8.00 D = 126; so we would expect a final pachymetry of 514 (470 +340-170-126 = 514). The final pachymetry was 380 μm, therefore 135 μm less. If we consider the possibility that the final hyperopia is due to a refractive treatment about 7 D greater than the diopters set, we will have a further ablation of 111 μm that would bring the theoretical final value to 404 μm, very close to the 380 μm that were actually measured.

The patient had a LASIK enhancement with the donor cornea was completely peeled back and was positioned with a very tight continuous suture (to reduce the hyperopia). Three weeks after this treatment, the UCVA was 20/70 and the BCVA was 20/40 with a refraction of -1.00 – 3.50 X 50. The topography indicated keratometry values of 43.51 D (Figure 16C-3) with irregular astigmatism so it was decided to remove the suture.

Figure 16C-1. Dense corneal haze following PRK.

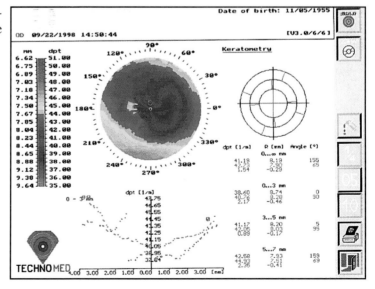

Figure 16C-2a. Irregular astigmatism after previous PRK and haze OD.

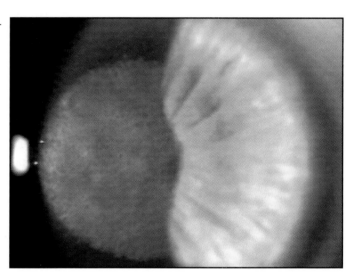

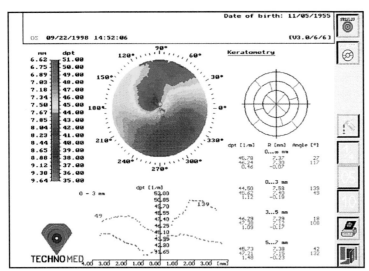

Figure 16C-2b. Irregular astigmatism after PRK OS.

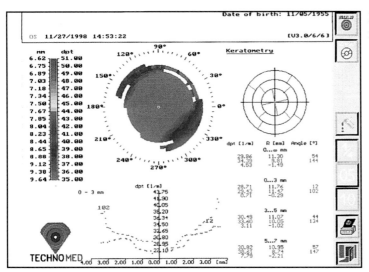

Figure 16C-3. Excessive corneal flattening after ELLK.

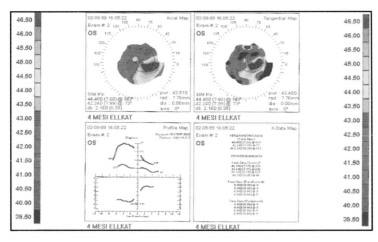

Figure 16C-4. Corneal steepening after suture placement with ELLK.

Editor's Notes

This case demonstrates the complexities associated with performing homoplastic lamellar keratoplasty to correct anterior corneal difficulties from surface ablations. The original PRK procedure that was performed for over -10 D spherical equivalent corrections in both eyes resulted in severe confluent haze associated with irregular astigmatism and a loss of BCVA. While haze can be treated with repeat PRK, the significant regression in the left eye would have made this difficult. Furthermore, the stromal thickness was considerably reduced in both eyes. There would be a significant risk of haze recurrence because of the large prescription that was corrected originally with PRK. Nevertheless, one option in this case for the right eye would have included further surface ablation with the use of haze modulating agents (topical steroids, thiotepa, or mitomycin) after the procedure for up to 4 months. The corneal thickness in the right eye approached 362 μm. We generally try to leave at least 300 μm of corneal stroma following the PRK procedure, therefore there is some tissue available for further surface ablation of the haze.

The lamellar keratoplasty in the left eye demonstrates the complexities that can occur with this type of procedure. The use of PTK to create a stromal bed along the creation of the stromal pouch represents a very ingenious way that Lucio Buratto, MD, has devised to insert the lamellar graft. The combination of the PTK to remove the haze and created the stromal bed followed by the lamellar graft with the excimer ablation on the stromal surface has introduced a number of variables into the refraction equation which resulted in the patient becoming hyperopic.

Another option in this case would be to place a properly sized lamellar disk in the stromal bed after the PTK ablation to create the stromal bed. This disk may attach sufficiently to allow a sutureless technique. Rather than performing the refractive ablation immediately, this could be left to stabilize and the refraction evaluated. Once the refractive error had stabilized, the graft could be lifted and the ablation performed on the stromal surface, as described in this case. With the replacement of this disk, the accuracy should be greatly enhanced.

CASE D, ELLKAT TO TREAT MYOPIA IN REFRACTIVE KERATOCONUS

Lucio Buratto, MD, and Sergio Belloni, MD

Main Concern: Keratoconus
Patient Age: 30

INITIAL PREOPERATIVE INFORMATION

	OD	OS	COMMENTS
Preoperative Refraction		-3.0 – 7.0 X 150	keratoconus OS
BCVA		20/100	
Topography Details		keratoconus	
SimK Values		51.92/46.87	
Pachymetry		430 µm	

PROCEDURES PERFORMED

	OD	OS	COMMENTS
1. Date/type		2/20/98 ELLKAT	
Laser/keratome/plate		117/PTK/homoplastic graft	

CURRENT POSTOPERATIVE INFORMATION

	OD	OS	COMMENTS
Time Postoperative		10 months	excellent results
Postoperative Refraction		pl – 1.0 X 170	
BCVA		20/22.5	
UCVA		20/25	
Topography Details		central steepening	
SimK Values		45.12/42.99	
Pachymetry		507 µm	
Visual Complaints		none	
Medications		none	
Refractive Correction		none	

A 30-year-old female patient had bilateral keratoconus diagnosed in October 1997. The patient did not tolerate corrective contact lenses and used them for just a few hours each day.

Under biomicroscopic examination, the epithelial condition of the more advanced keratoconus in the left eye was good, OD (Stage II) OS (Stage IV), there was inferior paracentral sagging, absence of central scarring, and the endothelial cell count was 2500 cells/mm2 under the reflecting microscope.

A refractive examination with a corneal lens showed visual acuity of 20/20 OD and 20/25 OS. The measurement of the central pachymetry was 460 µm OD, 430 µm OS.

Analysis of the keratometric map showed:

> OD: paracentral sagging, astigmatism of 1.59 D (dK) with the most refractive axis at 96°
> OS: paracentral sagging, astigmatism greater than 5 D (dK 5.05) with the most refractive
>   axis at 35° (Figure 16D-1).

ELLKAT (Excimer Laser Lamellar Keratoplasty of Augmented Thickness) was performed in OS on February 2, 1998.

The operation involved:
- ablation of the patient's superficial corneal tissue using the excimer laser
- positioning of a lamella of donor cornea from the Eye Bank on the host cornea
- suturing of the lamella to the host cornea.

In detail, the ELLKAT technique involves performing the ablation with the PTK technique on the host cornea with no refractive objective (Technolas Keracor 117) with removing the epithelium, for a depth of about 200 µm for a diameter of 7 mm (Figure 16D-2). Epithelium, Bowman's and part of the stroma are removed by this laser treatment and this also removes part of the altered corneal tissue, preparing the corneal bed to receive the homoplastic lamella. The ablation simultaneously provokes a certain degree of corneal flattening. In the depth of the ablation, at the peripheral extremities, using a disk knife the surgeon creates a circular, uniform pouch in a peripheral direction. The depth is homogeneous and the pouch extends for 360° for a pouch depth of 2 to 2.5 mm (Figure 16D-3). The donor cornea obtained from the eye bank had a diameter of 9 mm and a thickness of 350 µm. It was removed from the donor bulb using a microkeratome. It was delivered to us in a dehydrated state. It was rehydrated and washed carefully with a filtered salt solution.

The homoplastic flap was created with parallel faces and therefore lacks dioptric power. The patient was myopic, so the homoplastic flap was treated on the stromal face with the excimer laser (Keracor 117 Chiron Technolas)(correction of 4 D with a 6.5 D optic zone for a depth of 75 µm) (Figure 16D-4); a multizone treatment was performed with a minimal optic zone of 4 mm and a maximum of 6 mm. The lamella is positioned on the host bed with a spatula and fixed with sutures (Figure 16D-5). It is sutured with eight single sutures; the insertion of the lamella is performed in a clockwise direction. A further eight suture points are placed followed by a running suture (Figure 16D-6). All placed under strict keratoscopic control (Figure 16D-7).

On the first postoperative day, the flap was well centered, transparent, with slight edema and widespread areas of disepithelialization. There were folds in the Descemet membrane, folds of the limbus, and sutures under tension. On day 5, the edema was reduced, and epithelialization had occurred.

The UCVA was 20/100 OS with no change for the BCVA. The central pachymetry was 530 μm and the keratometric map showed astigmatism of 2 D (dK 2.32) which appeared to be irregular with the more refractive axis at 130° (Figure 16D-9).

After 6 weeks the flap was transparent. The UCVA was 20/50 and the BCVA was 20/30 with a refraction of plano − 4.0 X 30. The central pachymetry was 504 μm. The keratometric map (Figure 16D-10) showed astigmatism of 3 D (dK 3.51) with the more refractive axis at 128 (map dating April 3, 1998).

After 4 months, The biomicroscopic picture had improved considerably, the sutures were still under tension, the flap was crystal clear, two of the suture points at 10 and 5 o'clock were removed on the 130° axis (Figure 16D-11, 12 and 13); the keratometric map following removal of the suture at 10 o'clock shows astigmatism of 5 D (dK 5.30) with the most refractive axis at 115°; the keratometric map following the removal of a suture point at 5 o'clock shows an astigmatism of 5 D (dK 5.35) with the most refractive axis at 90°. The UCVA was 20/50 and the BCVA was 20/30 with refraction of pl − 4.0 X 100. The cycloplegic refraction was +1.0 − 4.25 X 13. The central pachymetry was 507 μm. The endothelial count with the reflecting microscope was 2500 cells/mm².

After 10 months, the biomicroscopic aspect showed a crystal clear flap, the residual 6 suture points and one running suture. The endothelial count and corneal thickness were unchanged.

The UCVA was 20/25 and the BCVA was 20/22.5 with the refraction of plano − 1.0 X 170. The cycloplegic refraction was + 0.25 − 3.0 X 16. The keratometric map showed (Figure 16D-14) regularization of the astigmatism (dK 2.13) with the most refractive axis at 79°. The central pachymetry was now 506 μm.

This particular clinical case highlighted how the ELLKAT technique for the treatment of keratoconus associated with myopia can be a valid alternative to perforating keratoplasty in the more precocious stages of keratoconus evolution. We feel that this technique is useful if the keratoconus is not in the advanced stages (only in stages 1 and 2) and if there are no deep corneal opacities (200 to 300 μm). Keratectomy on the patient's cornea with the excimer laser produces precise thicknesses, diameters and positions with surfaces that are optically smooth and homogeneous. The lamella can be treated refractively with the excimer laser on the stromal face of the flap in order to correct the preexisting myopia or the myopia induced by the keratoconus.

Compared to the PK, this technique only replaces the superficial layers of the cornea; it is an operation with lower intra- and postoperative risks; the general and topical therapy is greatly reduced; the suture remains in position for a shorter time, only 3 to 6 months compared with at least 1 year in PK. Selective removal of the suture points is possible which allows better management of the corneal astigmatism; visual stability is faster and postoperative astigmatism is lower.

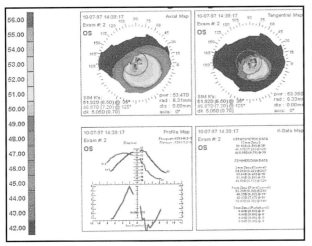

Figure 16D-1. The preoperative keratometric map shows paracentral sagging with astigmatism of 5 D (dK 5.05) with the most refractive axis at 35°.

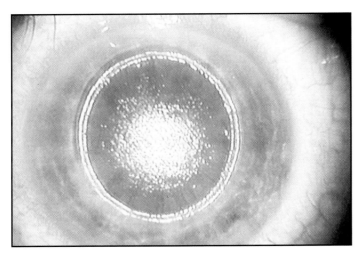

Figure 16D-2. The cornea following excimer laser ablation; the ablation is about 200 μm deep and has a diameter of 7 mm.

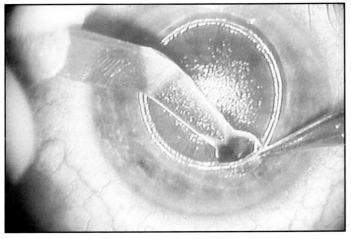

Figure 16D-3. Creation of a circular 360° pouch using a disk knife.

Figure 16D-4. The donor cornea, removed using the microkeratome, has a thickness of about 300 μm. It is treated on the stromal face with the excimer laser for the correction of the myopic defect.

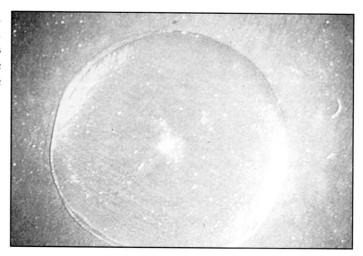

Figure 16D-5. Positioning of eight single sutures with the insertion of the lamella in the pouch.

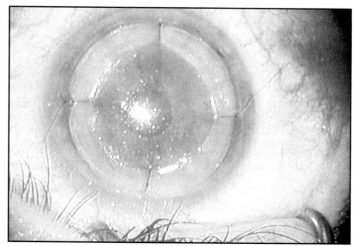

Figure 16D-6. Positioning of eight single sutures with the insertion of the lamella in the pouch.

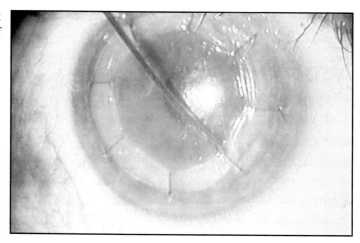

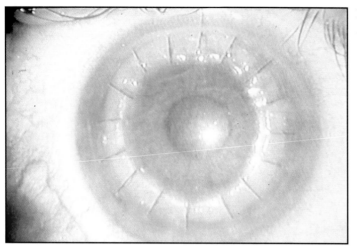

Figure 16D-7. Completion of the sutures.

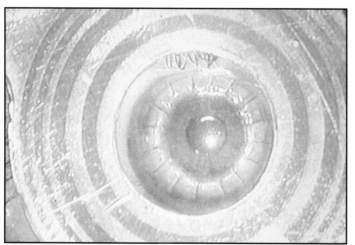

Figure 16D-8. Keratoscopic control of the sutured lamella.

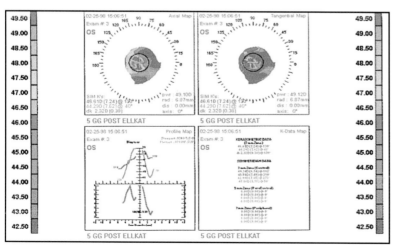

Figure 16D-9. The keratometric map on day 5 postoperative shows irregular astigmatism of 2 D (dK 2.32) with the most refractive axis at 130°.

Figure 16D-10. The keratometric map 45 days postoperative, shows astigmatism of 3 D (dK 3.51) with the most refractive axis at 128°.

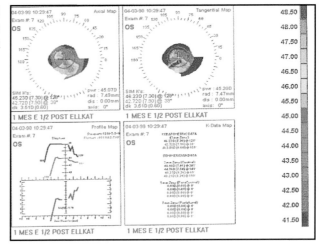

Figure 16D-11 The keratometric map, 4 months postoperative, shows astigmatism of 4.2 D (dK 4.28) with the most refractive axis at 117°.

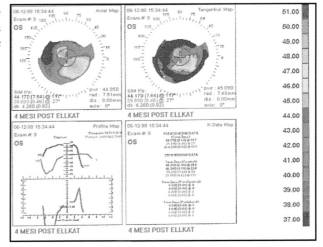

Figure 16D-12. Keratometric map following the removal of the suture point at 10 o'clock.

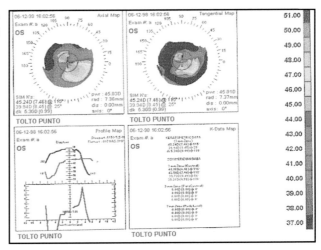

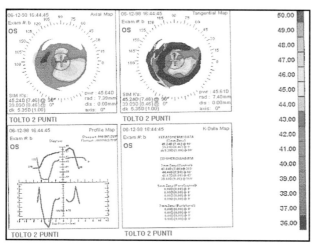

Figure 16D-13. Keratometric map following the removal of the suture point at 5 o'clock.

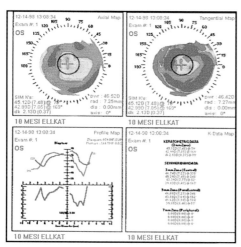

Figure 16D-14. Keratometric map, 10 months after surgery, shows astigmatism of 2 D (dK 2.13) with the most refractive axis at 79°.

Editor's Notes

This case demonstrates an ingenious technique for the correction of keratoconus. By using a PTK ablation, the stromal bed is created on the keratoconic cornea. A stromal pouch is created and the lamellar graft is then slipped into the stromal pouch. The refractive error can be treated underneath the stromal pouch. Although sutures were required to secure the lamella in position, this did allow a decrease in the time for visual rehabilitation and the patient had minimal astigmatism after the procedure.

This technique attempts to address the main problem of keratoconus (stromal thinning) by replacing the anterior stroma. Since it is only the anterior cornea replaced, the recovery is quicker and postoperative astigmatism is reduced. A variation of this could be used for Fuch's dystrophy or pseudophakic keratopathy when the problem is related to endothelial deficiencies. The posterior cornea could be replaced while the anterior cornea is preserved with a flap technique, improving visual rehabilitation and reducing induced astigmatism. Hopefully these concepts can be used to improve the results and rehabilitation of corneal transplant surgery to the levels achieved in refractive and cataract surgery.

17

BIOPTICS

BIOPTICS - SUMMARY NOTES

Indications
- high myopia (> 12.0 D)
- high hyperopia (> 6.0 D)
- refractive stability

Risks
- endothelial damage with anterior chamber IOL (ACIOL)
- dislocation of IOL
- crystalline lens/IOL touch with posterior chamber IOL (PCIOL)
- pupillary block glaucoma
- pigmentary dispersion glaucoma
- retinal detachment

Preoperative
- ensure refractive stability
- regular topography
- age less than 50 years
- no cataract present
- keratectomy prior to ACIOL insertion
- wait at least 1 month after implantation for LASIK

Phakic IOL Procedure
- preoperative or surgical iridectomy
- excellent pupillary dilation for implantable contact lens (ICL) insertion
- avoid phakic IOL/crystalline lens contact
- check IOP after insertion

LASIK Procedure
- minimize suction time
- treat residual sphere and cylinder

Postoperative
- check IOL centration
- enhance (as in primary LASIK)

CASE A, CATARACT AFTER ICL IMPLANTATION

Jose Güell, MD

Main Concern: Cataract and ICL Implantation

INITIAL PREOPERATIVE INFORMATION

	OD	OS	COMMENTS
Preoperative Refraction	-23.0 – 20 X 170	-22.0 + 20 X 180	extreme myopia
BCVA	20/80	20/60	
SimK Values	45 X 48	46.50 X 48	

PROCEDURES PERFORMED

	OD	OS	COMMENTS
1. Date/type	2/97 ICL	2/97 Artisan IOL	no complications
2. Date/type	4/97 LASIK	4/97 LASIK	no complications
Laser/keratome/plate	117/ACS/160	117/ACS/160	
3. Date/type	7/98 phaco IOL		cataract
Laser/keratome/plate	STAAR model CC 4203 VF +8.00		

CURRENT POSTOPERATIVE INFORMATION

	OD	OS	COMMENTS
Time Postoperative	1 month	16 months	reduced BCVA OU
Postoperative Refraction	-1.50 – 1.00 X 90	n/a	unchanged from
BCVA	20/80	20/50	preoperative levels
Topography Details	n/a	n/a	
SimK Values	n/a	n/a	
Pachymetry	n/a	n/a	
Visual Complaints	n/a	n/a	

The following are visual acuities we took of this patient.

		UCVA	Rx	BCVA	KM
June 1997	OD	20/80	pl – 050 X 150	20/80	near vision OU
	OS	20/50	plano		

		UCVA	Rx	BCVA	KM
February 1998	OD	20/200	plano/pinhole	20/80	45.73 X 46.42
	OS	20/50	plano		45.48 X 45.79

BMC: diffuse anterior subcapsular cataract OD

		UCVA	Rx	BCVA	KM
August 1998	OD	20/80	-150 – 100 X 90	20/60	
	OS	30/50			

From my point of view, a diffuse anterior subcapsular opacification of the ICL might be due to:
- constant or transitory (with pupillary dilation) but continuous trauma over the lens capsule
- metabolic changes secondary to the interposition of a plastic surface between the anterior capsule and the aqueous humor
- chronic subclinical inflammation

After cases like this, with no relevant surgical trauma and good positioning of the ICL over the lens capsule, we must consider lens opacification as an important and possibly frequent complications after implantation of an ICL in this location.

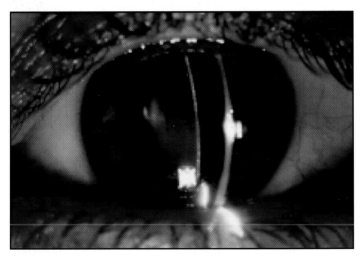

Figure 17A-1. Slit and retroillumination views of the diffuse anterior subcapsular cataract.

Figure 17A-2. Slit and retroillumination views of the diffuse anterior subcapsular cataract.

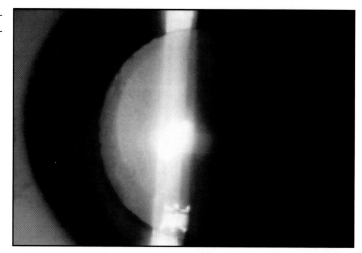

Figure 17A-3. ICL extraction.

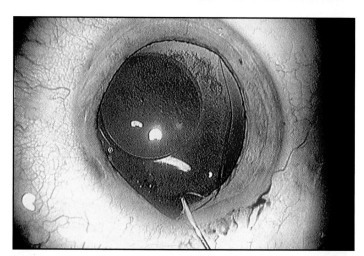

Figure 17A-4. "In-the-bag" low powered STAAR IOL implantation.

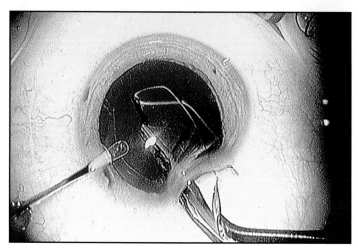

Editor's Notes

This case illustrates some important points with regards to the correction of extreme myopic errors. Generally 23.0 D of myopia is not correctable with LASIK and therefore other options must be considered. The two other main options would be phakic IOLs and clear lens extraction. Clear lens extraction is an effective option, however there is the associated risk of retinal detachment and a loss of accommodation. Therefore, phakic IOLs may be a more attractive option for patients in the prepresbyopic age group. This patient was interesting in that a posterior chamber STAAR ICL was placed OD and an Artisan iris/claw IOL was placed OS. The right eye developed a cataract despite atraumatic insertion of the ICL.

LASIK was then performed after the phakic IOL implantation to correct the residual refractive error and astigmatism. This bioptics technique was originally described by Roberto Zaldivar, MD. Jose Güell, MD, has described a modification of this technique, in which the flap is cut prior to the insertion of the Artisan iris claw phakic IOL. Since the suction and keratectomy do not need to be performed after the IOL is inserted, the risk of the anterior chamber IOL/endothelial cell touch during the flattening of the cornea for keratectomy is eliminated. Dr. Zaldivar simply performs LASIK after the posterior chamber IOL has been inserted and the refractive is stable. Dr. Zaldivar's bioptics technique does not require an initial keratectomy cut as the ICL is positioned in the posterior chamber and therefore not in danger of hitting the endothelial cells during the keratectomy.

It is important to note that patients that have had phakic IOL implantation and develop a cataract can be successfully treated with the removal of the phakic IOL, the cataract, and insertion of a posterior chamber IOL in the same way that we perform modern cataract surgery. These patients could then have enhancement LASIK following their cataract surgery and still end up with an excellent UCVA. Of course, accommodation would be lost and annual retinal exams would be required to identify any peripheral retinal pathology that could lead to retinal detachment.

Case B, Bioptics for Extreme Myopia

Roberto Zaldivar, MD, Susana Oscherow, MD, and Giselle Ricur, MD

Main Concern: Extreme Myopia OD
Patient Age: 29

Initial Preoperative Information

	OD	OS	Comments
Preoperative Refraction	-21.50 – 1.50 X 90		extreme myopia
UCVA	cf at 20 cm		
BCVA	20/60		
Topography Details	n/a		
SimK Values	43.88 D@141°		
	43.60 D@51°, dk: 0.28 D		
Pachymetry	550 μm		
Other	IOP: 15 mmHg		
	Endothelial Cells: 2498		

Procedures Performed

	OD	OS	Comments
1. Date/type	8/10/98 2 iridotomies		60° apart
Laser	Argon/Yag		
2. Date/type 8/13/98	ICL implantation		
	STAAR ICL -20 D		
3. Date/type	1 month later		
	LASIK enhancement		

Current Postoperative Information

	OD	OS	Comments
Time Postoperative	6 months		
Postoperative Refraction	-0.75 D		
UCVA	20/40		
BCVA	20/30		
SimK Values	40.50/40.00, dk 0.50 D		
Visual Complaints	none		
Medications	none		
Refractive Correction	none		
Other	slit lamp exam: cornea: OK		
	ICL: centered, vault 1/8, IOP:15 mm Hg		

The quest for improved optical quality and refractive outcomes in extreme emmetropes has grown stronger as we close in on the millennium.

Until recently, extreme refractive errors were out of reach with procedures such as CLE, LASIK or ICL alone. Loss of accommodation, increased risks of retinal detachment or macular edema, compromise of both corneal integrity and quality of scotopic vision, as well as residual spherical or astigmatic errors were common limitations encountered with these procedures.

So, we started working on a technique that could address two optical systems. In 1996, LASIK and ICL were combined into a refractive procedure we termed bioptics. Both, the corneal plane (LASIK) and the ciliary sulcus plane (ICL), were addressed with this procedure and anticipated post-ICL residual refractive errors were dealt with the LASIK portion of the bioptics procedure. Thus, there were two optical systems (hence *bi*optics) each addressed with an individual refractive procedure.

The blend of their advantages and magnification of their qualities was the outcome. ICL lenses with large optical zones (close to 5 mm) and lower powers, such as -15.0 or -16.0 D, were combined with a LASIK procedure intended for small optical corrections that allowed for optical zones of 5.5 and 6 mm and transitional zones of up to 7 mm. This permitted optimization of both systems' optical zones and enhanced the results. Corneal integrity was preserved and the quality of scotopic vision was minimally unaltered. Precision and efficacy were surprising with marked increase in patient's UCVA and gains in BCVA.

Postoperative management is similar to both techniques, individually. Our previous experience with both ICL and LASIK showed us the way in managing both entities separately. In bioptics, patients are exposed to known and so far unknown risks of both procedures described (ICL and LASIK). Preliminary results of ongoing long-term follow-up studies are revealing acceptable rates of stability and security that will hopefully confirm the benefits of the bioptics procedure.

Indications of this procedure are: myopic patients with spherical equivalents of -15.0 D or greater, patients with high levels of preoperative astigmatism (greater than 2.0 D), hyperopes over +5.0 D, and patients in whom lens power availability is a problem.

The following case (Figures 17D-1 and 2) represents a clear example of a bioptics indication. An extreme myopic patient with a spherical equivalent refraction of -22.25 D cannot be treated with ICL or LASIK alone, yet combining both procedures permitted this patient to increase her UCVA from count fingers at 20 cm before surgery to 20/40 6 months after the bioptics procedure was performed. Her preoperative BCVA of 20/60 improved to 20/30 postoperatively with a cylinder refraction of -0.50 X 75°.

IOP readings and crystalline densitometry have revealed normal findings. Patient satisfaction has been quite well-expressed and today, this patient's lifestyle (she works as an accountant) bears no trace of the lifestyle led 6 months ago (Figure 17D-3).

For extreme myopia, bioptics offers the precision not found yet with any other refractive procedure. Visually handicapped patients can benefit from an excellent visual prognosis.

Further studies are needed to evaluate the results of the bioptics procedure in the correction of extreme hyperopia and mixed astigmatism.

Suggested Reading

Davidorf JM, Zaldivar R, Oscherow S. Posterior chamber phakic intraocular lens for hyperopia of +4 to +11 diopters. *J Refract Surg.* 1998; 14:306-311.

Davidorf JM, Zaldivar R, Oscherow S. Results and complications of laser in-situ keratomileusis by experienced surgeons. *J Refract Surg.* 1998; 14:114-122.

Davidorf JM, Zaldivar R, Oscherow S, Ricur G. Posterior chamber phakic intraocular lens implantation for moderate to extreme myopia and hyperopia. *Operative Techniques in Cataract and Refractive Surgery.* 1998; 1:135-141.

Machat J, Slade S, Probst L. *The Art of LASIK.* 2nd ed. Thorofare, NJ: SLACK Incorporated; 1999.

Zaldivar R. Intraocular contact lens. In: Buratto L, Brint SF. ed. *LASIK: Principles and Techniques.* Thorofare, NJ: SLACK Incorporated; 1998.

Zaldivar R, Davidorf JM, Oscherow S. Posterior chamber phakic intraocular lens for myopia of -8 to -19 diopters. *J Refract Surg.* 1998; 14:294-305.

Zaldivar R, Oscherow S, Ricur G. Implantable contact lens. In: Fine H, ed. *Clear Corneal Lens Surgery.* Thorofare, NJ: SLACK Incorporated; 1999.

Figure 17B-1. Videographic image showing ICL implantation through a 2.8-mm clear corneal incision. The ICL is unfolded slowly inside the anterior chamber.

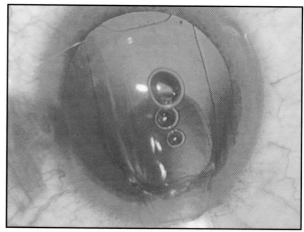

Figure 17B-2. Videographic image showing the ICL centered, as seen before pupil constriction. Positioning holes can be observed at the 12 and 6 o'clock positions.

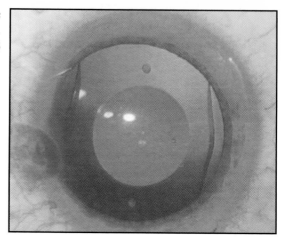

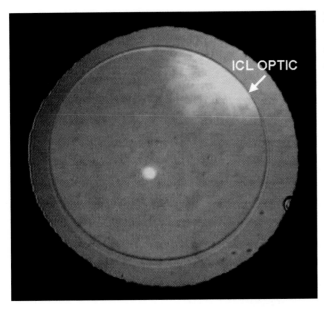

Figure 17B-3. Infrared image (Nidek EAS 1000; Nidek Co. LTD., Aichi, Japan) of the cornea 6 months after the bioptics procedure. The optic rim can be clearly seen.

Editor's Notes

This case illustrates the tremendous potential of the bioptics concept devised by Roberto Zaldivar, MD. In this technique, a phakic IOL is inserted in the eye and LASIK is performed following this procedure to correct any residual refractive error. Dr. Zaldivar's preferred phakic IOL is the STAAR posterior chamber ICL. The patient has achieved an excellent refractive result of -0.75 from the enormous preoperative error of over -22 D. The UCVA is 20/40, and the patients BCVA has improved from 20/60 to 20/30. This is perhaps the most significant result as the patient's day-to-day functioning and driving ability have substantially improved

This procedure offers a tremendous opportunity for those patients with extreme refractive errors who cannot be corrected by LASIK, as well as a chance to avoid the undesirable optical side effects from the small zone LASIK ablations. Nevertheless, this intraocular technique is early in the learning curve and will require further evaluation before the long-term safety can be determined.

CASE C, BIOPTICS FOR EXTREME MYOPIA AND ASTIGMATISM

Roberto Zaldivar, MD, Susana Oscherow, MD, and Giselle Ricur, MD

Main Concern: Extreme myopia OS
Patient Age: 37

INITIAL PREOPERATIVE INFORMATION

	OD	OS	COMMENTS
Preoperative Refraction		-14.75 – 2.50 X 60	
BCVA		20/20	
UCVA		cf at 20 cm	
Topography Details		n/a	
SimK Values		42.37/42.12	
Pachymetry		518 μm	
Other		IOP: 16 mmHg	
		Endothelial Cells: 2318	

PROCEDURES PERFORMED

	OD	OS	COMMENTS
1. Date/type		8/18/98 2 iridotomies	60° apart
Laser		Argon/Yag	
2. Date/type		8/20/98 ICL implantation	
Laser		STAAR ICL –20 D	
3. Date/type		9/28/98 LASIK	
Laser/keratome/plate		Nidek EC 5000/160 μm	

CURRENT POSTOPERATIVE INFORMATION

	OD	OS	COMMENTS
Time Postoperative		6 months	
UCVA		20/20	
BCVA		20/20	
Visual Complaints		none	
Medications		none	
Refractive Correction		none	
Other:		slit lamp exam: cornea OK	
		ICL: centered, vault 1/6	
		IOP: 15 mmHg	

As introduced in the previous case, bioptics is a combined procedure (ICL implantation and LASIK 1 month later) that offers treatment for patients that have extreme refractive errors. With the bioptics procedure, patients are exposed to known and so far unknown risks of the refractive procedures performed in this technique (ICL and LASIK).

Previous reports have described the complications inherent to the ICL procedure, including pupillary block, IOP spikes, anterior capsular opacities, broken, flipped or decentered implants, and the risk of endophthalmitis as with all intraocular procedures.

LASIK complications described in the literature include irregular astigmatism, night halos and glare, infection, and possible keratectasia.

Retinal complications, such as retinal tears, retinal detachments, retinal hemorrhage or edema are known complications when addressing extreme myopes with surgical procedures. So far, our studies have been unable to demonstrate if the bioptics procedure truly increases these retinal risks.

This case demonstrates that the complications a bioptics procedure can endure are those relevant to the techniques used: ICL and LASIK.

An uneventful ICL implantation (Figures 17C-1 and 2) in a high myopic patient (pre-ICL spherical equivalent refraction of -16.00 D) passed on to the second stage of the bioptics procedure with a LASIK ablation to treat the ICL residual cylinder (-0.50 X 178°). Postoperative slit lamp examination (15 min) revealed the presence of flap edema and superficial keratitis which was treated with ocular lubricants. Day 1 examination (Figure 17C-3) revealed a flap with central striae. The flap was lifted and the interface rehydrated with subsequent repositioning of the flap. Ulterior follow-up examinations proved uneventful and the patient today presents an UCVA of 20/20.

Untreated epithelial edema may lead to striae formation the following day due to "shrinkage" of the edematous epithelium, with no flap misalignment present. They are usually delicate and present where the corneal edema was. When diagnosed, these striae usually resolve uneventfully if the flap is refloated within the first 24 hours.

Another cause of striae, with undisturbed flap alignment, are those following an inflammatory process or the presence of sands of the Sahara. They may be irregular in shape or thickness and may be localized in almost any part of the flap, presenting no specific pattern. They too must be treated with lifting of the flap and interface hydration.

A discussion can be held on whether or not diagnosis of flap edema during immediate postoperative control should lead to a precocious administration of topical lubricants, steroids, or anti-inflammatory nonsteroid drugs.

In our experience, in cases of confirmed inflammatory processes or Sands of the Sahara, steroids should be applied frequently and intensive lubrication of the cornea is essential in order to avoid striae formation.

Suggested Reading

Davidorf JM, Zaldivar R, Oscherow S. Posterior chamber phakic intraocular lens for hyperopia of +4 to +11 diopters. *J Refract Surg.* 1998; 14:306-311.

Davidorf JM, Zaldivar R, Oscherow S. Results and complications of laser in-situ keratomileusis by experienced surgeons. *J Refract Surg.* 1998 14:114-122.

Davidorf JM, Zaldivar R, Oscherow S, Ricur G. Posterior chamber phakic intraocular lens implantation for moderate to extreme myopia and hyperopia. *Operative Techniques in Cataract and Refractive Surgery.* 1998; 1:135-141.

Machat J, Slade S, Probst L. *The Art of LASIK.* 2nd ed. Thorofare, NJ: SLACK Incorporated; 1999.

Zaldivar R. Intraocular contact lens. In: Buratto L, ed. *LASIK Principles and Techniques.* Thorofare, NJ: SLACK Incorporated; 1998.

Zaldivar R, Davidorf JM, Oscherow S. Posterior chamber phakic intraocular lens for myopia of -8 to -19 diopters. *J Refract Surg.* 1998; 14:294-305.

Zaldivar R, Oscherow S, Ricur G. Implantable contact lens. In: Fine H, ed. *Clear Corneal Lens Surgery.* Thorofare, NJ: SLACK Incorporated; 1999.

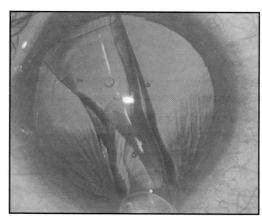

Figure 17C-1. Videographic image showing folded ICL being injected into the anterior chamber of the eye through a 2.8 mm clear corneal incision.

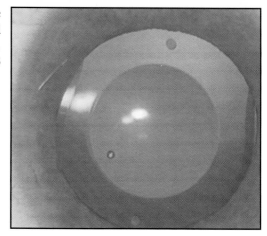

Figure 17C-2. Videographic image showing the unfolded ICL centered, with the footplates behind the iris plane, as seen before pupil constriction. Positioning holes can be observed at 12 and 6 o'clock positions.

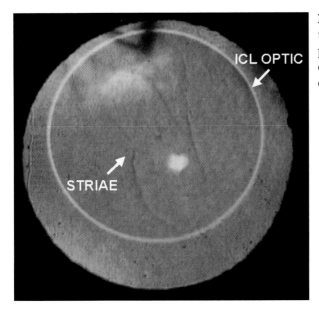

Figure 17C-3. Infrared image of the cornea the day after the LASIK stage of the bioptics procedure. The presence of central striae are clearly seen as well as the rim of the ICL optic.

Editor's Notes

When using a combined procedure such as bioptics, we benefit from the advantages of both procedures. These advantages are the accuracy of LASIK and the power of the ICL implantation. However, we also suffer from the disadvantages of both procedures, which includes both their complications. The authors have outlined the common complications with ICLs as well as LASIK. In this case, LASIK flap striae occurred that was felt to be related to the corneal edema.

Complications with LASIK can generally be corrected. Correction of flap striae involves refloating the corneal flap with the additional steps of hydration of the flap and stretching and smoothing the flap in cases of severe striae that have been present for extended periods of time. Complications of ICLs, including pupillary glaucoma, pigmentary dispersion glaucoma, anterior subcapsular cataract, and the intraocular complications of cataract surgery, are generally a little more difficult to treat. One possible solution involves removing the ICL.

INDEX

*F*or your information...

This book and many others on numerous different topics are available from SLACK Incorporated. For further information or a copy of our latest catalog, contact us at:

Professional Book Division
SLACK Incorporated
6900 Grove Road
Thorofare, NJ 08086 USA
Telephone: 1-856-848-1000
1-800-257-8290
Fax: 1-856-853-5991
E-mail: orders@slackinc.com
WWW: http://www.slackinc.com

We accept most major credit cards and checks or money orders in US dollars drawn on a US bank. Most orders are shipped within 72 hours.

Contact us for information on recent releases, forthcoming titles, and bestsellers. If you have a comment about this title or see a need for a new book, direct your correspondence to the Editorial Director at the above address.

If you are an instructor, we can be reached at the address listed above or on the Internet at **educomps@slackinc.com** for specific needs.

Thank you for your interest and we hope you found this work beneficial.